PCEP

Perinatal Continuing Education Program

Neonatal Care

4th Edition

BOOK 3

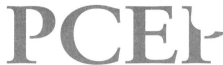

American Academy of Pediatrics

DEDICATED TO THE HEALTH OF ALL CHILDREN®

American Academy of Pediatrics Publishing Staff

Mary Lou White, *Chief Product and Services Officer/SVP, Membership, Marketing, and Publishing*

Mark Grimes, *Vice President, Publishing*

Heather Babiar, MS, *Senior Editor, Professional/Clinical Publishing*

Jason Crase, *Senior Manager, Production and Editorial Services*

Theresa Wiener, *Production Manager, Clinical and Professional Publications*

Peg Mulcahy, *Manager, Art Direction and Production*

Linda Smessaert, *Director, Marketing*

Published by the American Academy of Pediatrics
345 Park Blvd
Itasca, IL 60143
Telephone: 630/626-6000
Facsimile: 847/434-8000
www.aap.org

Information about obtaining continuing medical education and continuing education credit for book study may be obtained by visiting www.cmevillage.com.

Several different approaches to specific perinatal problems may be acceptable. The PCEP books have been written to present specific recommendations rather than to include all currently acceptable options. The recommendations in these books should not be considered the only accepted standard of care. We encourage development of local standards in consultation with your regional perinatal center staff.

The American Academy of Pediatrics is an organization of 67,000 primary care pediatricians, pediatric medical subspecialists, and pediatric surgical specialists dedicated to the health, safety, and well-being of all infants, children, adolescents, and young adults.

While every effort has been made to ensure the accuracy of this publication, the American Academy of Pediatrics does not guarantee that it is accurate, complete, or without error.

The recommendations in this publication do not indicate an exclusive course of treatment or serve as a standard of medical care. Variations, taking into account individual circumstances, may be appropriate.

Statements and opinions expressed are those of the authors and not necessarily those of the American Academy of Pediatrics.

Any websites, brand names, products, or manufacturers are mentioned for informational and identification purposes only and do not imply an endorsement by the American Academy of Pediatrics (AAP). The AAP is not responsible for the content of external resources. Information was current at the time of publication.

The publishers have made every effort to trace the copyright holders for borrowed materials. If they have inadvertently overlooked any, they will be pleased to make the necessary arrangements at the first opportunity.

This publication has been developed by the American Academy of Pediatrics. The contributors are expert authorities in the field of pediatrics. No commercial involvement of any kind has been solicited or accepted in the development of the content of this publication.

Every effort has been made to ensure that the drug selection and dosages set forth in this publication are in accordance with the current recommendations and practice at the time of publication. It is the responsibility of the health care professional to check the package insert of each drug for any change in indications or dosage and for added warnings and precautions.

Every effort is made to keep *Perinatal Continuing Education Program* consistent with the most recent advice and information available from the American Academy of Pediatrics.

Please visit www.aap.org/errata for an up-to-date list of any applicable errata for this publication.

Special discounts are available for bulk purchases of this publication. Email Special Sales at nationalaccounts@aap.org for more information.

Printed in the United States of America

5-315/0721   1 2 3 4 5 6 7 8 9 10

PC0028

ISBN: 978-1-61002-498-3

eBook: 978-1-61002-499-0

Cover design by Peg Mulcahy

Publication design by Peg Mulcahy

Library of Congress Control Number: 2020943714

Perinatal Continuing Education Program (PCEP), 4th Edition

Textbook Editorial Board

Editors

Editor in Chief, Neonatology
Robert A. Sinkin, MD, MPH, FAAP
Charles Fuller Professor of Neonatology
Department of Pediatrics
University of Virginia Children's Hospital
Vice Chair for Academic Affairs
Division Head, Neonatology
Charlottesville, VA

Editor in Chief, Obstetrics
Christian A. Chisholm, MD, FACOG
Medical Director for Outpatient Clinics, Labor,
  and Delivery
Vice Chair for Medical Education
Professor of Obstetrics and Gynecology
Division of Maternal-Fetal Medicine
Department of Obstetrics and Gynecology
University of Virginia School of Medicine
Charlottesville, VA

PCEP Editorial Board Members

Melissa F. Carmen, MD
Associate Professor of Pediatrics
Division of Neonatology
University of Rochester
Rochester, NY

Susan B. Clarke, MS, NPD-BC, RNC-NIC, CNS
NRP Instructor Mentor
Master Trainer, Helping Babies Survive
Affiliate Faculty, Center for Global Health
Colorado School of Public Health
University of Colorado Anschutz Medical Campus
Aurora, CO

Robert R. Fuller, MD, PhD
Associate Professor
Division of Maternal-Fetal Medicine
Department of Obstetrics and Gynecology
University of Virginia School of Medicine
Charlottesville, VA

Ann Kellams, MD, FAAP
Professor, Department of Pediatrics
Vice Chair for Clinical Affairs and Director of
  Breastfeeding Medicine Services
University of Virginia
Charlottesville, VA

Sarah Lepore, MSN, APRN, NNP-BC
University of Virginia Children's Hospital
Neonatal Intensive Care Unit
Charlottesville, VA

Peter D. Murray, MD, MSM, FAAP
Assistant Professor of Pediatrics
Division of Neonatology
University of Virginia Children's Hospital
Charlottesville, VA

Susan Niermeyer, MD, MPH, FAAP
Professor of Pediatrics
Section of Neonatology
University of Colorado School of Medicine
Colorado School of Public Health
Aurora, CO

Barbara O'Brien, MS, RN
Director, Oklahoma Perinatal Quality Improvement
  Collaborative
University of Oklahoma Health Sciences Center
Oklahoma City, OK

Chad Michael Smith, MD, FACOG
Medical Director, Oklahoma Perinatal Quality
  Improvement Collaborative
Vice President, Medical Affairs, Mercy Hospital
  Oklahoma City
Oklahoma City, OK

Jonathan R. Swanson, MD, MSc, FAAP
Professor of Pediatrics
Chief Quality Officer for Children's Services
Medical Director, Neonatal Intensive Care Unit
University of Virginia Children's Hospital
Charlottesville, VA

Sharon Veith, MSN, RN
Assistant Professor of Nursing
School of Nursing
University of Virginia
Charlottesville, VA

Santina Zanelli, MD
Associate Professor of Pediatrics
Division of Neonatology
University of Virginia Children's Hospital
Charlottesville, VA

Continuing Education Credit

Accreditation and Designation Statements

In support of improving patient care, this activity has been planned and implemented by the American Academy of Pediatrics and the University of Virginia School of Medicine and School of Nursing is jointly accredited by the Accreditation Council for Continuing Medical Education (ACCME), the Accreditation Council for Pharmacy Education (ACPE), and the American Nurses Credentialing Center (ANCC) to provide continuing education for the health care team.

AMA PRA Category 1 Credit

The University of Virginia School of Medicine and School of Nursing designates this enduring material (PI CME) for a maximum of 56.5 *AMA PRA Category 1 Credits*.™ Physicians should claim only the credit commensurate with the extent of their participation in the activity.

ANCC Contact Hours

The University of Virginia School of Medicine and School of Nursing awards 56.5 contact hours for nurses who participate in this educational activity and complete the post-activity evaluation.

AAPA Category 1 CME Credit

This activity is designated for 56.5 AAPA Category 1 CME credits. Approval is valid for 3 years. PAs should only claim credit commensurate with the extent of their participation.

Credit is awarded upon passing book exams, not individual educational unit posttests. Possible credits: Book 1, 14.5; Book 2, 16; Book 3, 17; Book 4, 9. To obtain credit, register online at www.cmevillage.com, choose Courses & Programs, then E-Learning, and scroll down to the PCEP program. Click on the PCEP program link and navigate to https://med.virginia.edu/cme/learning/pcep/pcep-book-exam-certificate/ and pass the book exams.

Disclosure of Faculty Financial Affiliations

The University of Virginia School of Medicine and School of Nursing as a Joint Accreditation Provider adhere to the ACCME *Standards for Integrity and Independence in Accredited Continuing Education*, released in December 2020, as well as Commonwealth of Virginia statutes, University of Virginia policies and procedures, and associated federal and private regulations and guidelines. As the accredited provider for this CE/IPCE activity, we are responsible for ensuring that health care professionals have access to professional development activities that are based on best practices and scientific integrity that ultimately supports the care of patients and the public.

All individuals involved in the development and delivery of content for an accredited CE/IPCE activity are expected to disclose relevant financial relationships with ineligible companies occurring within the past 24 months (such as grants or research support, employee, consultant, stock holder, member of speakers bureau, etc). The University of Virginia School of Medicine and School of Nursing employ appropriate mechanisms to resolve potential conflicts of interest and ensure the educational design reflects content validity, scientific rigor, and balance for participants. Questions about specific strategies can be directed to the University of Virginia

School of Medicine and School of Nursing of the University of Virginia, Charlottesville, Virginia.

The faculty, staff, and planning committee engaged in the development of this CE/IPCE activity in the Joint Accreditation CE Office of the School of Medicine and School of Nursing have no financial affiliations to disclose.

Disclosure of Discussion of Non-FDA-Approved Uses for Pharmaceutical Products and/or Medical Devices

As a Joint Accreditation provider, the University of Virginia School of Medicine and School of Nursing, requires that all faculty presenters identify and disclose any off-label or experimental uses for pharmaceutical and medical device products.

It is recommended that each clinician fully review all the available data on new products or procedures prior to clinical use.

BOOK 3

Neonatal Care

For more information, see the other books in the Perinatal Continuing Education Program (PCEP) series

Unit 1: Oxygen

Objectives

In this unit you will learn to

A. Identify babies who require supplemental oxygen.

B. Administer oxygen as a drug while understanding its benefits and hazards.

C. Operate the appropriate equipment for the controlled delivery of oxygen.

D. Monitor a baby's oxygenation.

Unit 1 Pretest

Before reading the unit, please answer the following questions. Select the *one best* answer to each question (unless otherwise instructed). Record your answers on the test and check them with the answers at the end of the book.

1. Which of the following procedures is the best way to measure the concentration of arterial oxygen?
   A. With an oxygen analyzer
   B. From an arterial blood gas sample
   C. Check the liter-per-minute flow of oxygen.
   D. From a warmed capillary blood sample

2. A baby with respiratory distress is breathing 45% oxygen and has an arterial blood oxygen tension of 96 mm Hg. What adjustments in oxygen should be made for this baby?
   A. Change the inspired oxygen to room air.
   B. Change the inspired oxygen to 40%.
   C. Change the inspired oxygen to 50%.
   D. No changes in oxygen therapy for this baby

3. A baby's eyes may be damaged from periods of too much
   A. Bilirubin in the blood
   B. Carbon dioxide in the air
   C. Oxygen in the blood
   D. Oxygen in the air

4. Which of the following procedures is the best way to gauge the amount of oxygen a baby needs?
   A. Arterial blood gas measurements
   B. Cyanosis of the trunk and mucous membranes
   C. Degree of respiratory distress
   D. Venous blood gas measurements

5. Which of the following babies is least likely to require supplemental oxygen?
   A. A preterm baby with respiratory distress and heart rate of 80 beats per minute
   B. A 5-day-old who appears dusky all over
   C. An extremely preterm baby in the delivery room with a 5-minute Apgar score of 2
   D. A preterm baby with an arterial blood oxygen tension (Pao_2) of 60 mm Hg

6. Which of the following techniques is the best way to regulate the amount of oxygen a baby receives?
   A. Administer oxygen alone and regulate the liter-per-minute flow.
   B. Control the time the baby receives supplemental oxygen.
   C. Hold the oxygen source closer to or farther away from the baby's face.
   D. Use an oxygen blender.

(*continued*)

Unit 1 Pretest (*continued*)

7. **True** **False** A baby found in mother's room with bluish-colored tongue and lips requires immediate oxygen therapy.

8. **True** **False** Arterial blood gas samples are not needed if continuous pulse oximetry is used.

9. **True** **False** Lung damage is a possible consequence of high inspired oxygen concentration over time.

10. **True** **False** Capillary blood gas measurements are a reliable way to determine a baby's blood oxygen level.

11. **True** **False** Oxygen from a tank that has been in a warm room for more than 24 hours does not need to be heated or humidified.

12. **True** **False** A pulse oximeter uses light to estimate the degree to which hemoglobin is saturated with oxygen.

13. **True** **False** Pulse oximetry is most sensitive in the detection of low blood oxygen.

Both too little and too much oxygen can be harmful.

- *Too little oxygen in the blood can cause damage to the brain and other vital organs.*
- *Too much oxygen in the blood can cause damage to the eyes and other organs.*
- *Too much inspired oxygen can cause damage to the lungs.*

1. How much oxygen does a baby need?

Oxygen is essential for survival, but oxygen can also be toxic in excess. Tissues require oxygen to metabolize normally. However, during metabolism involving oxygen, chemical reactions release toxic substances (oxygen free radicals) that can cause tissue injury. Free radicals are even more injurious to tissues that have already experienced a period of oxygen deprivation from asphyxia or hypoperfusion, such as that which may occur during a complicated pregnancy and delivery. Air-breathing mammals normally produce enzymes and other molecules that scavenge oxygen free radicals before they can produce significant injury. The fetus, however, develops in a very low-oxygen environment and has not yet fully developed free radical scavengers until born at term. Therefore, a baby who is preterm, has acquired a serious infection, has experienced an asphyxial event, has respiratory disease, or is otherwise compromised experiences particularly high risk from exposure to too little or too much oxygen.

When a healthy fetus is born and undergoes transition from receiving oxygen via the placenta to using the lungs to extract oxygen from the air, the amount of oxygen dissolved in the plasma and bound to hemoglobin in arterial blood increases dramatically over a period of approximately 10 minutes after birth. This increase occurs because the amount of oxygen available in the air being breathed by the baby is substantially greater than the amount of oxygen transferred across the placenta from the mother's circulation. If the baby's lungs are compromised, normal increase in blood oxygenation may not occur, and the baby may become oxygen deprived unless the concentration of oxygen is increased from the 21% contained in room air to some greater percentage. Conversely, if the concentration being breathed by the baby is excessive, arterial blood oxygenation can easily become too high. Hypoxemia (low blood oxygen) or hyperoxemia (high blood oxygen) can be harmful, so it is very important that a sick baby's arterial blood oxygen be maintained in the range normally found in a healthy baby who is breathing room air.

2. How is the amount of oxygen measured?

Oxygen concentration should be measured in the baby's inspired air and in the baby's blood (Figure 1.1).

  A. Inspired oxygen concentration
  Inspired oxygen concentration is frequently abbreviated as FIO_2 (fraction of inspired oxygen) and is the amount of oxygen a baby breathes. The FIO_2 is measured with an oxygen analyzer, which is a sensor placed near the baby's nose (Figure 1.1) or in-line with a device for delivering positive pressure. Most analyzers provide a constant readout of the oxygen concentration.

Fraction of inspired oxygen (FIO_2) is the fraction of oxygen in the space being measured. This can also be expressed as a percentage. Ambient or "room" air contains 21% oxygen, which is equivalent to FIO_2 of 0.21. Oxygen-enriched air has a higher FIO_2 than 0.21, up to 1.00, which means 100% oxygen. In this unit, percentages are used.

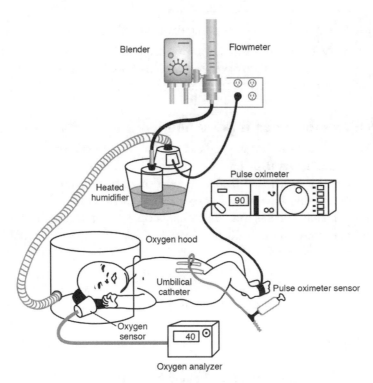

Figure 1.1. Equipment Needed for Administering Oxygen (blender, flowmeter, heated humidifier, oxygen hood), Measuring Delivered Oxygen (oxygen analyzer), and Measuring Baby's Blood Oxygen Level (umbilical catheter, pulse oximeter)

B. Arterial blood oxygen levels

Oxygen is carried in blood attached to hemoglobin in red blood cells and dissolved in plasma. The amount bound to hemoglobin (oxyhemoglobin) is expressed as Spo_2 and measured in percentage of saturation, and concentration in plasma is expressed as Pao_2, measured in millimeters of mercury (mm Hg).

 Arterial blood must be used for Pao_2 determinations.

Venous and capillary blood do not give accurate measurements of oxygenation.

1. Oxyhemoglobin saturation

When there is no oxygen bound to hemoglobin, it is "0% saturated"; when the hemoglobin is carrying as much oxygen as possible, it is "100% saturated."

Hemoglobin changes color, from blue to red, as it becomes increasingly saturated with oxygen. A pulse oximeter detects the color of the blood and gives a reading expressed as the percentage of saturation. It does this by shining a tiny light through the skin and registering the color of the light coming back from the skin (which is determined by the color of blood in the arteries), and thus estimating oxygen saturation, without requiring a blood sample to be drawn.

The desired level of oxyhemoglobin saturation in a baby is generally 85% to 95%. Many neonatologists will advise using the 88% to 92% saturation range as a target but will set oximeters to sound an alarm if the level decreases below 85% or increases above 95%.

2. Arterial blood oxygen dissolved in plasma

Arterial blood oxygen levels are shown as the PaO_2 value from arterial blood gas measurements. The blood to be analyzed is usually drawn from an umbilical artery catheter (see Unit 3, Umbilical Catheters, in this book), a peripheral arterial catheter, or a peripheral arterial stick (see Skill Unit: Monitoring Oxygen, Peripheral Arterial Blood Gas Sampling, in this unit). If an arterial catheter cannot be inserted, monitor oxygenation with continuous pulse oximetry until transport to a higher level of care can be arranged. The desired level of PaO_2 in any baby (sick, well, preterm, or post-term) is generally 45 to 65 mm Hg.

Babies with varying degrees of lung disease will require different levels of FIO_2 to maintain the desired arterial blood oxygen level. For example, a baby with severe respiratory distress syndrome may require 100% oxygen to maintain a PaO_2 between 45 and 65 mm Hg, while a baby with mild respiratory distress syndrome may require only 30% oxygen to maintain a PaO_2 between 45 and 65 mm Hg.

Note: There is disagreement among experts as to the appropriate range of PaO_2 and oxyhemoglobin saturation. Know the acceptable range for your hospital. Also, the target range will be different immediately after birth. (See Book 1: Maternal and Fetal Evaluation and Immediate Newborn Care, Unit 5, Resuscitating the Newborn.)

3. How does oxyhemoglobin saturation (SpO_2) compare to arterial blood oxygen (PaO_2) level?

Oxygen tension (or partial pressure) in a blood sample (PaO_2) can range from 0 to approximately 500 mm Hg; oxyhemoglobin saturation (SpO_2) can range from 0% to 100%. When SpO_2 is higher than 95%, the hemoglobin is almost fully saturated with oxygen, and a small increase in saturation can correspond to a large increase in PaO_2. If SpO_2 saturation is higher than approximately 95%, PaO_2 could be acceptable (45–65 mm Hg) or undesirably high (>65 mm Hg) (Table 1.1).

Table 1.1. Approximate Relationship of SpO_2 and PaO_2	
Oxyhemoglobin Saturation (SpO_2)	**Arterial Blood Oxygen (PaO_2)**
0%–85%	0–45 mm Hg
85%–95%	45–65 mm Hg
95%–100%	65–500 mm Hg

Oxyhemoglobin saturation as measured with a pulse oximeter is most valuable for detecting a low blood oxygen level.

Percentage of saturation is not a sensitive measure when PaO_2 is high.

The approximate relationship of PaO_2 and oxyhemoglobin saturation is shown in Table 1.1 and Figure 1.2.

The shaded area of Figure 1.2 shows the approximate relationship between 85% to 95% oxyhemoglobin saturation and 45 to 65 mm Hg arterial blood oxygen level for a slightly preterm baby during the first few days after birth.

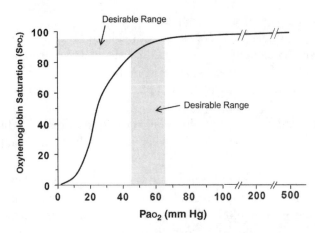

Figure 1.2. Relationship of PaO_2 and SpO_2

For some babies, simultaneous measurements of PaO_2 and SpO_2 may give results different than those predicted by the graph. The precise relationship of oxygen saturation and PaO_2 is affected by several factors, such as age since birth, the presence of acidosis, characteristics of hemoglobin (eg, methemoglobin, hemoglobin S), and whether the baby has undergone a blood transfusion.

4. What is the best way to monitor a baby's oxygenation?

A baby's blood oxygen level will frequently fluctuate from minute to minute, particularly if the baby is distressed or undergoing any sort of procedure. A pulse oximeter can be used to monitor these changes, so you will know quickly when the baby's oxygenation is persistently out of the desirable range and requires attention. However, because pulse oximeters only report SpO_2, which has a variable relationship to PaO_2, the baby's PaO_2 should be measured intermittently with a sample of arterial blood. Watch for oximeter readings to stabilize to know the best time to obtain an arterial blood sample that reflects the baby's resting state (not changes that may occur with crying or stress during procedures, for example).

The best way to monitor a baby's blood oxygen is to

• Follow trends or changes in SpO_2 with a pulse oximeter.
and

• Measure PaO_2 intermittently from samples of arterial blood.

5. When does a baby need supplemental oxygen?

Babies require oxygen therapy when the concentration of oxygen in arterial blood is low, and the oxygen needs of a sick baby vary over time. Therefore, the only sure way to determine if a baby is receiving the correct amount of oxygen is to measure SpO_2 continuously with pulse oximetry and to periodically measure PaO_2 via an arterial blood gas sample.

In emergency situations, a baby may need oxygen immediately. First, give oxygen; then measure the SpO_2 or PaO_2 as soon as possible. The following signs show that a baby needs oxygen:

A. Need for resuscitation

When a baby's respiratory rate and heart rate are very slow or have stopped, ventilation must be improved immediately to help restore the baby's vital signs. Oxygen concentrations required during assisted ventilation may range from 21% (room air) to as high as

100%, as guided by pulse oximetry. (See Book 1: Maternal and Fetal Evaluation and Immediate Newborn Care, Unit 5, Resuscitating the Newborn.)

B. Central cyanosis

Generally, with central cyanosis, a baby's body will look blue. This overall color change may be dramatic or much less obvious. The best clinical sign of central cyanosis is a bluish appearance of the lips, the inside of the mouth, and the conjunctival surface of the eyelids. Central cyanosis indicates that the baby needs immediate oxygen therapy. However, studies have shown that clinical assessment of cyanosis is inconsistent; therefore, if a baby receives oxygen therapy for more than a brief period, the baby's SpO_2 or PaO_2 must be measured.

C. Respiratory distress

Some babies have difficulty breathing and will require extra oxygen for long periods. (See Unit 2, Respiratory Distress, in this book.) For these babies, it is extremely important to ensure adequate ventilation, use continuous oximetry, and measure arterial blood oxygen levels (PaO_2) frequently to avoid the hazards of too much or too little oxygen. Continuous transcutaneous monitoring of both PaO_2 and $PaCO_2$ may be available in some critical care settings.

6. How much oxygen do you administer to a baby?

A. Resuscitation

The priority during resuscitation should be to establish ventilation and a normal heart rate. (See Book 1: Maternal and Fetal Evaluation and Immediate Newborn Care, Unit 5, Resuscitating the Newborn.) Guidelines recommend starting the resuscitation of a term newborn with no supplemental oxygen (room air) and beginning resuscitation of preterm babies (<35 weeks) with a low concentration of supplemental oxygen (eg, 21%–30%). In either case, FIO_2 should be adjusted to match reference arterial saturation values, as guided by oximetry values (SpO_2). Reference values for the few minutes after birth will be low, so the oximetry goal will also begin low and gradually increase to the 88% to 92% range (Figure 1.3). Some degree of cyanosis may also be normal during the first few minutes after birth. (See Book 1: Maternal and Fetal Evaluation and Immediate Newborn Care, Unit 5, Resuscitating the Newborn.)

B. Cyanosis

1. Immediate treatment

For cyanosis that appears in the nursery, decide on an initial oxygen concentration, depending on the degree of cyanosis. For example, if a baby is deeply cyanotic, choose a higher concentration (50%–100%). If the mucous membranes are only slightly dusky, choose a lower range (30%–40%) (ILCOR 2019 oxygen update).

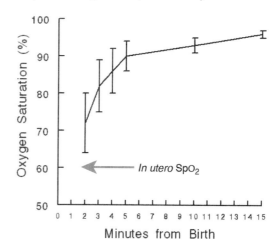

Figure 1.3. Preductal Oxygen Saturation Changes After Birth (Median and Interquartile Range)
Adapted with permission from Mariani G, Dik PB, Ezquer A, et al. *J Pediatr.* 2007;150(4):418–421.

Degree of cyanosis	slightly dusky mucous membranes $\longrightarrow$	increasing cyanosis $\longrightarrow$	deeply blue all over
Oxygen concentration	30% oxygen $\longrightarrow$	increasing oxygen $\longrightarrow$	100% oxygen

2. Adjust according to baby's response and SpO_2

Select the desired oxygen concentration for delivery to the baby, and attach a pulse oximeter as soon as possible. Adjust oxygen concentration up or down to achieve the desired saturation. Observe the baby for the disappearance of central cyanosis. Consider obtaining an arterial blood gas measurement.

C. Respiratory distress

Babies with respiratory distress need to be given oxygen only if they are cyanotic or have a low arterial blood oxygen concentration. The amount of oxygen required depends on the degree of cyanosis and how low the PaO_2 or SpO_2 values are.

It is possible for a baby to be in respiratory distress, *not* be cyanotic, and still have a low arterial blood oxygen value. These babies should receive continuous pulse oximetry monitoring and monitoring of arterial blood gas measurements and be given sufficient oxygen to keep arterial oxygenation within the reference range.

Use of a pulse oximeter should *not* replace periodic arterial blood gas measurements, which are also used to measure blood pH levels and carbon dioxide (CO_2) concentration, in addition to blood oxygen concentration. A pulse oximeter, appropriately applied with results checked against an arterial blood gas level, is helpful in providing continuous *estimates* of arterial blood oxygen levels and should reduce the number of arterial blood measurements that are needed.

7. When does a baby *not* need supplemental oxygen?

A. Acrocyanosis (only hands and feet blue)

Acrocyanosis without central cyanosis is *not* an indication for oxygen to be administered. This condition may be caused by reasons other than lack of oxygen (eg, cold stress, poor peripheral blood flow).

B. Prematurity without respiratory distress or cyanosis

Preterm babies should *not* be given supplemental oxygen unless they have central cyanosis, a low pulse oximetry level, or a low arterial blood oxygen level as measured with arterial blood gas analysis.

C. Babies with cyanotic congenital heart disease

During the first week or so after birth, some babies with certain types of congenital heart malformation will worsen if given high concentrations of supplemental oxygen. Use of supplemental oxygen and saturation targets for such babies should be determined by a pediatric cardiologist.

8. How should oxygen be given? (Figure 1.4)

The concentration of oxygen in room air is 21%. To deliver supplemental oxygen (22%–100%)

• Deliver oxygen blended with air by using equipment that will prevent fluctuations in oxygen concentration.

10

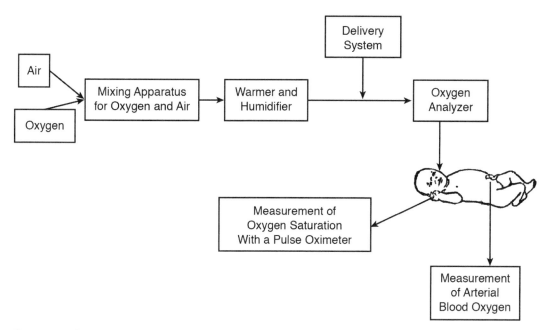

Figure 1.4. Components Required for Administering and Measuring Oxygen

- Heat and humidify the oxygen/air mixture to the baby's neutral thermal environment temperature. (See Book 1: Maternal and Fetal Evaluation and Immediate Newborn Care, Unit 7, Thermal Environment.)
- Measure inspired oxygen (FIO_2) precisely and continuously.
- Monitor oxyhemoglobin saturation (SpO_2) continuously via pulse oximetry.
- Measure the concentration of oxygen in the baby's blood (PaO_2) intermittently.

A. Blend oxygen and air

Oxygen from a wall outlet or tank is 100% oxygen, regardless of the liter-per-minute flow rate. The only way to achieve less than 100% oxygen is to mix the oxygen with air. Air for blending with oxygen is obtained from a wall outlet, compressed air tank, or electrical air compressor. An oxygen blender automatically regulates this blending of oxygen and compressed air to provide a specified and adjustable oxygen concentration. Blenders, however, are not always precise. An oxygen analyzer should be used to check the exact concentration of oxygen being delivered to a baby.

 The flow rate of oxygen does not determine the concentration of oxygen inspired by a baby.

The amount of oxygen and air blended together determine inspired oxygen concentration (FIO_2).

B. Heat and humidify oxygen and air

Oxygen and air directly from wall outlets or tanks are cold and dry, even if a tank itself is warm. Oxygen and air must be warmed to avoid chilling the baby. Regulation of the temperature of the oxygen/air mixture is just as important as strict regulation of the baby's environmental temperature (neutral thermal environment). Oxygen and air must also be humidified, to avoid drying the baby's mucous membranes and airways.

C. Prevent fluctuations in oxygen concentration

Fluctuations in F_{IO_2} can affect vascular resistance and the amount of blood flow through the lungs, resulting in even greater fluctuations in the amount of oxygen in the baby's arterial blood.

 If F_{IO_2} is lowered rapidly, the arteries to the lungs may constrict. This can seriously reduce blood flow to the lungs and result in a much lower Pa_{O_2} level. A consistently low Pa_{O_2} level, regardless of the cause, may lead to brain and other tissue damage.

The equipment used to deliver oxygen to babies who do not require assisted ventilation includes

1. Oxygen hood

An oxygen hood is made from clear plastic material and is placed over a baby's head. It has an inlet on one side for the oxygen/air mixture to enter and an opening on the opposite side to fit over the baby's neck.

During the acute phase of illness, the most effective way to maintain constant F_{IO_2} for a baby who does not require assisted ventilation is to use an oxygen hood.

 Giving oxygen by nasal cannula does not permit monitoring of the oxygen concentration delivered. The baby breathes a combination of room air along with oxygen from the cannula, and this combination can vary with deep or shallow respirations. Worsening or improving respiratory status can be detected more easily when F_{IO_2} is measured directly in an oxygen hood.

2. Oxygen mask

With an oxygen mask, the concentration of oxygen a baby receives will vary, depending on the concentration administered and how far the mask is held from the baby's nose. There is no way to precisely measure the amount of oxygen the baby receives if the mask is not held snugly to the face. When the mask is held tightly to the face, pressure builds up in the mask, and oxygen is administered with continuous positive airway pressure (CPAP). (See Book 4: Specialized Newborn Care, Unit 3, Continuous Positive Airway Pressure.) Free-flow oxygen may be delivered with a separate oxygen mask, a flow-inflating bag and mask, or a T-piece resuscitator during resuscitation, but none is reliable for providing constant oxygen for more than a few minutes. Free-flow oxygen cannot be reliably provided from a self-inflating bag.

3. Nasal cannula

Once newborns are stable beyond transition, extubated, or weaned from CPAP, it may be more convenient for them to receive oxygen via nasal cannula. However, oxygen concentration is not as stable, heating and humidification are less, and the cannula will partially obstruct the baby's airway. The size of the cannula should be no more than 50% of the nasal opening, so as not to obstruct the nares. Using a heated, high-flow nasal cannula is another method of providing distending airway pressure; it may be an alternative to CPAP, with the caveat that the amount of pressure being administered is variable and unreliable.

Delivery of oxygen directly to an incubator is *not* recommended. When oxygen is delivered in this way, the concentration cannot be precisely controlled. If a baby requires oxygen therapy beyond the period of stabilization, an oxygen hood or nasal cannula should be considered. See the skill units at the end of this unit for details.

9. How can you use a pulse oximeter to adjust inspired oxygen?

While it is important to correct too-low or too-high PaO_2 values quickly to prevent tissue damage, rapid and extreme fluctuations in PaO_2 can also be hazardous. A pulse oximeter can help guide you to change the FIO_2 as quickly as possible without causing rapid fluctuations in PaO_2. Saturations may decrease during procedures, making it necessary to pause in the procedure or increase FIO_2 temporarily to maintain saturations in the desired range, as measured with oximetry.

Self-test A

Now answer these questions to test yourself on the information in the last section.

A1. What is the only certain way to know if a baby is receiving too much or too little oxygen?
   A. Measure the arterial blood oxygen level (SpO_2 or PaO_2).
   B. Observe the baby for degree of cyanosis.

A2. Name 3 situations in which supplemental oxygen may be needed.
_____
_____
_____

A3. What should you do before or soon after starting to administer supplemental oxygen?
_____

A4. What are the general principles of delivering oxygen?
_____
_____
_____
_____
_____

A5. What monitoring should be used if a baby continues to require supplemental oxygen for more than a brief period?
_____

A6. If monitoring shows too much oxygen in the baby's blood, what damage could result?
_____

A7. If monitoring shows too little oxygen in the baby's blood, what damage could result?
_____

A8. When do you administer oxygen to a baby in respiratory distress?
   A. Only if the baby is cyanotic
   B. Only if the arterial blood oxygen value or oximeter reading is low
   C. If the baby has central cyanosis or has a low arterial blood oxygen value or oximeter reading

A9. A baby has an FIO_2 of 0.50, a PaO_2 of 75 mm Hg, and an SpO_2 of 95%. What is the inspired oxygen for this baby?
   A. 50%
   B. 75 mm Hg
   C. 95%

A10. A baby is receiving 35% inspired oxygen, has a PaO_2 of 60 mm Hg, and has an SpO_2 of 90%. What describes the oxygen level in the baby's blood?
   A. 35%
   B. 60 mm Hg
   C. 60 mm Hg and 90% saturation

A11. Which of the following techniques is the best way to obtain blood for blood oxygen measurement?
   A. From an umbilical artery catheter
   B. From an umbilical venous catheter
   C. From a heel stick

A12. The reference arterial blood oxygen level in a baby is between ____ and ____ mm Hg.

A13. If oxygen needs to be administered for longer than a brief period, how much should a baby receive?
   A. Not more than 40%
   B. Enough to keep the baby pink
   C. Enough to keep arterial blood oxygen between 45 and 65 mm Hg

A14. Pulse oximeters are used to measure the amount of oxygen
   A. In plasma
   B. Bound to hemoglobin
   C. In inspired air

Check your answers with the list that follows the Recommended Routines. Correct any incorrect answers and review the appropriate section in the unit.

10. When do you obtain an arterial blood gas measurement?

If an oximeter is used, wait until the baby is relatively calm and oximeter readings have been stable, without wide fluctuations, for several minutes. Then obtain an arterial blood sample, as described in the skill units. Even if the oximeter reads consistently within reference range, if a baby has acute lung disease and is receiving supplemental oxygen, Pao_2 should be measured from an arterial blood sample.

11. What are reference arterial blood gas values, and how are capillary and venous blood gas values used?

Reference values for blood gas measurements are dependent on gestational and postnatal age.

A. Arterial blood gas measurements
   Reference arterial values:

pH level:	7.30–7.40
$Paco_2$:	40–50 mm Hg
Pao_2:	45–65 mm Hg

   Reference ranges for newborns reflect slightly higher $Paco_2$ and lower pH levels than those for adults. This unit focuses on how to provide oxygen therapy and assess and monitor a baby's oxygenation. Values for CO_2 and pH are given here so different types of samples can be compared. Further discussion of the interpretation of pH and CO_2 concentration in assessing a baby's ventilation status or need for assisted ventilation is given in Unit 2, Respiratory Distress, and Unit 9, Identifying and Caring for Sick and At-Risk Babies, in this book.

B. Capillary blood gas measurements
   Blood gas measurements obtained from capillary blood give close estimates of arterial blood pH and CO_2 concentration *if* the samples have been obtained using the proper technique. However, arterial blood oxygen concentration cannot be estimated accurately from capillary oxygen concentration. Capillary blood gas measurements should not be used to assess a baby's oxygenation.

Capillary measurements may be useful to assess a baby's need for assisted ventilation based on pH and P_{CO_2} values in an emergency and when it has not been possible to obtain an arterial blood gas sample. Capillary blood gas measurements, coupled with use of pulse oximetry, are also used in older babies who continue to require oxygen but do not have umbilical arterial catheters in place. (See Book 4: Specialized Newborn Care, Unit 7, Continuing Care for At-Risk Babies.)

Reference capillary values: pH level: 7.25–7.35, with proper technique

P_{CO_2}: 45–55 mm Hg, with proper technique

P_{O_2}: Unreliable

C. Venous blood gas measurements

Blood gas measurements obtained from venous blood also give close, but slightly lower, estimates of arterial blood pH level and slightly higher CO_2 concentration. The sampling technique is simpler than it is for capillary samples. Blood obtained from any venipuncture will provide reliable estimates.

As with capillary blood gas measurements, venous blood gas values cannot be used to assess oxygenation; however, venous blood gas values may be useful in an emergency, when it has not been possible to obtain an arterial sample, to estimate the baby's ventilation on the basis of pH level and P_{CO_2} values.

Reference venous values: pH level: 7.25–7.35

P_{CO_2}: 45–55 mm Hg

P_{O_2}: Unreliable

 Only arterial blood gas measurements and oximetry provide accurate information about a baby's oxygenation.

12. What are the problems related to oxygen therapy?

The chances of developing complications from too much or too little oxygen can be lessened by

- *Monitoring oxyhemoglobin saturation*
- *Obtaining frequent arterial blood gas measurements*
- *Making appropriate changes in inspired oxygen (F_{IO_2}) promptly*

A. Too little oxygen in the blood: brain damage

If a baby does not receive enough oxygen, permanent brain damage may occur. Other organs, such as the kidneys or gastrointestinal tract, may also be damaged.

B. Too much oxygen in the blood: eye damage

Preterm babies may have serious eye damage if they have too much oxygen in their blood for prolonged periods. This condition is called *retinopathy of prematurity* (ROP).

Eye damage can occur, even if F_{IO_2} is relatively low. A baby with normal lungs receiving supplemental oxygen at a concentration as low as 28% may have a Pa_{O_2} as high as 150 mm Hg.

Although preterm babies with high blood oxygen concentrations for prolonged periods are at risk for developing ROP, many other factors are also implicated in ROP development.

The more preterm the baby, the more severe the ROP is likely to be. All extremely preterm babies, regardless of the amount or duration of exposure to supplemental oxygen, and any preterm baby who received supplemental oxygen for a substantial period, should undergo an eye examination to rule out ROP. (See Book 4: Specialized Newborn Care, Unit 7, Continuing Care for At-Risk Babies.)

 One of several factors that causes retinopathy of prematurity is high concentrations of oxygen in the blood.

C. Too much oxygen to the lungs: lung damage
Lung damage may result from being exposed to high concentrations of oxygen in the inspired air over time.

D. Rapidly changing inspired oxygen
Rapid decreases in F_{IO_2} can cause a sharp decrease in Pa_{O_2} level. This may worsen a baby's condition. Higher F_{IO_2} may then be needed to maintain the baby's Pa_{O_2} between 45 and 65 mm Hg. If movement of a baby is essential (eg, to weigh a baby, to obtain a radiograph), continue to give the baby oxygen via mask during the *entire* procedure.

 Do not remove oxygen from an oxygen-dependent baby for even a brief period. Maintain oxygenation by using mask oxygen, and monitor the baby with oximetry.

Self-test B

Now answer these questions to test yourself on the information in the last section.

B1. What may happen when a baby who requires additional oxygen is removed from oxygen for a brief period?

_____

B2. **True**   **False**   A baby who has an arterial blood oxygen level of 90 mm Hg with an inspired oxygen concentration of 22% requires continued supplemental oxygen.

B3. A baby's SpO_2 level is 90%, while the baby is breathing 45% oxygen. The concentration of inspired oxygen should
    A. Be lowered
    B. Be increased
    C. Not be changed at this time

B4. Which 2 organs are most likely to be damaged from too little blood oxygen?
    A. Brain
    B. Eyes
    C. Lungs
    D. Kidneys

B5. Which organ is most likely to be damaged from too much blood oxygen?
    A. Brain
    B. Eyes
    C. Lungs
    D. Kidneys

B6. Which organ is most likely to be damaged from supplemental inspired oxygen (even with normal blood oxygen) over a long period?
    A. Brain
    B. Eyes
    C. Lungs
    D. Kidneys

B7. A baby has an oxyhemoglobin saturation of 84% with an inspired oxygen concentration of 37%. What should you do?
    A. Increase the inspired oxygen concentration until the oxyhemoglobin saturation is between 85% and 95%.
    B. Check that the oximeter probe is correctly attached.
    C. Both of the above

B8. A baby has an FiO_2 of 0.50, a PaO_2 of 35 mm Hg, and an SpO_2 of 80%. How should you adjust the baby's inspired oxygen concentration?
    A. Increase it
    B. Decrease it
    C. No change

B9. Fill in the following chart for the reference values for arterial, venous, and capillary blood gas samples. Refer to the previous sections if necessary.

Arterial Blood	**Venous Blood**	**Capillary Blood**
PaO_2: _____	PO_2: _____	PO_2: _____
$PaCO_2$: _____	PCO_2: _____	PCO_2: _____
pH: _____	pH: _____	pH: _____

Check your answers with the list that follows the Recommended Routines. Correct any incorrect answers and review the appropriate section in the unit.

OXYGEN

Recommended Routines

All the routines listed below are based on the principles of perinatal care presented in the unit you have just finished. They are recommended as part of routine perinatal care.

Read each routine carefully and decide whether it is standard operating procedure in your hospital. Check the appropriate blank next to each routine.

Procedure Standard in My Hospital	Needs Discussion by Our Staff	Recommended Routine
_____	_____	1. Periodically check oxygen delivery equipment to ensure • A precise and adjustable concentration from 22% to 100% can be achieved. • Oxygen can be humidified and warmed to a precise and adjustable temperature. • Blended oxygen and pulse oximetry are available in the delivery room.
_____	_____	2. Establish a routine for monitoring inspired oxygen concentration (FIO_2) continuously for every baby who receives supplemental oxygen.
_____	_____	3. Establish a routine for pulse oximeter use, including • Assessment for initiation of oxygen therapy • Continuous oximetry monitoring for any baby receiving oxygen therapy • Adjusting FIO_2 based on oximeter readings • Obtaining arterial blood gas samples intermittently, after oximeter readings have stabilized, following a significant change in FIO_2 or worsening of the baby's clinical condition
_____	_____	4. Establish a policy that will allow sufficient oxygen to be given to keep a cyanotic baby pink, followed by immediate attachment of the oximeter to maintain SpO_2 in the 88% to 92% range.

_____   _____

5. Establish a system that ensures an ophthalmologist with experience with retinopathy of prematurity performs a dilated funduscopic examination for
   - Babies born at 30 weeks' gestational age or less or with a birth weight less than 1,500 g (<3 lb 5 oz)

   or

   - Babies with a birth weight of 1,500–2,000 g (3 lb 5 oz to 4 lb 6 oz) or a gestational age >30 weeks believed to be at risk for retinopathy of prematurity

   Examinations should begin at
   - 31 weeks' postmenstrual age for babies born at 22–27 weeks' gestational age

   and

   - 4 weeks' chronological age for babies born at 27 to 30 weeks' gestational age and more (See Book 4: Specialized Newborn Care, Unit 7, Continuing Care for At-Risk Babies.)

Self-test Answers

These are the answers to the Self-test questions. Please check them with the answers you gave and review the information in the unit wherever necessary.

Self-test A

A1. A. Measure the arterial blood oxygen level (SpO_2 or PaO_2).

A2. Central cyanosis

Resuscitation (21%–100% oxygen, depending on the baby's condition and response)

Respiratory distress with low arterial oxygenation (SpO_2 or PaO_2)

A3. Attach a pulse oximeter.

A4. Use an oxygen blender to provide the desired concentration.

Warm and humidify the oxygen/air mixture to the baby's neutral thermal environment temperature.

Prevent fluctuations in oxygen concentration (use an oxygen hood).

Measure the inspired concentration precisely (use an oxygen analyzer).

Measure the baby's blood oxygen concentration with an oximeter and intermittently by obtaining an arterial blood oxygen level.

A5. Monitor the oxyhemoglobin saturation and the arterial blood oxygen level.

A6. Damage to vital tissues, particularly the eyes

A7. Brain damage, as well as damage to other vital organs

A8. C. If the baby has central cyanosis or has a low arterial blood oxygen value or oximeter reading

A9. A. 50%

A10. C. 60 mm Hg and 90% saturation

A11. A. From an umbilical artery catheter

A12. The reference arterial blood oxygen level in a baby is between *45* and *65* mm Hg.

A13. C. Enough to keep arterial blood oxygen between 45 and 65 mm Hg

A14. B. Bound to hemoglobin

Self-test B

B1. If oxygen concentrations are lowered rapidly, even for a few minutes, the arteries to the lungs may constrict, reducing oxygen flow to the body, resulting in a low arterial blood oxygen level. The arteries may stay constricted, even after the inspired oxygen concentration is increased, causing the baby to become sicker.

B2. False.   *Reason:* Arterial blood oxygen of 90 mm Hg is higher than the desired range of 45 to 65 mm Hg. Therefore, the inspired oxygen concentration should be lowered. Inspired oxygen concentration of 22% can be lowered only to 21%, because that is the oxygen concentration in room air. Continued supplemental oxygen, therefore, is not required.

B3. C. Not be changed at this time. (SpO_2 is in an acceptable range.)

B4. A. Brain

D. Kidneys

B5. B. Eyes

B6. C. Lungs

B7. C. Both of the above. (First, look at the baby. If the baby's clinical appearance remains the same, check to be sure the oximeter is functioning correctly. Check for a disconnection in the oxygen delivery system. If the baby's clinical appearance has deteriorated or the oximeter is operating correctly but the percentage of saturation remains low, immediately increase the inspired oxygen concentration.)

B8. A. Increase it. (Increase the inspired oxygen concentration to keep the arterial blood oxygen level between 45 and 65 mm Hg and the oxyhemoglobin saturation between 88% and 92%.)

B9.
Arterial Blood	Venous Blood	Capillary Blood
Pao_2: 45–65 mm Hg	Po_2: Unreliable	Po_2: Unreliable
$Paco_2$: 40–50 mm Hg	Pco_2: 45–55 mm Hg	Pco_2: 45–55 mm Hg*
pH: 7.30–7.40	pH: 7.25–7.35	pH: 7.25–7.35*

*Only if proper technique is used to collect the sample. If the heel is not warmed or there is not a steady flow of blood during collection of the sample, the values obtained are likely to be incorrect and misleading.

Unit 1 Posttest

After completion of each unit, there is a free online posttest available at www.cmevillage.com to test your understanding. Navigate to the PCEP pages on www.cmevillage.com and register to take the free posttests.

Once registered on the website and after completing all the unit posttests, pay the book exam fee ($15) and pass the test at 80% or greater to earn continuing education credits. Only start the PCEP book examination if you have time to complete it. If you take the book examination and are not connected to a printer, either print your certificate to a .pdf file and save it to print later, or come back to www.cmevillage.com at any time and print a copy of your educational transcript.

Credits are only available by book, not by individual unit within the books. Available credits for completion of each book examination are as follows: Book 1: 14.5 credits; Book 2: 16 credits; Book 3: 17 credits; and Book 4: 9 credits.

For more details, navigate to the PCEP webpages at www.cmevillage.com.

Administering Oxygen

The following 3 skill subunits will teach you how to use the equipment needed to deliver a desired amount of oxygen to a baby. You will learn how to calibrate an oxygen analyzer, measure environmental oxygen concentration, use an oxygen blender, and heat and humidify oxygen.

Study these skill units; then attend a skill practice and demonstration session.

To master the skills, you will need to demonstrate each of the following steps correctly:

Measuring Oxygen Concentration
1. Follow the manufacturer's directions for calibrating the analyzer.

2. Place the oxygen analyzer in the hood to measure the oxygen concentration.

Blending Oxygen and Compressed Air

Heating and Humidifying an Oxygen/Air Mixture
1. Set up heating/humidifying equipment.

2. Adjust the temperature of the heater/humidifier.

3. Connect the oxygen/air source to the equipment.

4. Determine the liters-per-minute flow rate and FIO_2 on the blender.

5. Establish the precise oxygen concentration.

6. Monitor the oxygen hood temperature.

The following drawing shows the equipment necessary for administering oxygen to a baby:

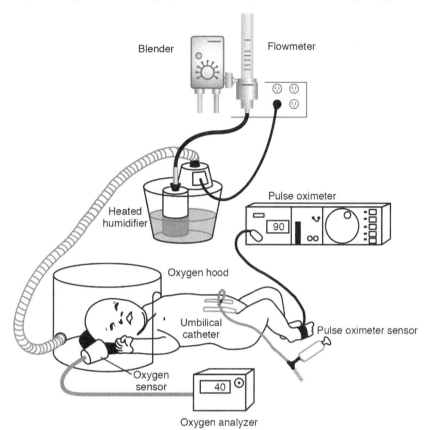

Measuring Oxygen Concentration

It is important to know the type of oxygen analyzer in use in your nursery and how to operate, calibrate, and maintain it. For example,

- Some analyzers require batteries. Know when and how the batteries should be changed.
- Some analyzers require the sensor unit be changed periodically. Know when and how to do this.
- Many analyzers require periodic recalibration, but the frequency of recalibration varies. Know when and how to calibrate the analyzer according to manufacturers' recommendations.

Measuring the Baby's Inspired Oxygen Concentration

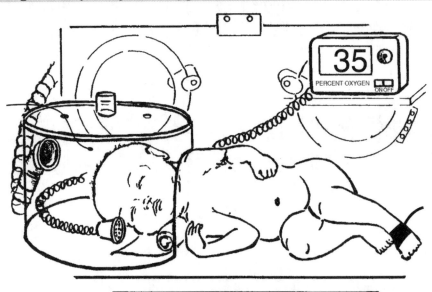

Oxygen hoods come in various sizes and shapes and are made from various materials. Whatever type is used in your nursery, be sure a baby's head fits completely inside the hood. There are also several types of *oxygen analyzers*. Many have a digital display of oxygen concentration. Thermometers are sometimes contained in a flexible wire that fits within the oxygen delivery tubing. Whatever type of *thermometer* is used, be sure it measures the temperature of the oxygen/air mixture at a point near the baby.

1. After calibrating the oxygen analyzer, put the sensor inside the baby's oxygen hood. Place the sensor near the baby's nose, as newborns are obligate nose breathers.

   Oxygen concentration will vary slightly in different places inside the oxygen hood. It is important to check oxygen concentration near the baby's nose.

2. If possible, leave the oxygen sensor in the oxygen hood for continuous monitoring of inspired oxygen concentration. Some monitors have alarms that will signal if the oxygen concentration decreases.

   If continuous monitoring is not possible, oxygen concentration should be measured and recorded at least every hour.

What Can Go Wrong?

1. The analyzer shows a decrease in oxygen concentration in the oxygen hood.

   Check to ensure

   - Tubing is connected and flow rates are set as ordered.
   - Sensor is not wet, giving a false reading.
   - Analyzer calibrates properly and batteries (if needed) are fresh.
   - No excess water is in the tubing between the heating/humidifying device and the oxygen hood.
   - Sensor does not need to be replaced.

2. The baby is in oxygen alone (no compressed air), but the analyzer reads only 94%.

   This may be OK. Because the analyzer was calibrated in 100% dry oxygen, it may only read a maximum of 94% in humidified oxygen.

PERINATAL PERFORMANCE GUIDE

Blending Oxygen and Compressed Air

When only oxygen is delivered to an oxygen hood, it will result in the baby breathing 100% oxygen, regardless of the liter-per-minute flow rate.

Flow rate of oxygen (expressed in liters per minute) regulates only the speed of oxygen flow, not the concentration. Oxygen directly from a wall outlet or tank is always 100% oxygen.

Oxygen must be blended with compressed air to deliver less than 100% oxygen.

The concentration of oxygen in room air is 21%. Any oxygen concentration between 22% and 99% may be achieved by blending varying amounts of compressed air with 100% oxygen.

ACTIONS	REMARKS
Preparing to Mix Oxygen and Air	
1. Collect the proper equipment.	The equipment listed is shown in the illustration at the beginning of these skill units.
• Oxygen source • Compressed air source • Blender	Oxygen and compressed air may come from wall outlets or separate tanks. If you are using tanks, check how much gas is left in each tank. If there is any question, get a new tank before embarking on transport. Portable air compressors may also be used to provide compressed air.
• Heater/humidifier for oxygen/air mixture	Many commercial units are available that will heat and humidify oxygen at the same time.

• Oxygen hood
• Oxygen analyzer
• Temperature probe that can be placed in the baby's oxygen hood or integrated into delivery tubing
• *Sterile* water for the humidifier
• Oxygen and air high-pressure tubing to connect blender to oxygen and air sources
• Tubing
  — Small diameter → to connect blender to heater/humidifier
  — Large diameter → to connect heater/humidifier to oxygen hood
	An oxygen hood is necessary to keep a constant oxygen concentration around a baby's face.

26

ACTIONS   **REMARKS**

Preparing to Mix Oxygen and Air (continued)

2. Connect tubing and set up heating/
   humidifying system.

Adjust the temperature of the heater/
humidifier to the baby's neutral thermal
environment range. (See Book 1: Maternal
and Fetal Evaluation and Immediate Newborn Care, Unit 7, Thermal Environment.)

Achieving Approximate Oxygen Concentration

3. Make sure an oxygen analyzer is in
   good working condition. Calibrate it
   as necessary.

See the previous skill unit section, Measuring
Oxygen Concentration.

4. Decide what oxygen concentration you
   want to deliver (eg, 65% oxygen)

5. Set the flowmeter and dial the desired
   oxygen concentration on the blender.

Generally, a 6 to 10 L/min flow is adequate.
Different flows may be specified for hoods of
different design to avoid carbon dioxide
buildup. If transporting the patient by using
portable tanks, use lower flows to conserve
oxygen and air sources.

Adjusting Oxygen Concentration

6. Measure the oxygen concentration inside
   the oxygen hood by placing the analyzer
   sensor near the baby's nose.

7. Turn the dial on the blender up or down
   until the desired concentration is achieved.

   After making each adjustment, wait a
   moment, until the display is stable, before
   making another adjustment.

A properly calibrated and maintained analyzer is more accurate than a blender. Adjust
the blender dial up or down until the analyzer registers the desired concentration, even
if that means the percentage of oxygen
shown on the blender dial is slightly above
or below the concentration registered by the
oxygen analyzer.

8. Recheck and record the FIO_2 in the baby's
   oxygen hood a few minutes after each adjustment and at least once every hour.

ACTIONS	REMARKS

What Can Go Wrong?

1. The baby's $PaCO_2$ increases.

Check the flow rate; adjust it to higher than 8 L/min to be sure the baby is not rebreathing exhaled air. An increasing $PaCO_2$ level may also mean the baby's lung disease is getting worse, and you should consider the need for assisted ventilation.

2. Oxygen concentration as measured by the analyzer is different from the concentration set on the blender dial.

Check that all tubes are connected. Remove condensed water from tubes. Check analyzer functioning and recalibrate or change the sensor. If the difference persists and is not too great, consider the analyzer to be correct.

3. The baby's body temperature becomes too high or too low.

Check that the temperature of the oxygen hood is adjusted to the baby's neutral thermal environment. If the baby is cool, check that flow rate of the oxygen/air mixture is not too high. A high flow rate could cool a baby by means of convective heat loss.

4. The baby's blood oxygen concentration (PaO_2) or oxygen saturation (SpO_2) level decreases quickly, or the baby's color becomes blue.

First, increase the oxygen concentration in the oxygen hood or temporarily ventilate the baby with a bag, mask, and oxygen until the baby is pink (and oxygen saturation is stable between 88% and 92%). Check to see that all the tubing is properly connected. Consider the possibility of a pneumothorax and obtain a portable chest radiograph. Monitor the baby's oxygenation and provide other therapy as appropriate.

PERINATAL PERFORMANCE GUIDE

Heating and Humidifying an Oxygen/Air Mixture

ACTIONS   REMARKS

Deciding to Heat and Humidify an Oxygen/Air Mixture

1. Do you anticipate the admission of a baby who may require oxygen therapy?

   Yes: Set up the equipment used in your nursery for heating and humidifying an oxygen/air mixture.

   No: Make sure clean equipment for heating and humidifying an oxygen/air mixture is available at all times.

Preparing to Heat and Humidify an Oxygen/Air Mixture

2. Collect the proper equipment.
   - Heater for oxygen/air mixture
   - Humidifier for the oxygen/air mixture
   - Temperature probe, which can be placed in the oxygen hood or in-line in the delivery system, at a point near the baby
   - *Sterile* water for the humidifier
   - Tubing, oxygen hood, oxygen analyzer, and other equipment needed for oxygen therapy (see previous sections)

The heater must have a range of temperature settings. Although there are some humidifiers that only humidify without heating an oxygen/air mixture, these units are *not* desirable. Heated humidifiers work by heating the water used for humidification and increasing the amount of water vapor that can be carried in the oxygen/air mixture.

Do *not* use tap water to fill the humidifier. Tap water contains numerous bacteria that would multiply in the warmed water.

Heating and Humidifying an Oxygen/Air Mixture

3. Use sterile water to fill the humidifying container to the "full" line.

   or

   Connect a bag of sterile water to the heater/humidifier with IV tubing.

It is important to keep the water level between the "full" and "refill" marks. A heater will not work properly unless there is sufficient water in the humidifying container. More water may need to be added periodically (frequency depends on the brand of heater/humidifier).

Some units have a connection port for IV tubing so that sterile water fills the humidifier continuously and the system does not need to be opened to add water.

4. Plug in the heater.

ACTIONS	REMARKS

Heating and Humidifying an Oxygen/Air Mixture (continued)

5. Adjust the temperature setting on the heater to a medium setting.

Some heaters may be set in degrees. If this is the case for your heater, set the temperature to a midpoint in the baby's NTE range. (See Book 1: Maternal and Fetal Evaluation and Immediate Newborn Care, Unit 7, Thermal Environment.)

6. Connect the heating/humidifying unit between the blender and oxygen hood.

7. Ensure that the temperature probe and heater wire(s) are placed appropriately in the circuit.

The temperature of the oxygen/air mixture will drop several degrees as it passes through the tubing between the heating/humidifying unit and the oxygen hood. It is important to repeatedly measure the temperature of the baby.

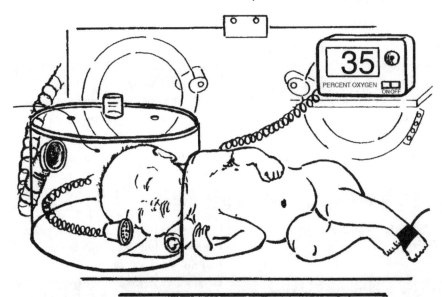

Note: The illustration is designed to show the equipment needed for oxygen delivery and monitoring, not all components of a baby's care.

8. Adjust the blender to the desired oxygen concentration.

See the previous skill unit section, Blending Oxygen and Compressed Air.

9. Regulate the heating adjustment until the temperature inside the oxygen hood is within the baby's NTE range.

   Temperature inside the oxygen hood will be determined by the temperature of the oxygen/air mixture, not by the temperature of the incubator or radiant warmer.

For some heaters, this may require careful, frequent monitoring and readjustment.

Some heaters have a servo control mechanism. If this is the case, place the probe near the baby and set the heater temperature to a midpoint in the baby's NTE range.

ACTIONS   **REMARKS**

Maintaining a Heating/Humidifying System

10. Change the heating/humidifying unit and tubing periodically. This will reduce the possibility of bacteria growing within the system. Frequency of the change depends on the type of system you are using.

    To change a heating/humidifying system,

    a. Set up a clean, alternate heating/ humidifying unit and tubing by following steps 1 through 9.

    b. Heat the water in the clean heating/ humidifying system.

    c. Quickly disconnect the old unit and connect the clean, alternate unit. Do this very quickly so the baby's oxygen is not interrupted for more than a few seconds.

    Plan ahead so the water can be heated to the appropriate temperature and the switch between "clean" and "dirty" equipment can be made quickly.

If the heater/humidifier needs to be opened to add sterile water to the water reservoir, it may need to be changed more often (usually every 24 hours) than a system that is closed with a continuous drip of sterile water to maintain water level. Devices that contain heating wires within the delivery tubing minimize water condensation within the tubing and, thus, allow less chance for bacterial growth.

In-line heating wires and a closed system generally mean the system needs to be changed much less frequently (usually every 48–72 hours or longer).

It is important to maintain the temperature of the oxygen/air mixture in the baby's oxygen hood at a constant, appropriate temperature. A baby's whole body can be chilled or overheated if the temperature of the oxygen/ air mixture is lower or higher than the baby's NTE. (See Book 1: Maternal and Fetal Evaluation and Immediate Newborn Care, Unit 7, Thermal Environment.)

What Can Go Wrong?

1. The temperature of the oxygen/air mixture may become too cold.

   This will markedly increase the baby's oxygen and caloric requirements. Keep the temperature in the oxygen hood within the baby's NTE range.

2. The temperature of the oxygen/air mixture may become too hot.

   This will severely stress the baby and increase the body temperature. Keep the temperature in the oxygen hood within the baby's NTE range.

3. The humidifier may run dry.

   The unit will not be able to heat the oxygen/ air mixture or provide humidity, and the baby's mucous membranes will become dry. Check the water level frequently.

ACTIONS	REMARKS

What Can Go Wrong? (continued)

4. Contamination may result from inadequate cleaning of nondisposable heating/humidifying equipment or interruption of closed heating/humidifying systems.	Change the heating/humidifying equipment as recommended, according to the type of system used, to avoid infections. Be sure all nondisposable equipment is cleaned thoroughly between uses. Avoid interruption of closed heating/humidifying systems.

Abbreviations: IV, intravenous; NTE, neutral thermal environment.

SKILL UNIT

Monitoring Oxygen

You learned in the previous skill unit how to measure and adjust the concentration of the oxygen that a baby breathes. Now, you need to monitor the concentration of oxygen that reaches the baby's blood. Estimating blood oxygen saturation (Spo_2) continuously is most easily achieved with a pulse oximeter. The oximetry skill was described in Book 1: Maternal and Fetal Evaluation and Immediate Newborn Care, Unit 4, Is the Baby Sick? Recognizing and Preventing Problems in the Newborn.

You also need to measure oxygen concentration (Pao_2) directly in arterial blood samples, which can be obtained from a peripheral or a central artery and sent to the laboratory for blood gas analysis. The following skill describes obtaining arterial blood from a peripheral artery. In Unit 3, Umbilical Catheters, in this book, you will learn how to insert an umbilical arterial catheter and use it to obtain multiple arterial blood gas samples.

Peripheral Arterial Blood Gas Sampling

Not everyone will be required to perform the skill. However, all staff members should study the skill unit and learn the technique to assist with the procedure.

Study this skill unit; then attend a skill practice and demonstration session.

To master the skills, you will need to demonstrate each of the following steps correctly:
1. Be aware of the risks associated with any arterial puncture.
2. Collect and prepare the appropriate equipment.
3. Locate the radial artery and cleanse the site for puncture.
4. Perform the puncture and obtain an arterial blood sample (by using an infant mannequin or an actual baby in need of an arterial puncture).
5. Apply appropriate pressure to the puncture site for an appropriate length of time.

ACTIONS	REMARKS
Deciding to Obtain a Peripheral Blood Gas Sample	

1. Obtain a peripheral ABG sample if the baby needs a blood gas determination and does not have a UAC in place.	This may be done • When it is anticipated that a baby will require supplemental oxygen for only a few hours • To check a baby's ventilation and oxygenation status before undertaking an umbilical catheterization procedure • When UAC insertion has been unsuccessful or it was necessary to remove the catheter
Use a UAC (see Unit 3, Umbilical Catheters, in this book) whenever possible to obtain frequent blood gas samples.	There are several reasons ABG samples taken from a UAC are preferred to peripheral ABG samples. • A sample obtained with a needle may cause the baby to cry vigorously and, therefore, give a falsely low PaO_2 value or a falsely high or low $PaCO_2$ value. • Peripheral ABG samples may be difficult to obtain. • A peripheral puncture is more stressful for the baby than sampling obtained from an umbilical catheter. • Certain complications may develop as a result of a needle puncture. • Venous blood, not arterial blood, may be obtained with a peripheral sample.

ACTIONS   REMARKS

Deciding to Obtain a Peripheral Blood Gas Sample (continued)

2. Be aware of the risks and complications associated with peripheral arterial punctures.

   Possible complications include

   - *Hematoma* (a swollen, black-and-blue mark caused by bleeding from the vessel into the surrounding tissue)

Proper technique will minimize the occurrence of these complications and allow the same puncture site to be used repeatedly.

A hematoma may result from

- Repeated punctures and excessive probing with the needle to find the artery
- Inadequate pressure applied to the artery after the procedure is completed

A hematoma may cause

- Tissue or nerve damage due to pressure
- Difficulty in obtaining additional arterial samples from that site by obscuring the artery

   - *Nerve damage*

Nerves often run parallel to arteries and may be damaged if punctured repeatedly. Pressure from a hematoma may also cause nerve damage.

   - *Thrombus formation* (blood clot attached to the wall of a blood vessel)

A thrombus may develop after numerous punctures into the same spot in an artery. This can cause partial or complete blockage of the blood flow.

   - *Embolus* (blood clot, air bubble, or other plug carried by the bloodstream)

An embolus can lodge in a blood vessel, obstruct the blood flow in that vessel, and thereby cut off the blood supply to the tissues the artery perfuses. Thrombi and emboli can cause severe tissue damage.

   - *Arterial spasm*

Any artery that has been punctured may "clamp down" or constrict completely. This may or may not have serious consequences, depending on the amount of collateral circulation (blood flow to the same tissues but through different vessels) and the length of time the artery is in spasm.

   - *Infection*

This may be a superficial soft-tissue infection, such as that which might occur as a result of any needle puncture. If the bone is penetrated, osteomyelitis (bone infection) can occur. Although this is rare, osteomyelitis can be extremely difficult to treat and may cause severe, permanent damage.

ACTIONS   REMARKS

Deciding to Obtain a Peripheral Blood Gas Sample (continued)

3. Be aware of the advantages and special hazards associated with the puncture site chosen. These are listed and illustrated on the following pages.

ABG determinations are often extremely important for determining therapy. Always try to obtain a sample from the lowest-risk site first. If this is unsuccessful, however, it may be necessary to obtain an ABG sample from a site associated with more risk.

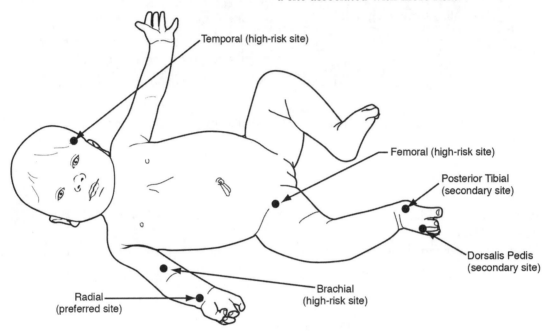

Deciding to Obtain a Peripheral Blood Gas Sample (continued)

Preferred Sites

Radial Artery (preferred site)

Advantages

- No large veins nearby; therefore, almost 100% assurance that any blood obtained is arterial.

- Good collateral circulation via the ulnar artery.

- Position of the artery is stable, making it relatively easy to penetrate the artery.

Hazards

- Hazards for all arterial punctures

Posterior Tibial Artery (secondary site)

Advantages

- Good collateral circulation.

- No large veins nearby; therefore, relative assurance that any blood obtained is arterial.

- The position of the artery is stable, making it relatively easy to penetrate the artery.

Hazards

- Hazards for all arterial punctures

- The possibility of posterior tibial nerve damage

Dorsalis Pedis Artery (secondary site)

Advantages

- Good collateral circulation

Hazards

- Hazards for all arterial punctures

- A small artery; therefore, difficult to puncture

The radial artery is the recommended site for peripheral ABG sampling in newborns.

The ulnar artery is rarely used, and it should only be used after ensuring that collateral circulation is intact by performing the Allen test (https://www.youtube.com/watch?v= yajMvWnTFO4). A modified Allen test is shown at https://www.youtube.com/ watch?v=gdgomN6TsuE.

A video for arterial blood sampling in the newborn can be found at https://www.bing. com/videos/search?q=arterial+blood+gas+ sampling+in+newborn&&view=detail& mid=42685C62B960E1DC106842685C62B 960E1DC1068&&FORM=VRDGAR.

ACTIONS	REMARKS

Deciding to Obtain a Peripheral Blood Gas Sample (continued)

High-Risk Sites

Brachial Artery

Advantages

- Collateral circulation via 3 small arteries

Hazards

- Hazards for all arterial punctures
- A deeper artery, not easily stabilized, tends to roll when puncture is attempted
- A high likelihood of obtaining venous blood
- Possibility of median nerve damage

Because collateral circulation is not ensured, brachial artery puncture should be avoided.

Temporal Artery

Advantages

- Easily palpated, stable artery

Hazards

- Hazards for all arterial punctures.
- Thrombus or embolus could cut off blood supply to area(s) of the brain.

Temporal arteries should be AVOIDED as sampling sites in newborns.

Femoral Artery

Advantages

- A large artery in stable position; therefore, penetrated relatively easily

Hazards

- Hazards for all arterial punctures.
- No collateral circulation because the femoral artery divides below the groin; therefore, arterial spasm, thrombus, or embolus occurring at the groin can damage the entire leg.
- Traumatic damage or infection of the hip joint.
- A high likelihood of obtaining venous blood from the femoral vein, which runs parallel with the artery.

This site should be AVOIDED for arterial punctures in newborns.

If complications occur, consequences are often extremely serious.

Preparing for a Radial Artery Puncture

Note: The radial artery is the most commonly used site for peripheral ABG sampling (see a procedural video at https://www.youtube.com/watch?v=4LSlOx4uaBg). With care, this site may be used repeatedly, with little chance of adverse consequences. The steps that follow are therefore restricted to the technique for radial artery puncture.

ACTIONS   REMARKS

Preparing for a Radial Artery Puncture (continued)

4. Collect the following equipment:

   - Preheparinized syringe
   - Appropriate disinfectant skin preparation
   - Sterile gauze pad
   - A 23–25-gauge scalp vein (butterfly) needle or a 23–25-gauge venipuncture needle

Many hospitals have replaced butterfly needles with small catheters that are introduced into the blood vessel over introducing needles. Other hospitals only have safety catheters, where the needle snaps into a protective sheath after the catheter enters the vessel. The details of these devices are not described in this program.

5. Check that collateral circulation is sufficient by
   - Elevating the baby's hand
   - Occluding the radial and ulnar arteries at the wrist
   - Massaging the palm toward the wrist
   - Releasing occlusion of the ulnar artery, looking for color to return to the baby's hand

In addition to the equipment listed, a second person is usually needed to draw blood into the syringe once the artery has been punctured.

Preheparinized syringes are commercially available and contain powdered heparin. Syringes containing 50 units of heparin are preferable to those containing 100 units.

Return of color in less than 10 seconds indicates adequate collateral circulation; return in more than 15 seconds signifies inadequate collateral supply, and arterial puncture should not be performed.

RADIAL ARTERIAL BLOOD SAMPLING

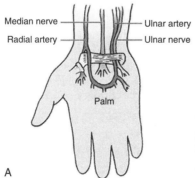

A

The radial artery is preferred for sampling procedures. Its superficial location is easy to palpate and puncture, and there are no immediately adjacent nerves or veins that may be injured or accidentally punctured.

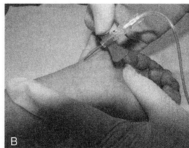

B

Hold the wrist in a position of supination and slight extension. Insert the needle at a 30° to 45° angle while applying continuous, gentle suction with the plunger. Advance the needle until the radial artery is punctured and blood is returned or until resistance is met.

From Santillanes G, Claudius I. Pediatric Vascular Access and Blood Sampling Techniques. In: *Roberts and Hedges' Clinical Procedures in Emergency Medicine and Acute Care.* 6th ed. Elsevier; 2013.

ACTIONS   **REMARKS**

Performing a Radial Artery Puncture

6. Hold the baby's wrist in extension.

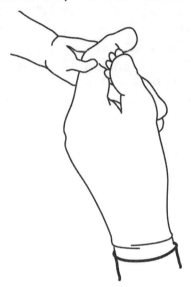

The wrist should be neither flexed nor hyper-extended. The artery is most easily penetrated when the wrist is held in a neutral position. A second person holds the baby and withdraws blood into the syringe when the puncture is successful. It is generally less awkward, however, if the person performing the puncture also holds the baby's hand.

7. Using your index finger, palpate the baby's wrist for the radial pulse.

The best place to feel the radial pulse is on the thumb side of the baby's wrist, just above the first wrist crease. Transillumination can also help locate the artery. Special devices for transillumination of blood vessels are commercially available.

8. Clean the baby's wrist with disinfectant skin preparation.

9. Open the sterile gauze pad.

10. Remove the needle or rubber cap from the heparinized syringe and save it for later capping of the syringe.

11. Place the heparinized 1-mL syringe (without cap or needle attached) on the sterile gauze pad.

12. Take the sheath off the butterfly needle, and take the cap off the tubing.

The tubing should be uncapped so blood can flow into the tubing as soon as the artery is punctured.

ACTIONS   REMARKS

Performing a Radial Artery Puncture (continued)

13. Grasp both "wings" of the butterfly needle and quickly insert it into the spot
where the artery was palpated. (See the
following illustration.)

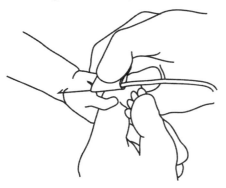

A 45° angle with the tip of the needle entering the skin at the first wrist crease should be
used. The bevel may be positioned downward at an angle of 15° to 25° in small,
preterm newborns.

14. If blood is not immediately seen in the
butterfly tubing, withdraw the needle
slowly. Stop withdrawing the instant
blood is seen in the tubing.

You may have gone through both sides of
the artery and need to withdraw the needle
until it is within the vessel.

15. If no blood enters the tubing, continue to
withdraw the needle until it almost exits
from the skin.

16. Palpate the artery again and reinsert the
needle in another quick thrust.

Try not to make tiny jabbing advances of the
needle. These are rarely successful and tend
to cause more tissue damage than decisive,
"clean" insertions of the needle.

17. If you have made several unsuccessful attempts at puncturing the artery, withdraw
the needle completely and start the procedure over again with a fresh butterfly
needle.

The butterfly needle you were using may
have become plugged with tissue during the
puncture attempt(s).

18. As soon as blood is seen in the butterfly
tubing, the second person should attach
the heparinized syringe to the tubing.

Blood should be seen pulsating or flowing
very rapidly within the tubing. This is evidence of a good arterial sample.

19. The second person then *gently* pulls back
on the syringe while the first person holds
the butterfly needle steady in the artery.

If the blood stops flowing, it may be necessary for the first person to reposition the
needle slightly.

41

ACTIONS

REMARKS

Performing a Radial Artery Puncture (continued)

20. Withdraw blood into the tubing and syringe until the necessary volume has been obtained.

As with any laboratory test for a baby, obtain only the minimum amount of blood required for the test. There is 0.3-mL volume in 12 inches of butterfly needle tubing. Many blood gas machines require 0.3 mL or less for analysis.

21. The second person then places the gauze pad on the baby's wrist and presses firmly as soon as the first person withdraws the butterfly needle.

22. Aspirate any blood remaining within the butterfly tubing into the syringe.

23. Disconnect and discard the butterfly needle and tubing from the syringe.

24. All air bubbles should now be removed from the syringe, so that only blood remains within the syringe.

If air bubbles are allowed to remain within the syringe, they might affect oxygen and carbon dioxide levels in the blood. The Pao_2 result would be falsely high, and the $Paco_2$ result would be falsely low.

25. Cap the syringe with a rubber stopper or clean the needle and the needle cover.

26. If there will be a delay of more than 10 to 15 minutes between the times the sample is collected and analyzed, the syringe should be placed in ice.

Metabolism of the blood cells continues within the syringe. If there is a delay between sample collection and analysis, metabolism could result in a falsely low Pao_2 value. When the sample is chilled by being placed in ice, the metabolic rate is brought almost to a standstill and will not affect the results.

27. The second person should continue to hold the puncture site for a minimum of 3 minutes.

Pressure is generally required for a minimum of 3 minutes but may be needed for 5 minutes or longer in very sick babies.

Pressure should be firm and constant but not so hard as to occlude blood flow to the baby's hand. The baby's hand should remain pink and not turn white or purple. Firm, steady pressure will prevent the baby from losing any unnecessary blood and also prevent formation of a hematoma.

Abbreviations: ABG, arterial blood gas; UAC, umbilical arterial catheter.

ACTIONS   REMARKS

What Can Go Wrong?

1. You may not obtain any blood.

Consider the following actions:

- Try a new needle, because the first one may have become clogged with body tissue.
- Take a short break from the procedure, and then start from step 1 of the skill, perhaps by using the baby's other wrist. Do *not* persist in numerous fruitless attempts, because they will only traumatize the wrist and stress the baby.
- Ask someone else to attempt the procedure. Sometimes asking another team member to make a fresh attempt will result in a better outcome.

2. You may obtain venous blood rather than arterial blood.

In well-oxygenated babies with normal blood pressure, arterial blood will

- Be a brighter, more vivid red color than venous blood.
- Flow more rapidly than venous blood.
- Sometimes pulsate within the butterfly tubing.

In sick babies with low arterial oxygen concentration or low blood pressure, it may be impossible to detect any differences between the appearance of venous and arterial blood. The best way to be sure you have obtained arterial blood is to select a puncture site where there is little chance of penetrating a vein. Obtaining a venous blood gas level can be helpful in estimating pH, P_{CO_2}, and bicarbonate levels but is of no value in estimating the state of oxygenation.

3. Hemorrhage from the site may occur.

Someone should apply continuous pressure to the puncture site for a minimum of 3 minutes, or as long as required for the bleeding to stop. Do *not* apply a pressure bandage, because this may be too tight and may severely restrict circulation or be too loose and allow the baby to bleed into the bandage. Do *not* leave the baby unattended until you are certain bleeding has stopped. Pressure may be required for 5 minutes or longer in very sick babies who have a tendency toward prolonged clotting time. Observe the site after pressure is released to be certain bleeding does not restart.

ACTIONS	REMARKS

What Can Go Wrong? (continued)

4. The baby's hand may turn white during or immediately after the procedure.

This indicates that the artery has gone into spasm, cutting off all blood flow to the hand.

*Immediately wrap the **opposite** arm and hand in a warm compress.* This is done to dilate blood vessels in that hand and hopefully cause a sympathetic response with dilation of the vessels in the affected hand.

Do **not** wrap the **affected** hand. If the affected arm and hand were wrapped, the warmth of the compress would increase the metabolic demands of the tissues, thereby increasing the need for blood flow in an area where circulation is already compromised.

5. A hematoma may develop.

This is due to bleeding under the skin and results from repeated punctures and excessive probing with the needle or inadequate pressure applied to the puncture site. Again, apply pressure to the wrist as soon as the needle is withdrawn and maintain firm, steady pressure until the bleeding has stopped completely. If a hematoma develops, it will make it much more difficult to obtain additional blood samples from that site.

6. The puncture site may become infected.

Use careful aseptic technique. Use a new butterfly needle every time you completely withdraw the needle from the skin and make another insertion.

Unit 2: Respiratory Distress

Unit 2 Pretest

Before reading the unit, please answer the following questions. Select the *one best* answer to each question (unless otherwise instructed). Record your answers on the test and check them with the answers at the end of the book.

1. To determine if a baby is cyanotic, which of the following body parts is the best part of the baby's body to examine?
   - **A.** Nail beds
   - **B.** Feet
   - **C.** Lips
   - **D.** Nose

2. A baby's respiratory rate is 70 breaths per minute. This breathing pattern is called
   - **A.** Normal
   - **B.** Tachypnea
   - **C.** Apnea
   - **D.** Flaring

3. What causes respiratory distress syndrome in the newborn?
   - **A.** Congenital malformation of the upper airway
   - **B.** Polycythemia (thick blood)
   - **C.** Pneumothorax
   - **D.** Surfactant deficiency

4. Which of the following babies is not at increased risk for respiratory distress?
   - **A.** Baby born in a taxicab during the winter
   - **B.** A term baby whose nails are meconium stained
   - **C.** A 38-week, appropriate-for-gestational-age baby whose mother's membranes had been ruptured for 6 hours before delivery
   - **D.** A baby with a 5-minute Apgar score of 2

5. A baby has respiratory distress. You note asymmetrical movement of the chest, with breath sounds louder on the left side. Which of the following actions is most appropriate for this baby?
   - **A.** Obtain an electrocardiogram.
   - **B.** Obtain a chest radiograph.
   - **C.** Position the baby with the right side down.
   - **D.** Insert an oral airway.

6. If a preterm baby stops breathing for 10 seconds, this is considered
   - **A.** Expected, unless accompanied by bradycardia or cyanosis
   - **B.** Unexpected and requiring immediate treatment

(*coninued*)

Unit 2 Pretest (*continued*)

7. Which of these may be a cause of apnea? (Choose the letter that identifies the correct answers.)
   1. Imbalance in blood chemistry, such as low blood glucose, calcium, or sodium level
   2. Infections
   3. Low blood volume
   4. Temperature change, such as when a cold baby is being warmed
   A. 2, 3
   B. 3, 4
   C. 1, 2, 4
   D. 1, 2, 3, 4

8. A baby with respiratory distress has an apneic spell. What should you think about this?
   A. Apnea is expected in babies with respiratory distress.
   B. Apnea shows the baby is getting worse quickly.

9. What percentage of babies weighing less than 1,000 g (<2 lb 3 oz) will have at least 1 apneic spell?
   A. <20%
   B. 50%
   C. 75%
   D. >90%

10. When a baby is assisted with ventilation for an apneic spell, it is important to _____ the rate of assisted breathing before stopping assistance.
    A. decrease
    B. increase
    C. not change

11. **True   False**   Three hours after birth, a baby shows mild grunting and nasal flaring. This is probably expected.

12. **True   False**   Babies frequently cannot breathe through their mouths by themselves.

13. **True   False**   A baby in respiratory distress who is grunting probably has poor lung compliance ("stiff lungs").

14. Which of the following babies is at highest risk for developing a pneumothorax?
    A. Term baby with congenital heart disease
    B. Term baby whose mother had hydramnios
    C. Preterm baby with respiratory distress syndrome
    D. Preterm baby requiring an exchange transfusion

(continued)

Unit 2 Pretest (*continued*)

15. A baby with a pneumothorax is least likely to develop
   A. High blood pressure
   B. Sudden cyanosis
   C. Abdominal distension
   D. Shift in location of heart sounds

16. The possible consequences of a pneumothorax include all of the following conditions, except
   A. Hypoxia
   B. Intraventricular hemorrhage
   C. Anemia
   D. Acidosis

17. Approximately _____ of healthy term newborns will develop a pneumothorax.
   A. 0.1%
   B. 1.0%
   C. 5.0%
   D. 10.0%

18. **True   False**   A pneumothorax should be considered anytime there is a sudden deterioration in a baby's condition, even if the baby is recovering from an illness.

Part 1: Respiratory Distress

Objectives

In Part 1 of this unit you will learn to

A. Identify babies at risk for respiratory distress.

B. Identify babies with respiratory distress.

C. Understand the causes of neonatal respiratory distress.

D. Understand the principles of therapy for babies with respiratory distress.

E. Take appropriate emergency actions for babies with respiratory distress.

1. What are the signs of neonatal respiratory distress?

The 5 signs of respiratory distress in the newborn are

- Tachypnea (rapid breathing)
- Retractions—intercostal and subcostal
- Nasal flaring
- Grunting
- Cyanosis

A. Tachypnea

A normal newborn respiratory rate may be erratic, with brief periods of very rapid respirations mixed with periods of no breathing for a few seconds (periodic breathing). For this reason, when vital signs are obtained in a newborn, respirations should be counted for a full minute.

Sustained respirations greater than 60 breaths per minute are outside the normal range. This is called *tachypnea.*

B. Retractions

These may be seen each time a baby inhales. The skin between the ribs (intercostal) or below the ribs (subcostal) is pulled in as the baby tries to expand lungs that may be stiffer than normal.

C. Nasal flaring

The nostrils widen with each inspiration as the baby attempts to move more air into the lungs.

D. Grunting

This is one of the most important signs of respiratory distress in the newborn. It is heard during the expiratory phase of the breathing cycle in a baby with decreased pulmonary compliance ("stiff lungs"). In an attempt to hold open the alveoli (air sacs in the lungs), a baby will exhale against a partially closed glottis (upper airway). The resulting noise may be heard as a grunt or even a whine or cry repeated with each expiration. Occasionally, the grunt may be heard only with a stethoscope on the chest. Grunting is the baby's attempt to produce positive end-expiratory pressure.

E. Cyanosis

Central cyanosis indicates a low blood oxygen level outside of the normal range. Absence of cyanosis, however, is *not* a reliable indicator of oxygenation within the normal range.

It is not uncommon for a baby to show tachypnea, grunting, flaring, or retractions, but without cyanosis, and still have low arterial blood oxygen concentration (partial pressure of oxygen, Pao_2). In addition, an extremely anemic baby may *not* show cyanosis despite having a low blood oxygen level.

Healthy newborns may have a ruddy skin color, which is sometimes mistaken for cyanosis. In addition, acrocyanosis (blue hands and feet) may be seen in a newborn and is not, by itself, an indicator of respiratory distress or low blood oxygen level. Central cyanosis involves a more generalized blueness or duskiness and can best be determined by observing mucous membranes, such as the lips, and confirming blood oxygen saturation (Spo_2) with a pulse oximeter. (See Unit 1, Oxygen, in this book.)

A pink baby may still have a low Spo₂ or Pao₂ level.

Mucous membranes should be used to judge the presence or absence of cyanosis.

If cyanosis is suspected, check the blood oxygen level with arterial blood gas analysis or pulse oximetry.

2. When is it expected and unexpected for a baby to show signs of respiratory distress?

During the first hour after delivery, mild tachypnea, retractions, flaring, or grunting may occasionally be seen in a healthy baby who will not later exhibit respiratory distress. This is because the baby is absorbing lung fluid and the circulation is adjusting to the extrauterine environment.

Central cyanosis is *never* normal and always requires prompt investigation and treatment. Likewise, severe or worsening tachypnea, retractions, flaring, or grunting within the first hour after birth also requires investigation.

Signs of respiratory distress are present

- *Whenever tachypnea, retractions, flaring, or grunting persist beyond 1 hour after birth*
- *Anytime severe or worsening tachypnea, retractions, flaring, or grunting develop*
- *Anytime cyanosis or a low Spo₂ is present*

Self-test A

Now answer these questions to test yourself on the information in the last section.

A1. What are the 5 signs of respiratory distress?

_____
_____
_____
_____
_____

A2. What part of a baby's body should you examine to determine if the baby is cyanotic?

_____

A3. Thirty minutes after birth, a baby is pink but shows mild grunting and nasal flaring. You check the baby's vital signs, and they are within reference range. What would you do next?
   A. Observe the baby for the next 30 minutes.
   B. Act now to treat respiratory distress.
   C. Attach a pulse oximeter and observe the baby.

A4. Two hours after birth, a baby shows mild grunting and nasal flaring. Is this expected, or are these signs of respiratory distress?

_____

A5. Three hours after birth, a 1,900-g (4 lb 3 oz) baby develops mild grunting, intercostal retractions, and nasal flaring and has a respiratory rate of 80 breaths per minute but is pink all over. It is 4:00 am. What should you do?

Yes **No**

_____ _____ Assist the baby's breathing with bag-and-mask ventilation.
_____ _____ Check the baby's vital signs.
_____ _____ Attach a cardiac monitor to the baby.
_____ _____ Feed the baby to prevent hypoglycemia.
_____ _____ Attach a pulse oximeter to the baby.

Check your answers with the list that follows the Recommended Routines. Correct any incorrect answers and review the appropriate section in the unit.

3. What are the causes of neonatal respiratory distress?

There are many causes of neonatal respiratory distress. They may be divided into

- *Obstructive problems* (a mechanical obstruction preventing air from getting into the lungs or preventing lung expansion)
- *Primary disorders of the lung*
- *Miscellaneous non-pulmonary problems*

A. Obstructive problems
   1. Anything that obstructs the airway, from the nose to the alveoli, will result in respiratory distress.
      Babies breathe through their noses and seldom through their mouths. In general, babies are able to breathe through their mouths only when they are crying. When at rest, babies may suffocate if their nasal airways become obstructed.
      - Some babies with airway obstruction may produce an inspiratory or expiratory noise called *stridor*.
      - *Mucus* in the nasal passageways is a common cause of respiratory distress. Babies with esophageal atresia may choke on normal oral and pulmonary secretions.
      - A *misplaced phototherapy mask* or *misplaced continuous positive airway pressure* (CPAP) apparatus may also obstruct the nose.
      - Other less common causes of respiratory distress include congenital abnormalities of the airway, such as *choanal atresia* (congenital obstruction of the nasal passageways), *Pierre Robin sequence* (or syndrome) (congenitally small mandible, which causes the tongue to obstruct the pharynx), and *vocal cord paralysis*.
   2. Conditions that restrict lung expansion within the chest cavity will result in respiratory distress.
      - The most common of these is a *pneumothorax*. This is a rupture in the lung tissue that allows air to leak from the lungs and become trapped in the space between the lungs and the rib cage (pleural space), thus forming a large "bubble" that inhibits the lungs from expanding with inhalation.
      - A rare cause of restricted lung expansion is *diaphragmatic hernia*. This is a congenital defect in the diaphragm that allows the abdominal contents to enter the chest cavity, thus compressing the lungs and greatly restricting their ability to expand normally with inhalation.

- Fluid collection in the chest cavity (*pleural effusion*) may also compress the lung. Fluid collection in the abdomen (*ascites*) or a large *abdominal mass* may interfere with downward movement of the diaphragm and limit expansion of the lungs.

B. Primary disorders of the lung

1. The most common primary lung disorder is *respiratory distress syndrome* (RDS). This is caused by an immaturity of the lungs. The mature lung produces substances called *surfactants* that coat the alveoli and allow them to remain open during exhalation. Without surfactants, alveoli collapse during exhalation and are difficult to open with the next breath. As a result of this surfactant deficiency, the lungs are stiff and difficult to inflate.

 Respiratory distress in the neonate has many causes, only one of which is respiratory distress syndrome.

Respiratory distress syndrome is caused by lack of lung surfactant.

2. Other primary lung problems include

- *Aspiration syndrome:* This occurs when a fetus aspirates amniotic fluid into the lungs. This is particularly severe when the amniotic fluid contains meconium or blood that is inhaled. A newborn may aspirate fluid at delivery or later with feedings in the nursery or the mother's room.
- *Bacterial or viral pneumonia:* The baby's lungs may become infected before birth (the mother or fetus may or may not show signs of infection).
- *Transient respiratory distress of the newborn* or transient tachypnea of the newborn: Some babies, particularly those born without maternal labor, may have delayed absorption of lung fluid after birth. These babies may have mild to moderate signs of respiratory distress.
- *Hypoplastic (abnormally small) lungs:* These may be the result of prolonged severe oligohydramnios as a result of rupture of the membranes before 20 weeks of gestation or of inadequate fetal urine production due to abnormal formation of the kidneys or severe obstruction of the urinary tract.

C. Miscellaneous non-pulmonary problems

Respiratory distress also may result from non-pulmonary problems, such as

1. Blood flow to the lungs (too much or too little)

Decreased blood flow to the lungs may result from *hypotension* (which may be due to blood loss or sepsis), *congenital heart disease,* or *severe hypoxia and acidosis* (which may cause blood vessels supplying the lungs to constrict). Increased blood flow to the lungs can also be caused by *congenital heart disease* or a persistent *patent ductus arteriosus.*

2. Increased demand for oxygen

Cold stress increases the body's demand for oxygen. For acutely ill babies, *excessive handling* and *oral feedings* may also increase oxygen demands.

3. Concentration of red blood cells above or below the normal range

Anemia may result from blood loss or hemolytic disease. Regardless of the cause of anemia, there are a decreased number of red blood cells to carry oxygen to the muscles and organs.

Polycythemia (an excess of red blood cells) may cause the blood to become too thick to move easily through the lungs and may result in respiratory distress.

4. Hypoglycemia, which may present with apnea

5. Nervous system injury or intracranial bleeding
Nervous system injury, such as *phrenic nerve injury* (sometimes accompanied by Erb-Duchenne paralysis), can cause poor diaphragmatic function or intracranial bleeding from associated hypoxic-ischemic injury.

6. Maternal medication during labor
Some maternal medications administered during labor, such as *magnesium,* may suppress newborn respiratory activity.

 Many times, correction of underlying non-pulmonary problems can significantly diminish or completely eliminate a baby's respiratory distress.

Self-test B

Now answer these questions to test yourself on the information in the last section.

B1.   **True**   **False**   Babies usually breathe through their noses. They usually cannot breathe through their mouths.

B2.   What causes respiratory distress syndrome?
   A. A blockage in the airway between the nose and lungs
   B. Immaturity of the baby's lungs and resulting lack of surfactant needed to keep alveoli open
   C. Inhalation of amniotic fluid into the lungs
   D. Low blood volume
   E. Thick blood

B3.   What causes respiratory distress? (Choose as many as needed.)
   A. A blockage in the airway between the nose and lungs
   B. Immaturity of the baby's lungs and resulting lack of surfactant needed to keep alveoli open
   C. Inhalation of amniotic fluid into the lungs
   D. Low blood volume
   E. Thick blood

B4.   List 2 obstructive causes of respiratory distress.
   _____
   _____

B5.   Besides respiratory distress syndrome, list 2 primary lung problems that cause respiratory distress.
   _____
   _____

B6.   List 3 non-pulmonary problems that may cause respiratory distress.
   _____
   _____
   _____

Check your answers with the list that follows the Recommended Routines. Correct any incorrect answers and review the appropriate section in the unit.

4. Which babies are prone to developing respiratory distress?

Observe the following babies closely and frequently for signs of respiratory distress:

A. Preterm babies

Lungs may be immature with insufficient surfactant, such that a baby may develop RDS. Preterm babies are also at increased risk for developing an infection, which may take the form of bacterial or viral pneumonia.

B. Babies after difficult births

Blood flow to the lungs may be decreased due to pulmonary vasoconstriction, a baby may have aspirated meconium, the diaphragm may be paralyzed due to phrenic nerve injury, or a pneumothorax may have resulted from resuscitative efforts.

C. Babies of women with diabetes mellitus

Regardless of gestational age, babies born to women with diabetes mellitus are delayed in their ability to produce surfactants and are therefore more likely to develop RDS.

D. Babies born by elective cesarean delivery

Delayed absorption of lung fluid (transient respiratory distress of the newborn) is more likely to occur in babies born by elective cesarean delivery than in babies delivered vaginally or whose mothers went through labor prior to cesarean delivery.

E. Babies with maternal risk factor(s) for infection

Babies born to women with fever, rupture of membranes for 18 hours or longer, or foul-smelling/cloudy amniotic fluid are at particular risk for developing bacterial pneumonia. Maternal history of group B β-hemolytic streptococcal cervical or rectal colonization or bacteriuria during pregnancy, or a baby previously infected with group B β-hemolytic streptococcus, increases the risk for neonatal group B β-hemolytic streptococcal infection.

See Book 2: Maternal and Fetal Care, Unit 3, Infectious Diseases in Pregnancy, and Unit 8, Infections, in this book, for more information about surveillance, as well as intrapartum and neonatal management of infectious risk factors.

F. Babies with meconium-stained skin

Meconium aspiration may have occurred. Meconium inactivates surfactant within alveoli.

G. Babies born to women with polyhydramnios

Polyhydramnios (excess amniotic fluid) may result from any of several causes. One cause is when fetuses are unable or too weak to swallow amniotic fluid. These babies may have esophageal atresia and tracheoesophageal fistula or central nervous system depression.

Hydrops fetalis (generalized fetal edema) is also associated with polyhydramnios. These babies may have respiratory distress from pulmonary edema, pleural or pericardial effusions, or severe ascites.

H. Babies with other problems

The increased oxygen needs of severely cold-stressed babies may lead to respiratory distress. If perinatal blood loss has occurred, respiratory distress can result from decreased blood flow to the lungs to pick up oxygen or from insufficient red blood cells to carry an adequate amount of oxygen from the lungs to perfuse the rest of the baby's body and organs. Thus, cold stress, hypovolemia, hypotension, or anemia and its associated complications may result in respiratory distress. (See Section 3C, Miscellaneous Non-pulmonary Problems, in this unit.)

5. What should be done to evaluate a baby who shows signs of respiratory distress?

Any baby with tachypnea, intercostal or subcostal retractions, nasal flaring, or grunting persisting beyond the first hour after birth, or with cyanosis at any time, should be given oxygen and other emergency treatment, as indicated by physical examination findings.

Based on physical findings, consider transillumination or chest radiography, pulse oximetry and arterial blood gas, screening tests, and evaluation for sepsis.

A. Review of maternal and labor and delivery history
Careful review of pregnancy history (eg, gestational age, ultrasonography results, oligohydramnios or polyhydramnios) and events during labor and delivery (eg, meconium staining, fetal distress, low Apgar scores) may give important insight into the possible cause of the distress.

B. Physical examination (See Table 2.1.)

Table 2.1. Physical Findings Associated With Respiratory Distress		
Observation	**Action**	**Comments**
1. Tachypnea (respiratory rate faster than 60 breaths/min)	• Check vital signs. • Obtain chest radiograph. • Review perinatal history.	Babies with severe distress may breathe slowly due to difficulty moving air in/out. Some may breathe very rapidly, but comfortably, without retractions or grunting. Use a process of elimination to rule out possible causes.
2. No air flow into lungs	• Suction mucus. • Reposition baby. • Attempt to pass a nasogastric tube, insert an oral airway (choanal atresia). • If Pierre Robin sequence, position the baby prone and, if needed, insert a large-bore catheter as a nasopharyngeal tube to prevent occlusion by the tongue.	Consider the possibility of obstruction due to **mucus, choanal atresia,** or **Pierre Robin sequence.**
3. Meconium staining	• Suction the upper airway as soon as the baby is born. • Consider suctioning below the vocal cords if the baby has respiratory depression at birth.	If amniotic fluid is meconium stained, **meconium** may be in the baby's airway (see Book 1: Maternal and Fetal Evaluation and Immediate Newborn Care, Unit 5, Resuscitating the Newborn). Non-vigorous newborns with meconium-stained fluid do not require routine intubation and tracheal suctioning. Initial steps may be performed at the radiant warmer. Meconium-stained amniotic fluid is a perinatal risk factor that requires the presence of one resuscitation team member with full resuscitation skills, including endotracheal intubation.

(*continued*)

Observation	Action	Comments
Table 2.1. Physical Findings Associated With Respiratory Distress (*continued*)		
4. **Decreased breath sounds on one side, asymmetrical chest movement,** or **cyanosis**	Transilluminate or obtain a chest radiograph.	Baby may have a **pneumothorax, pleural effusion,** or **diaphragmatic hernia.** Symmetrical breath sounds do not exclude these conditions.
5. **Grunting** (a predominant sign)	Obtain a chest radiograph.	This indicates the baby has **poor lung compliance** ("stiff lungs").
6. **Cyanosis** of mucous membranes	• Give oxygen. • **Confirm hypoxemia with pulse oximetry.** • Obtain a chest radiograph.	Assume that any baby with blue mucous membranes has a **low blood oxygen level.**
7. **Sunken abdomen**	• Pass a nasogastric tube to withdraw swallowed air and decompress the stomach. • Obtain a chest or abdominal radiograph. • Position the baby at a 45° head-up angle. • If in severe respiratory distress, intubate the trachea and assist with ventilation.	Babies with **diaphragmatic hernias** have sunken (scaphoid) abdomens because the intestines are located in the chest. Avoid distending the gastrointestinal tract with air.
8. **Pale baby, weak pulses,** or **poor peripheral perfusion**	Obtain blood pressure, hematocrit value, and white blood cell count with differential.	Babies with low blood pressure related to **blood loss** or **sepsis** may exhibit signs of respiratory distress (see Unit 4, Low Blood Pressure [Hypotension], and Unit 8, Infections, in this book).
9. **Excessive or particularly thick mucus**	• Suction the mucus. • Pass a nasogastric tube. • Obtain a chest radiograph. • Position the baby at a 45° head-up angle.	Babies with **esophageal atresia** may aspirate secretions. If atresia is present, a radiograph will show the nasogastric tube coiled in a blind esophageal pouch.

C. Transillumination and chest radiography (See also Skill Unit: Detecting a Pneumothorax.) *Transillumination* is the technique of holding a bright light against the body to detect a collection of air. The chest may be transilluminated to detect a pneumothorax.

A positive transillumination result may be sufficient evidence to insert a needle or tube into the chest to relieve a pneumothorax if other indications, such as vital signs or arterial blood gases, are rapidly deteriorating. If the baby's condition allows intervention to be delayed for a brief time, obtain a chest radiograph to confirm the presence and location of a pneumothorax before insertion of a needle or tube.

A follow-up chest radiograph should be obtained to assess the position of the chest tube or evacuation of the pneumothorax, as well as detection of other disorders, such as pneumonia or RDS.

D. Pulse oximetry and arterial blood gas

For a newborn who requires increased inspired oxygen for longer than a brief period or who has persistent respiratory distress

- Monitor oxygen saturation levels with a pulse oximeter.
- Determine arterial blood oxygen, pH, carbon dioxide, and bicarbonate levels. Oxygenation (PaO_2) and acid-base status (pH, $PaCO_2$, and bicarbonate levels) may be measured from blood drawn from an artery. Oxygenation may also be estimated with an oximeter, while acid-base status can only be measured from a blood sample.

 It is inadequate to measure only oxygenation without determining the acid-base status.

A baby may be severely acidotic or have a high carbon dioxide level that requires immediate treatment and still have oxygenation within the normal range.

E. Screening tests
- Hematocrit value
- Blood glucose screen
- White blood cell count and differential

F. Evaluation for sepsis or pneumonia

Some babies with respiratory distress may have bacterial pneumonia, which is indistinguishable from RDS on a chest radiograph. Many experts advise obtaining a blood culture and starting antibiotic therapy in any newborn with respiratory distress (see Unit 8, Infections, in this book). If the blood culture result is reported as negative at 36 to 48 hours, antibiotic therapy may then be discontinued.

6. What general support measures are indicated for any baby with respiratory distress?

General principles of therapy for any baby with respiratory distress include

A. Improve oxygen delivery to the lungs

This is most easily accomplished by increasing the oxygen concentration in the baby's environment (see Unit 1, Oxygen, in this book). Extreme care must be taken to avoid delivering excess or insufficient oxygen.

 Too little oxygen in the blood can cause brain damage. Over time, too much oxygen can cause damage to several body systems, particularly the eyes, brain, and lungs.

Appropriate oxygenation can be determined by measuring arterial blood gases or proper use of a pulse oximeter. Environmental oxygen should be regulated to maintain arterial blood oxygen levels of 45 to 65 mm Hg or 88% to 95% saturation.

Some babies with respiratory distress require ventilatory assistance beyond increased environmental oxygen. These babies

- Generally require more than 45% to 50% inspired oxygen to maintain arterial blood oxygen (PaO_2) between 45 and 75 mm Hg

or

- Have severe, recurring apnea

or

- Have evidence of respiratory failure or an arterial carbon dioxide concentration ($Paco_2$) greater than approximately 50 mm Hg

These babies may require CPAP or intermittent positive-pressure ventilation, depending on the cause and severity of respiratory distress. For babies with RDS, administration of surfactant may also be appropriate. These procedures and treatments require special equipment and expertise and are discussed in other units.

B. Improve pulmonary blood flow
Adequate pulmonary blood flow depends on

- Maintenance of arterial blood oxygen and oxygen saturation in a non-hypoxemic range
- Correction of acidosis
- An adequate circulating blood volume
- An adequate number of red blood cells

Hypoxemia and acidosis each constrict pulmonary blood vessels and, thus, decrease pulmonary blood flow, with a resultant further decrease in arterial blood oxygen levels.

The most common causes of *metabolic acidosis* include

- Insufficient arterial oxygen
- Poor tissue perfusion from low circulating blood volume or heart failure and low blood pressure
- Cold stress
- Infection

Metabolic acidosis is best treated by correcting the cause. Use of sodium bicarbonate ($NaHCO_3$) to temporarily improve acidosis is controversial and is *not* recommended without discussion with neonatal experts.

Severe *respiratory acidosis* (pH level less than 7.2, $Paco_2$ of at least 55–60 mm Hg) indicates respiratory failure. Sodium bicarbonate should *not* be used in this situation. In most cases, treatment for respiratory acidosis is assisted ventilation.

Low blood pressure may require treatment with a blood volume expander (eg, physiological [normal, 0.9%] saline solution at 10–15 mL/kg). A newborn in respiratory distress with a *low hematocrit value* (<35%) or who has a history of acute blood loss may require a blood transfusion (see Unit 4, Low Blood Pressure [Hypotension], in this book).

Babies with a *very high hematocrit value* can develop respiratory distress from viscous blood that becomes compacted in small pulmonary capillaries, with subsequent reduction in blood flow through the capillaries. Be sure blood is drawn from an artery or vein for determination of hematocrit value, as heel stick hematocrit values are frequently falsely high.

If a venous or arterial hematocrit value is greater than 65% to 70% and the baby has otherwise unexplained respiratory distress, a reduction exchange transfusion can be performed to lower the hematocrit level. This partial exchange transfusion is accomplished by removing some of the baby's blood and replacing it with normal saline solution. See Book 4: Specialized Newborn Care, Unit 2, Exchange, Reduction, and Direct Transfusions, and consult with regional perinatal center staff if a reduction exchange is considered.

C. Decrease oxygen consumption

You can do several things to minimize a baby's oxygen requirement by decreasing the baby's oxygen consumption. These measures include

- Providing an appropriate neutral thermal environment (See Book 1: Maternal and Fetal Evaluation and Immediate Newborn Care, Unit 7, Thermal Environment.)
- Warming and humidifying inspired oxygen/air mixture (See Unit 1, Oxygen, in this book.)
- Withholding oral feedings (Adequate hydration and some caloric requirements can be met with intravenous fluids.)
- Handling a baby as little as possible
  — Do not bathe the baby.
  — Do not perform an extensive physical examination.
  — Perform only essential procedures, with minimal, gentle handling.

These principles apply to the care of babies with acute respiratory distress during the first several days after birth. If a baby requires oxygen for a prolonged period, care practices may change somewhat, depending on the baby's gestational age, postnatal age, and condition.

Self-test C

Now answer these questions to test yourself on the information in the last section.

C1. List at least 3 groups of babies who are at risk for developing respiratory distress.

_____
_____
_____

C2. What should be done, in addition to a physical examination, for a baby showing signs of respiratory distress?

_____
_____
_____

C3. If grunting is the primary physical symptom, you would suspect the baby has _____. You would obtain a _____ to help evaluate the cause.

C4. If a catheter cannot be passed through the nose of a baby with respiratory distress, you would suspect the baby has _____. You would immediately insert _____ in the baby's mouth.

C5. If a baby with respiratory distress suddenly turns blue, you would suspect the baby has _____. You would perform a _____ and obtain a _____ to confirm the diagnosis.

C6. If a baby in respiratory distress soon after birth has a hematocrit value of 30%, the baby probably experienced _____. You should prepare to administer _____.

C7. If arterial PaO_2 is low, increase the baby's _____ to avoid damage to the baby's _____.

C8. If arterial PaO_2 is very high, you should _____ the amount of inspired oxygen to avoid damage to organs such as the _____ and _____.

C9. If arterial $Paco_2$ is high and pH level is low, you should
  A. Ventilate the baby.
  B. Give sodium bicarbonate.

C10. If arterial $Paco_2$ is within reference range and the pH level is low, you should consider
  A. Ventilating the baby
  B. Treating the underlying cause of acidosis

Check your answers with the list that follows the Recommended Routines. Correct any incorrect answers and review the appropriate section in the unit.

Part 2: Apnea

Objectives

In Part 2 of this unit you will learn

A. The definition of apnea

B. Which babies are likely to develop apnea

C. The causes of apnea

D. What to do for an apneic baby

1. What is apnea?

Apnea means cessation of breathing for longer than a 20-second period or for a shorter time if there is also bradycardia or cyanosis. Many healthy newborns will have brief breathing pauses or "periodic breathing," but these pauses are not apnea episodes.

Babies may have several different types of apnea.

- Central apnea, in which there is no or inadequate movement of the respiratory muscles due to absent or decreased signal from the brainstem
- Obstructive apnea, in which there is respiratory muscle activity but absent or inadequate air exchange due to airway obstruction
- Mixed central and obstructive apnea (the most common)

Traditional electronic respiratory monitoring indicates only absent respiratory muscle movement. Heart rate and oximetry monitors will indicate bradycardia or decrease in oxygen saturation associated with obstructive episodes.

2. Which babies are at risk for apnea?

A. Preterm babies

Thirty percent of all preterm babies weighing less than 1,800 g (<3 lb 15½ oz) will have at least one apneic spell. The chances of apnea occurring increase as the birth weight decreases. Essentially, all babies with a birth weight less than 1,000 g (<2 lb 3 oz) will have at least one apneic spell. Preterm babies, in addition to having central apnea from immature brains, are also at increased risk of obstructive episodes due to difficulty in maintaining their airway associated with head and neck positioning.

A preterm baby who is stable and doing well can suddenly have a severe apneic spell.

B. Babies with respiratory distress

Any newborn, regardless of birth weight, may develop apnea as a complication of respiratory disease.

When a baby with respiratory disease has an apneic spell, assume the baby's condition is worsening.

Active intervention is indicated (eg, increased oxygen administration, intubation, assisted ventilation, correction of acidosis, other measures as needed).

C. Babies with metabolic disorders

Low blood glucose, calcium, or sodium level can all result in apnea. Babies who are acidotic (low blood pH level from too much acid in their blood) may also become apneic.

D. Babies with infections

Apnea may be the first sign of sepsis or meningitis.

E. Cold-stressed babies who are being warmed
Cold babies are likely to have apneic spells as they are being warmed.

F. Over-warming
Over-warming a preterm baby in an incubator or under a radiant warmer may cause apnea.

G. Babies with central nervous system disorders
Babies with seizures may occasionally stop breathing during a seizure. Babies with central nervous system hemorrhage or rapidly progressing hydrocephalus may also develop apnea.

H. Babies with low blood volume or low hematocrit level
Babies with low blood volume or anemia may develop apnea as the first sign of their condition.

I. Babies who experience perinatal compromise
Babies may develop many of the problems mentioned previously (eg, metabolic disorders, central nervous system damage) after a period of hypoxia or acidosis. Apneic spells may also result.

J. Babies whose mothers received certain medications
Depressant drugs, such as narcotics or general anesthetics, given to a woman during labor will cross the placenta and may cause apnea in the baby.

3. How should apnea be anticipated and detected?

All the babies mentioned previously are at risk for developing apnea. They should undergo continuous electronic monitoring of heart rate and respirations. (See Book 1: Maternal and Fetal Evaluation and Immediate Newborn Care, Unit 4, Is the Baby Sick? Recognizing and Preventing Problems in the Newborn.) Those with respiratory problems or requiring supplemental oxygen should also be monitored with pulse oximetry. (See Unit 1, Oxygen, in this book.)

A. Heart rate monitor
Set the alarm to sound when the heart rate falls below 80 to 90 beats/min (100 beats/min for small or preterm babies).

B. Respiratory monitor
Set the alarm to sound when there is a 15- to 20-second period without respiratory effort.

C. Pulse oximeter
Set the pulse oximeter to alarm when oxygen saturations fall below 88% (or refer to your institution's policy on pulse oximeter saturation guidelines).

4. What should you do when a baby has an apneic spell?

A. Evaluate the cardiorespiratory monitor

An evaluation of the monitor screen will let you know if the electrocardiogram and respiratory signals are clear.

Many monitors will also show what preceded the apneic spell (eg, whether bradycardia or absence of chest movement came first).

B. Look at the baby

1. If the baby is blue and/or apneic

First, stimulate the baby to resume breathing. In many cases, this involves merely gently stroking or rubbing the baby's back or extremities. Babies will often quickly resume breathing after stroking them lightly. Sometimes, more vigorous rubbing of the skin may be needed.

If mild or moderate stimulation does not result in resumed respirations, do not persist in these efforts. Use a bag and mask or your institution's preferred method to assist the baby's ventilation until the heart rate is within normal range and spontaneous respirations resume.

You may need to decrease the rate of assisted ventilation and, at the same time, stimulate the baby before spontaneous breathing resumes. At times, assisted ventilation may remove some of the stimulus to breathe.

Use supplemental oxygen if cyanosis persists after assisted or spontaneous ventilation is established.

2. If the baby is pink, has a heart rate within normal range, and is breathing

In this case, the episode may represent a

• True apneic spell with spontaneous resumption of breathing by the baby

or

• Malfunction of the monitor (Check placement of the leads on the baby, monitor settings, and functioning.)

C. Record your observations and actions

5. What should you think of when a baby has an apneic spell?

As noted previously, apnea may be caused by many different disorders or may have no identifiable cause. However, all treatable causes must be considered before attributing the apneic spell to "apnea of prematurity."

The following actions are not indicated with every apneic spell. However, with the first spell, or if spells become more frequent or severe, all actions should be considered.

- If the baby has respiratory disease, it may be rapidly worsening. Obtain an arterial blood gas sample and increase respiratory support for the baby. Obtain a chest radiograph.
- Check the blood glucose level.
- Check if the baby aspirated milk or formula while feeding.
  - — Could the baby have aspirated while nipple feeding?
  - — Does the baby have a nasogastric or orogastric tube that may have slipped out of the stomach and allowed milk or formula to go into the lungs?
  - — Did the baby vomit and aspirate vomitus?
- Measure blood pressure.
- Check body and environmental temperature (including oxygen/air temperature if the baby is receiving supplemental oxygen).
- Check hematocrit/hemoglobin levels.
- Consider the possibility of sepsis or meningitis, review the recent feeding history, and assess the baby's vital signs, tone, and activity. Consider obtaining a white blood cell count and differential and blood and cerebrospinal fluid cultures and starting antibiotics.
- If a cause still has not been found, check serum calcium, sodium, and pH levels.
- Consider the possibility that the apneic spell was a type of seizure activity. Review the history for evidence of perinatal compromise and evaluate the baby's neurological status.

6. What should be done if the apnea is recurrent or severe?

Most preterm babies with apnea require no more intervention than occasional stimulation.

If spells occur frequently (more than a few each day), other therapies, such as CPAP, caffeine, or mechanical ventilation, may be required. These babies generally require long-term intensive care, and such treatments are not discussed in this unit.

7. When can apnea monitoring be discontinued?

Most experts agree that the chances of recurrent apnea are very small if all of the following conditions are true:

- Acute illness has resolved.
- The baby weighs more than 1,800 g (>4 lb) and has reached a gestational age of 35 weeks or older, although babies who were born at very low gestational age (eg, <28 weeks) are more likely to continue having apnea beyond 35 weeks' postmenstrual age.
- Baby has been apnea free for 5 to 7 consecutive days, unless the baby may require longer hospitalization or monitoring for other reasons.
  Note: These guidelines are intended to apply only to babies during the first few weeks after birth and should not be used for babies who stop breathing at several months of age (this would be considered an acute life-threatening event, formerly termed "near-miss sudden infant death syndrome").

See Book 4: Specialized Newborn Care, Unit 7, Continuing Care for At-Risk Babies, for more information about apnea monitoring and treatment in stable, growing preterm babies.

Self-test E

Now answer these questions to test yourself on the information in the last section.

E1. **True** **False** Whenever a preterm baby has an apneic spell, it is reasonable to assume it is due to "apnea of prematurity."

E2. If an apneic baby does not breathe spontaneously after mild to moderate tactile stimulation, what should you do next? _____

E3. List at least 6 screening procedures that should be considered for a baby who experienced an apneic spell.

_____
_____
_____
_____
_____
_____

E4. When can apnea monitoring be discontinued?

_____
_____
_____

Check your answers with the list that follows the Recommended Routines. Correct any incorrect answers and review the appropriate section in the unit.

Part 3: Pneumothorax

Objectives

In Part 3 of this unit you will learn

A. The definition of a pneumothorax

B. Which babies are at risk for developing a pneumothorax

C. How to detect a pneumothorax

D. The consequences of a pneumothorax

E. How to treat a pneumothorax

1. What is a pneumothorax?

A pneumothorax is a collection of air (*pneumo*) within the chest cavity (*thorax*). It results from a rupture in the lung tissue that allows air to leak outside the lung. This air forms a pocket between the lung tissue and chest wall, compressing the lung. For this reason, a pneumothorax is sometimes referred to as a "collapsed lung" or an "air leak."

The air pocket may become so large that it also causes a shift in the normal position of the heart. A pneumothorax in the baby's chest cavity on the left side shifts the heart toward the right, while a pneumothorax in the right side of the chest causes the heart to shift toward the baby's left side. The pneumothorax and shifted heart position can be seen on chest radiographs.

2. When does a pneumothorax occur?

A. Healthy babies

In healthy newborns, a pneumothorax may develop at delivery. This is due to the high inspiratory pressures the baby creates with the first few breaths. As noted previously, pneumothorax in an otherwise healthy baby is rarely symptomatic and should not be treated unless a baby develops clinically significant respiratory distress. Some providers have placed newborns in an oxygen hood containing 100% oxygen (described as a "nitrogen washout"); however, this is no longer recommended.

B. Sick babies

In sick babies, a pneumothorax may occur at the time of resuscitation or at any time during their illness. High CPAP and assisted ventilation pressures increase the risk for pneumothorax. A pneumothorax should be considered anytime there is a sudden deterioration in the baby's condition, even if the baby is recovering from an illness.

C. Babies with a pneumothorax

Development of one pneumothorax increases the chance of developing additional pneumothoraces on the same side as the original pneumothorax or on the opposite side.

A blocked chest tube may also lead to redevelopment of a pneumothorax in the already affected side.

3. Which babies are at risk for a pneumothorax?

Approximately 1% of all well, term newborns develop a spontaneous pneumothorax. Most of these babies show no signs or do not have any symptoms, and the pneumothorax resolves without treatment.

Much more frequently, babies with lung disease develop a pneumothorax as a complication of their lung disease. The risk increases with increasing severity of lung disease. A pneumothorax is most likely to occur in

A. Babies receiving positive-pressure ventilation

If a baby is receiving CPAP, the higher the CPAP pressure, the greater the risk of a pneumothorax. Likewise, if a baby is receiving assisted ventilation with a mechanical respirator or by bag and mask, the higher the pressure, the greater the risk of a pneumothorax. Higher than reference range pressures required to achieve adequate oxygenation increase the risk of a pneumothorax. Techniques for CPAP and assisted ventilation are discussed in separate units in Book 4: Specialized Newborn Care.

B. Babies with poor lung compliance

Whether they require CPAP or assisted ventilation, babies with poor lung compliance (stiff lungs) are at increased risk for developing a pneumothorax. For example, a baby with RDS requiring oxygen therapy via an oxygen hood, CPAP, or assisted ventilation is more likely to develop a pneumothorax.

C. Babies with aspiration syndrome

Aspiration of a foreign substance, such as meconium, blood, or amniotic fluid, places the baby at risk for development of a pneumothorax because the aspirated material creates a ball-valve effect in the small branches of the airway. When the baby inhales, airways expand slightly, and air and oxygen flow past these bits of foreign material and into the alveoli. However, during exhalation, airways collapse around the foreign matter. This means that the trapped gas keeps the alveoli abnormally inflated during exhalation. This process can continue until the alveoli are so overinflated that a rupture in the lung tissue occurs. Up to 50% of newborns with meconium aspiration syndrome can develop a pneumothorax.

D. Babies who required resuscitation

High ventilation pressures may be required during resuscitation of a sick baby. While it is always important to resuscitate a baby as quickly and effectively as possible, some babies will develop a pneumothorax as a result of the bag and mask or bag and endotracheal-tube ventilation that was required.

4. What are the signs of a pneumothorax?

In addition to risk factors, certain signs and arterial blood gas values are characteristic indicators that a baby has developed a pneumothorax. A baby may have one or several of the following findings:

A. Clinical findings
- Sudden onset of cyanosis.
- Increase or decrease in respiratory effort or rate.
- Breath sounds that are louder over one lung. However, because breath sounds radiate easily across the small chest of a newborn, a difference in breath sounds may be impossible to detect, even with a large pneumothorax.
- Shift in the location where the baby's heartbeat is best heard.
- One side of the chest becomes higher than the other. The pneumothorax may cause hyperexpansion of the affected side of the chest.
- Development of abdominal distension. The pneumothorax pushes the diaphragm down, compressing the abdominal organs and making the belly appear distended.
- Development of low blood pressure, when the blood pressure had been within normal range. Pressure from the pneumothorax on the major veins inhibits blood return to the heart, causing a decrease in circulating blood volume, which then results in lower blood pressure.
- Deterioration in appearance, with mottling of the skin and sluggish peripheral blood flow. (When the skin is pressed, the blanched area is slow to turn pink again.)

B. Oxygen saturation and arterial blood gas changes

When a pneumothorax occurs, oxygen saturation drops acutely, and arterial blood gas values change as the lung is unable to expand fully. Pressure from the pneumothorax compresses the alveoli in large areas of the lung and interferes with the normal exchange of oxygen and carbon dioxide.

If oxygen saturation and clinical changes are detected early enough, they may be seen before dramatic changes in arterial blood gas values occur. Typical changes in arterial blood gas values include

- Decrease in arterial oxygen (PaO_2) concentration
- Increase in arterial carbon dioxide ($PaCO_2$) concentration
- Decrease in blood pH level

Some babies may tolerate a pneumothorax well, with minimal symptoms. Other babies, even those with small air collections, may become acutely ill and unstable.

5. What should you do when you suspect a baby has developed a pneumothorax?

Several things will need to be done rapidly, depending on how sick the baby appears. Your first action should always be to maintain the baby's oxygenation. Then proceed to detect and treat the pneumothorax.

1. Quickly increase the baby's inspired oxygen concentration until the baby is pink. If not already in place, attach a pulse oximeter to the baby to monitor oxygenation. Adjust the baby's inspired oxygen concentration to maintain saturation within normal range (88%–95%).
2. If an umbilical arterial catheter is in place, obtain an arterial blood gas sample. Do *not* wait for the results before taking further action. Proceed with techniques to detect a pneumothorax.
3. Transilluminate the baby's chest. If the transillumination result is positive and the baby's clinical condition is unstable or deteriorating, you may need to insert a needle into the baby's chest and aspirate the pneumothorax as an emergency measure.
4. If the baby is stable, obtain a portable chest radiograph as soon as possible. After a pneumothorax is detected, several follow-up radiographs may also be needed to evaluate treatment (needle aspiration or chest tube insertion).
5. If an arterial blood gas sample could not be obtained earlier, obtain one now. Provide oxygen therapy and respiratory support as indicated by the arterial blood gas results. You will probably need to conduct several arterial blood gas analyses as the baby's condition changes and treatment is provided. Even if a pulse oximeter is being used, arterial blood gas analyses are necessary to monitor the baby's PaO_2, $PaCO_2$, pH, and serum bicarbonate levels and to adjust therapy accordingly.

6. How is a pneumothorax detected?

A. Transillumination

A baby's chest may be illuminated with a bright light to detect a pneumothorax (Figure 2.1). Light penetrates air better than tissue. Therefore, the area of the pneumothorax "lights up," creating a positive transillumination result. The transilluminator should be placed directly onto the chest wall and alternated between both sides of the chest to compare the degree of transillumination between the 2 sides. Normally, there is approximately a 1-cm (0.4-in) ring around the light. With a pneumothorax, the light will be much larger and may be asymmetric. It is also helpful to perform transillumination in a darkened room.

A large pneumothorax can be detected easily and quickly with transillumination, but a small pneumothorax may not be seen clearly. A small pneumothorax may still be present, even though a transillumination result is negative.

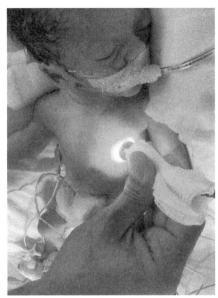

Figure 2.1. Transillumination for Detection of Pneumothorax
Reprinted with permission from Razak A, Mohanty PK, Venkatesh HA. Anteromedial pneumothorax in a neonate: 'The diagnostic dilemma' and the importance of clinical signs. *BMJ Case Reports.* 2014.

False-negative results can be seen with large newborns with increased skin thickness, as well. False-positive results can be seen in newborns with subcutaneous edema, pneumomediastinum, and pulmonary interstitial emphysema.

 Immediate treatment should be undertaken for a baby with a clearly positive transillumination result, whose condition is deteriorating. Do not wait for a chest radiograph.

B. Chest radiography
    If the baby's condition is stable or there is any question about transillumination, obtain a chest radiograph. The details of transillumination and radiograph interpretation for a pneumothorax are presented in the skill units.

7. What are the consequences of a pneumothorax?

A. Hypoxia and acidosis
    Pressure on the heart and lungs from the pneumothorax pocket of air may restrict adequate air movement to the lungs or blood flow from the heart.

B. Intraventricular hemorrhage
    - Decreased venous return to the heart from cerebral veins occurs as a result of compression by the pneumothorax on the heart and major blood vessels.
    - Hypercarbia (high blood carbon dioxide level) and peripheral arterial constriction usually accompany development of a pneumothorax, causing an acute increase in blood flow to the brain.

    Decreased venous drainage from the brain, together with increased blood flow to the brain, is thought to be responsible for the increased occurrence of intraventricular

73

hemorrhage in babies with pneumothorax. Because cerebral blood vessels of preterm babies are particularly fragile, preterm babies are at highest risk for intraventricular hemorrhage.

8. How is a pneumothorax treated?

If a pneumothorax is small and the baby is not in respiratory distress, no treatment is required. In these cases, the pneumothorax will gradually resolve spontaneously, over several hours.

If a baby is symptomatic, however, needle aspiration or chest tube placement may be used to relieve a pneumothorax.

A. Needle aspiration

If a baby's condition is deteriorating rapidly, a needle or percutaneous catheter is placed through the chest wall and into the collection of air. A stopcock and syringe are attached to the needle or catheter, and the air is aspirated. Needle aspiration is a temporary measure, performed in an emergency. It is usually followed by placement of a chest tube.

B. Chest tube placement

A chest tube may be inserted initially, if the baby's condition is relatively stable, or after needle aspiration of the pneumothorax. After insertion, a chest tube is attached to low, continuous suction by using a 3-chamber or preset valve system until the rupture in the lung heals and the air leak stops.

The step-by-step details of these 2 procedures are described in the skill units.

Self-test F

Now answer these questions to test yourself on the information in the last section.

F1. A pneumothorax is _____.

F2. Which babies are at highest risk for a pneumothorax?

_____

_____

_____

_____

F3. **True**   **False**   Breathing with a bag and mask during resuscitation should be strictly limited to prevent development of a pneumothorax.

F4. List at least 4 signs that a baby with a pneumothorax may develop.

_____

_____

_____

_____

F5. When a baby has a pneumothorax, you would expect the PaO_2 concentration to _____, the $PaCO_2$ to _____, and the blood pH level to _____.

F6. **True**   **False**   All term babies with a spontaneous pneumothorax should have a chest tube placed to relieve the pneumothorax.

F7. A pneumothorax
    A. Can be a life-threatening condition
    B. Is a minor complication of positive-pressure ventilation
    C. Occurs only in term newborns
    D. Occurs only in babies on ventilators
    E. Will always cause intraventricular hemorrhage

F8. What are 2 techniques used to treat a pneumothorax?

_____

_____

F9. **True**   **False**   If a pneumothorax is present, a transillumination result will always be positive.

F10. **True**   **False**   A chest radiograph should always be obtained before treatment of a pneumothorax.

Check your answers with the list that follows the Recommended Routines. Correct any incorrect answers and review the appropriate section in the unit.

RESPIRATORY DISTRESS

Recommended Routines

All the routines listed here are based on the principles of perinatal care presented in the unit you have just finished. They are recommended as part of routine perinatal care.

Read each routine carefully and decide whether it is standard operating procedure in your hospital. Check the appropriate blank next to each routine.

Procedure Standard in My Hospital	Needs Discussion by Our Staff	Recommended Routine
_____	_____	1. Establish a routine of using a pulse oximeter to monitor oxygenation of any baby with respiratory distress, starting from the time distress is first noted.
_____	_____	2. Establish a routine for obtaining the following information for any baby with respiratory distress: Immediately: • Vital signs (temperature, pulse, respirations, and blood pressure) • Pulse oximetry monitoring • Physical examination Within 30 minutes: • Portable chest radiograph • Arterial blood gas • Hematocrit level from venous or arterial (not capillary) blood • Blood glucose screening test or laboratory test • Blood culture or white blood cell count with differential
_____	_____	3. Establish a policy to allow sufficient oxygen to be given to keep a cyanotic baby pink until appropriate blood gas determinations are made.
_____	_____	4. Establish a policy of withholding baths and oral feedings from any acutely ill baby who has respiratory distress or receives supplemental oxygen.
_____	_____	5. Provide continuous electronic cardiorespiratory monitoring for all babies at risk for apnea.
_____	_____	6. Be prepared to provide immediate transillumination for any baby in your nursery.

_____ _____ 7. Establish a system for obtaining a chest radio-graph and conducting an arterial blood gas analysis within 30 minutes of the time a pneumothorax is suspected.

_____ _____ 8. Be prepared to provide immediate needle aspiration of a pneumothorax.

_____ _____ 9. Establish a policy that will ensure the presence of a sterile chest tube insertion tray and suction drainage system in the nursery at all times.

Self-test Answers

These are the answers to the Self-test questions. Please check them with the answers you gave and review the information in the unit wherever necessary.

Self-test A

A1. Tachypnea
Intercostal or subcostal retractions
Nasal flaring
Grunting
Cyanosis

A2. Mucous membranes (eg, lips)

A3. C. Attach a pulse oximeter and observe the baby.

A4. Tachypnea, retractions, nasal flaring, or grunting after 1 hour from birth indicates respiratory distress.

A5. This baby is now sick. You would

Yes	No	
___	_X_	Assist the baby's breathing with bag-and-mask ventilation.
_X_	___	Check the baby's vital signs.
_X_	___	Attach a cardiac monitor to the baby.
___	_X_	Feed the baby to prevent hypoglycemia.
_X_	___	Attach a pulse oximeter to the baby.

Self-test B

B1. True

B2. B. Immaturity of the baby's lungs and resulting lack of surfactant needed to keep alveoli open

B3. A, B, C, D, and E can each cause respiratory distress.

B4. Any 2 of the following causes:
- Mucus
- Mechanical obstruction, such as a misplaced phototherapy mask
- Choanal atresia
- Pneumothorax
- Diaphragmatic hernia
- Pierre Robin sequence

B5. Any 2 of the following problems:
- Aspiration syndrome
- Pneumonia
- Transient respiratory distress
- Hypoplastic lungs

B6. Any 3 of the following problems:
- Hypotension
- Congenital heart disease
- Cold stress
- Anemia
- Polycythemia
- Hypoxia and acidosis
- Hypoglycemia
- Babies with central nervous system injury
- Certain maternal medications administered during labor

Self-test C

C1. Any 3 of the following groups:
- Preterm babies
- Babies with difficult deliveries
- Babies born to women with diabetes mellitus
- Babies born by cesarean delivery
- Babies born to women with fever, prolonged rupture of membranes, foul-smelling amniotic fluid, or risk factors for group B β-hemolytic streptococcal infection
- Meconium-stained babies
- Babies born to women with polyhydramnios
- Babies with other problems, such as cold stress, hypotension, anemia, polycythemia

C2. Monitor with pulse oximetry.
Carefully review maternal, labor, delivery, and pregnancy history.
Obtain
— Arterial blood gas analysis
— Chest radiograph
— Hematocrit level
— Blood glucose screen
— White blood cell count and differential
Consider blood culture and antibiotics.

C3. If grunting is the primary physical symptom, you would suspect the baby has *poor lung compliance ("stiff lungs")*. You would obtain a *chest radiograph* to help evaluate the cause.

C4. If a catheter cannot be passed through the nose of a baby with respiratory distress, you would suspect the baby has *choanal atresia*. You would immediately insert *an oral airway* in the baby's mouth.

C5. If a baby with respiratory distress suddenly turns blue, you would suspect the baby has *a pneumothorax*. You would perform a *transillumination* and obtain a *chest radiograph* to confirm the diagnosis.

C6. If a baby in respiratory distress soon after birth has a hematocrit value of 30%, the baby probably experienced *perinatal blood loss*. You should prepare to administer *a blood transfusion*.

C7. If arterial PaO_2 is low, increase the baby's *inspired oxygen concentration* to avoid damage to the baby's *brain*.

C8. If arterial PaO_2 is very high, you should *decrease* the amount of inspired oxygen to avoid damage to organs such as the *eyes* and *lungs*.

C9. A. Ventilate the baby.

C10. B. Treating the underlying cause of acidosis

Self-test D

D1. False   *Reason:* Breathing pauses are expected in newborns. Apnea is when breathing stops for longer than 20 seconds or for a shorter period if accompanied by cyanosis or bradycardia.

D2. Yes

D3. Any 5 of the following problems:
- Preterm
- Rapidly worsening respiratory disease
- Metabolic disorder, such as low blood glucose, calcium, or sodium level or acidosis
- Sepsis or meningitis
- Rewarming of a cold-stressed baby
- Over-warming

- Central nervous system disorder
- Low blood volume or low hematocrit level
- History of severe hypoxia or acidosis
- Maternal depressant drugs during labor

D4. All babies at risk for apnea should be electronically *monitored (with heart rate and respiratory monitor and pulse oximetry).*

Self-test E

E1. False *Reason:* There are many causes of apnea. Each should be considered before deciding it is due to "apnea of prematurity."

E2. Use a bag and mask to breathe for the baby; administer oxygen if cyanosis is present and persists after ventilation is established.

E3. Any 6 of the following procedures:
- Arterial blood gas analysis
- Chest radiography
- Blood glucose screen
- Blood pressure check
- Baby's temperature, environmental temperature, and oxygen/air temperature (if supplemental oxygen is being used)
- Hematocrit level
- Evaluate for sepsis and meningitis.
- Evaluate for seizures; assess neurological status.
- Serum sodium, calcium, and pH levels
- Evaluate feedings for the possibility of milk aspiration.

E4. Acute illness has resolved.
Baby weighs 1,800 g (4 lb) or more and has reached a gestational age of 35 weeks or older. Baby has been apnea free for 5 to 7 consecutive days.

Self-test F

F1. A pneumothorax is *a collection of air within the chest cavity, between the lung and chest wall, that results from a rupture in the lung tissue, allowing air to leak outside the lung.*

F2. Babies receiving positive-pressure ventilation
Babies with poor lung compliance ("stiff lungs"), as seen with respiratory distress syndrome
Babies with aspiration syndrome
Babies requiring resuscitation

F3. False   *Reason:* High pressures may be needed to ventilate a baby adequately. The pressure needed should be given and not limited; however, unnecessarily high pressures should be avoided. You should be aware that a possible complication of assisted ventilation is a pneumothorax, but that possibility should not restrict resuscitation efforts.

F4. Any 4 or more of the following signs:
- Sudden onset of cyanosis or decreased Spo_2
- Increase or decrease in respiratory effort or rate
- Breath sounds louder over one lung
- Shift in location of heart sounds
- Unequal chest expansion
- Abdominal distension
- Low blood pressure, especially when it had been within normal range
- Deterioration in appearance with poor peripheral perfusion

F5. When a baby has a pneumothorax, you would expect the Pao_2 concentration to *decrease,* the $Paco_2$ to *increase,* and the blood pH level to *decrease.*

F6. False   *Reason:* Otherwise healthy babies who are in no respiratory distress do not need treatment for a spontaneous pneumothorax. Treatment is needed only if a pneumothorax becomes symptomatic.

F7. A. Can be a life-threatening condition

F8. Needle aspiration
Chest tube placement

F9. False   *Reason:* A small pneumothorax may not yield a clearly discernible ("positive") transillumination result. Also, as you will learn in the skill unit, a clearly positive transillumination result may be difficult to obtain in obese babies, in whom the light transmission may be obscured.

F10. False   *Reason:* You should not wait for a chest radiograph if the transillumination result is clearly positive and the baby's condition is rapidly worsening.

Unit 2 Posttest

After completion of each unit there is a free online posttest available at www.cmevillage.com to test your understanding. Navigate to the PCEP pages on www.cmevillage.com and register to take the free posttests.

Once registered on the website and after completing all the unit posttests, pay the book exam fee ($15) and pass the test at 80% or greater to earn continuing education credits. Only start the PCEP book exam if you have time to complete it. If you take the book exam and are not connected to a printer, either print your certificate to a .pdf file and save it to print later or come back to www.cmevillage.com at any time and print a copy of your educational transcript.

Credits are only available by book, not by individual unit within the books. Available credits for completion of each book exam are as follows: Book 1: 14.5 credits; Book 2: 16 credits; Book 3: 17 credits; Book 4: 9 credits.

For more details, navigate to the PCEP webpages at www.cmevillage.com.

SKILL UNIT

Detecting a Pneumothorax

These skill units will teach you how to detect a pneumothorax. Two techniques will be covered: transillumination and chest radiography. Not everyone will be required to learn how to transilluminate a baby's chest with a fiber-optic light or to interpret chest radiographs. However, all staff members should read this unit and attend a skill session to learn equipment, sequence of steps, and correct positioning of a baby to assist with these skills. A video of transillumination may be viewed at https://www.youtube.com/watch?v=0aQqcW6F9gw.

Note: The illustrations for these separate skill units are not meant to be linked to each other, although the baby appears similar throughout. Transillumination and chest tube insertion skills show left pneumothoraces, while a right pneumothorax is illustrated in the needle aspiration skill, and radiographs of left and right pneumothoraces are shown.

Study these skill units; then attend a skill practice and demonstration session. To master the skills, you will need to demonstrate each of the following skill steps correctly:

Transillumination
1. Position the "baby" (mannequin).
2. Set the transillumination light to the proper setting(s).
3. Darken the room.
4. Maintain the baby's therapy, such as oxygen delivery, thermal environment, and intravenous (IV) infusions.
5. Position the tip of the fiber-optic light on the baby's chest.
   - Midaxillary area
   - Midclavicular area

Chest Radiograph Evaluation
Anteroposterior view
1. Place the baby in a supine position.
   - In an incubator
   - Under a radiant warmer
2. Maintain the baby's therapy, such as oxygen delivery, thermal environment, and IV infusions.
3. Reposition the baby's tubes or wires, as necessary and appropriate.
4. Caution others within range of the x-ray beam to move or put on a lead apron.
5. Restrain the baby, if necessary.

Lateral decubitus view
1. Place the baby in a lateral decubitus position (with the side under suspicion placed "up").
   - In an incubator
   - Under a radiant warmer
2. Maintain the baby's therapy, such as oxygen delivery, thermal environment, and IV infusions.

3. Reposition the baby's tubes or wires, as necessary and appropriate.

4. Caution others within range of the x-ray beam to move or put on a lead apron.

5. Restrain the baby, if necessary.

6. Hold the x-ray plate in proper position. A lead apron should be worn by the individual holding the plate in position.

Note: While useful results depend on performing these skills correctly, interpretation of findings is not included in these checklists. Physicians, and selected nurses, may be asked to participate in a workshop for interpretation of transillumination and chest radiographic findings.

PERINATAL PERFORMANCE GUIDE

Transillumination

Transillumination of the neonatal chest is a technique widely used in neonatal intensive care units to confirm the diagnosis of pneumothorax, but most anesthesiologists may not be familiar with this technique. A high-intensity transilluminating portable light source with a flexible fiber-optic light probe is used. With ambient light dimmed, the probe is placed just superior to the nipple on the supine neonate's chest. It is then lifted and placed inferior to the nipple. The transilluminating light can be applied as long as necessary to each side of the chest since the probe remains cool. A pneumothorax appears as a translucent area in the chest cavity. Lung parenchyma is opaque. With a massive pneumothorax, the entire affected hemithorax lights up. The thinness of the neonate's chest and the very low density of air provide optimal conditions to detect pulmonary air leaks by transillumination in neonates (*J Anaesthesiol Clin Pharmacol.* 2016;32[3]:397-399).

A chest radiograph is obtained any time a pneumothorax is suspected. The benefit of transillumination is that it can be performed easily at the bedside and more quickly than radiography. This allows for immediate treatment of a large, life-threatening pneumothorax without waiting for radiographic evaluation.

ACTIONS	REMARKS
Anticipating the Need for Transillumination	

1. Is there a clinical indication that the baby might have developed a pneumothorax? • Sudden cyanosis or hypoxia • Increase in respiratory rate • Unequal breath sounds • Unequal chest size • Development of abdominal distension • Shift in location of heart sounds • Low blood pressure (especially if it had been within reference range) • Mottled skin with poor peripheral blood flow If yes, immediately • Connect an oximeter to the baby, if the baby is not already being monitored. • Prepare to transilluminate the baby's chest. • Obtain an arterial blood gas measurement.	When a pneumothorax first develops, a baby may show only one of these signs. Often, the most important initial sign is the sudden deterioration of a baby's condition. As the pneumothorax worsens, more changes may become evident. *Be sure to increase the baby's inspired oxygen concentration and provide other supportive therapy as necessary.* If a baby does not have an umbilical arterial catheter and a peripheral arterial blood gas analysis cannot be performed quickly, or if the baby's condition is deteriorating rapidly, it will be necessary to confirm and treat the pneumothorax immediately, before performing an arterial blood gas analysis. Some babies may require assisted ventilation or endotracheal intubation prior to chest tube insertion to stabilize their condition.

ACTIONS

REMARKS

Anticipating the Need for Transillumination (continued)

2. Do the blood gas or oximeter values suggest the occurrence of a pneumothorax?

   • Decrease in Pao_2 or Spo_2

   • Increase in $Paco_2$

   • Acidosis

   If yes, transilluminate the baby's chest.

These changes are typical during development of a pneumothorax. However, sometimes Pao_2 does not decrease and, at first, the $Paco_2$ level may increase only slightly.

Changes in blood gas values or Spo_2 may also reflect worsening lung disease. Blood gas values must be interpreted together with the baby's clinical appearance.

Whenever there is sudden clinical deterioration, a pneumothorax should be suspected, and transillumination should be performed or a chest radiograph should be obtained.

Transilluminating a Baby's Chest

3. Obtain the transillumination light.

A transillumination light is a high-intensity fiber-optic light that shines through the end of a flexible metal tube.

4. Position the baby supine.

5. Turn out the nursery lights and darken the room as much as possible.

6. Position the tip of the light firmly against the baby's chest at the midaxillary area between the fourth and sixth interspaces.

The surface of the fiber-optic light should be held flat against the baby's chest, pressed firmly but gently against the chest wall.

7. Turn on the fiber-optic light to its highest intensity setting.

   Shine the light first on one side of the baby's chest and then on the other.

Look for a difference in the amount of transillumination between the side with the suspected pneumothorax and the opposite side.

85

ACTIONS REMARKS

Transilluminating a Baby's Chest (continued)

8. Observe the area of the baby's chest that lights up. A large pneumothorax will show up as a bright area that extends throughout the air that is trapped outside of the lung but within the chest cavity. This is shown in the illustration (shown at right) as a shaded area on the baby's chest.

9. Move the transilluminating light to anterior parts of the chest and to the opposite side to look for positive transillumination results there, as well. When there is no pneumothorax, the light will form a narrow, symmetrical halo around the light source (shown below).

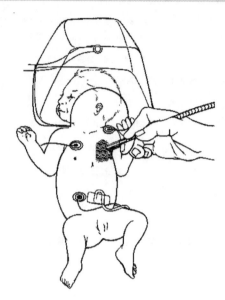

Transillumination Result Positive

Compare both sides. Although it is possible to have bilateral pneumothoraces, this is rare. Usually, a large pneumothorax will appear as lighting up of the affected side (shown above).

Transillumination of the unaffected side would show only a narrow halo around the light (shown at left).

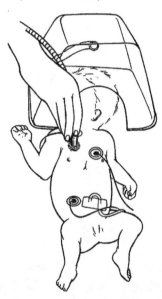

Transillumination Result Negative

10. Repeat steps 8 and 9 to double-check your findings and confirm with radiography.

ACTIONS	REMARKS

Interpreting Transillumination Findings

11. **Normal (negative transillumination result)**
    - The area that lights up will be a symmetrical ring or halo around the tip of the fiber-optic light and will generally not extend more than 1 cm (0.4 in) from the light source.
    - The size of the translucent area will be equal for both sides of the baby's chest.

Thin preterm babies will normally transilluminate more than full-term babies, even when there is no pneumothorax.

A clearly positive transillumination result may be difficult to obtain in babies born at term and in large-for-gestational-age babies. False-negative transillumination results can occur in infants with increased subcutaneous fat or edema. The thickened tissue, particularly in the case of edema, interferes with transillumination (https://www.indianpediatrics.net/feb2017/VID-20161006-WA0020.mp4).

12. **Abnormal (positive transillumination result)**
    - The translucent glow will be larger on one side of the chest than on the other.
    - The translucent area on the side with the pneumothorax will often have an irregular pattern.

The air collection of the pneumothorax lights up. Rarely, there will be a bilateral pneumothorax, in which both sides of the chest will have positive transillumination results.

13. **Suspicious**

    It is difficult to be sure if the area of translucent glow on one side of the chest is larger than that on the other side.

A large pneumothorax will almost always show a positive transillumination result. A small but clinically significant pneumothorax may not show a definitively positive transillumination result.

Using Transillumination Information

14. **Negative transillumination result**

    If the baby's clinical appearance or blood gas values still suggest a pneumothorax, obtain a chest radiograph.

Continue to provide oxygen therapy, assisted ventilation, and other supportive therapy as necessary.

15. **Positive transillumination result**

    If the baby's condition is deteriorating, relieve the pneumothorax immediately with needle aspiration or chest tube insertion.

    If the baby's condition is stable, you may wish to obtain a chest radiograph before chest tube insertion.

This is a life-threatening situation. If the baby's vital signs are deteriorating or adequate oxygenation cannot be achieved, immediate decompression of the pneumothorax is required. Do not wait for a chest radiograph.

16. **Suspicious**

    A baby with a suspicious transillumination result should always be evaluated with chest radiography.

If the baby's condition deteriorates, transilluminate the chest again. Also, be sure to investigate other causes of a marked deterioration in the baby's condition (eg, dislodged or occluded endotracheal tube).

87

ACTIONS	REMARKS

What Can Go Wrong?

1. The fiber-optic light may not be bright enough.

Be sure the light is always set on the highest intensity setting. Replace the batteries if necessary.

2. The room may not be dark enough.

It may not be possible to see the full area of translucent glow.

3. You may not be holding the tip of the light firmly enough against the baby's chest wall.

This will prevent complete transillumination, and a pneumothorax may be missed.

4. You may not be holding the tip of the fiber-optic light flat against the baby's chest.

When you transilluminate a baby's chest, shift the angle of the light slightly until the largest area of translucent glow is seen.

5. You may be holding the light under a skin fold and obtaining an excessive false transillumination result.

Be certain to place the tip of the fiber-optic light flat against the baby's chest.

   Note: Significant edema can also cause a false transillumination result.

6. You may insert a chest tube unnecessarily.

It is always best to confirm a positive transillumination result with chest radiography, unless the baby's condition is rapidly deteriorating.

PERINATAL PERFORMANCE GUIDE

Chest Radiography

Complete chest radiographic evaluation of a newborn will *not* be covered in this skill unit. A few key points that are important for radiographic evaluation and identification of a pneumothorax are presented. In almost all circumstances, obtaining an anteroposterior view of the chest is adequate. Lateral views are helpful occasionally; these are discussed where appropriate. Determination of chest tube placement with radiography is also covered.

ACTIONS	REMARKS
Preparing a Baby for Chest Radiograph	
1. Position the baby supine. The baby's shoulders, back, and hips should be flat, without rotation to the left or right.	Rotation will cause the body structures to appear distorted in size and malpositioned. Accurate evaluation cannot occur on a radiograph in which the baby is rotated.
2. Be sure that all components of the baby's care (eg, oxygen therapy, thermal environment, intravenous infusions) are maintained without interruption during the radiographic procedure.	If the baby is in an incubator, the radiograph can be obtained easily through the top of the incubator. This will not interfere with the evaluation of the chest radiograph. The small hole in the center of the top of most incubators will appear on the radiograph as a symmetric lucent circle. Because it is perfectly round, it is easily identified as an artifact and should not be confused with an abnormal finding. Ensure all "developmental aids" are removed from under the baby. These can interfere with image interpretation.
3. If possible, remove any tubes or wires that drape across the baby's chest.	Cardiac monitor leads attached to the anterior or posterior surface of a baby's chest may need to be removed during radiography and replaced as soon as the procedure is completed. Monitor leads attached to the sides of a baby's chest do not need to be removed for imaging.
4. Obtain the radiograph when the baby is quiet. Do not acquire a chest radiograph when a baby is crying vigorously.	Ideally, the radiograph should be obtained during inspiration, but this is difficult to do with a baby's rapid respiratory rate. Also, because of a baby's small breaths, little difference is seen between inspiratory and expiratory images. However, a radiograph obtained during forceful crying may appear as if the lungs are completely collapsed and will not allow accurate image interpretation.

Positioning a Baby for Chest Radiography

The following illustration shows the correct position of a baby for anteroposterior chest radiography. Note that the baby's shoulders, back, and hips are flat against the x-ray plate; the legs can be immobilized by using a flat cloth diaper or blanket; and oxygen therapy is maintained, as are all other components of the baby's care (not shown). Although not shown, a baby may remain inside an incubator for this procedure, with the radiograph obtained through the top of the incubator.

Once properly positioned, some very sick babies may not need to be restrained during imaging. If the baby is at all active, you should immobilize the baby's extremities. If needed, use restraints only during the very brief period when the radiograph is acquired.

If the x-ray beam is vertical (as shown here), there will be no detectable radiation beyond 6 feet. If the x-ray beam is horizontal (as shown later), a lead apron is necessary to shield staff and other patients in the beam's path.

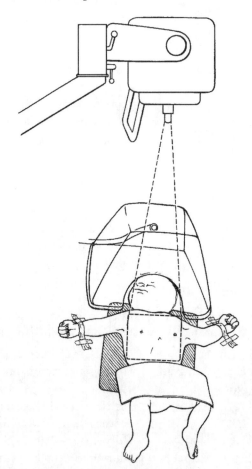

ACTIONS   **REMARKS**

Evaluating a Chest Radiograph for a Pneumothorax

6. Assess the chest radiograph for rotation of the baby. Do this by comparing the length of the anterior ribs on the left and right sides.

When the baby is not rotated on the image, the ribs will appear of equal length on both sides.

7. Assess the radiograph for any asymmetry between the right and left sides.

Asymmetrical findings generally indicate an abnormality and should be further evaluated.

8. Look for typical asymmetrical findings seen with a pneumothorax (see the radiograph below).

   • *Compression of the affected lung:* The edge of the lung should be clearly visible.

If the lungs are stiff, complete collapse of the lungs is unlikely; this feature may limit the degree of heart shift.

   • *Shift of midline structures:* This can occur in varying degrees.

Sometimes, there is a drastic shift in the heart location, while at other times, there is only a lucent curve above the heart as the pneumothorax crosses the midline.

   • *Downward displacement of the diaphragm* on the affected side.

This causes a clinical appearance of abdominal distension. Even without a pneumothorax, the left side of the diaphragm is usually slightly lower than the right side.

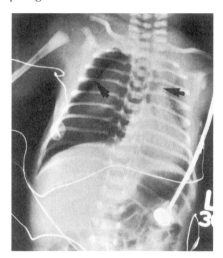

ACTIONS	REMARKS

Clarifying Questionable Findings

- *A hyperlucent area ringing the superior, lateral, and/or inferior edges of the lung.*
- *One lung field that is more lucent than the other (see the radiograph below).*

The area corresponds with the location of the pneumothorax air collection.

Because most radiographs are obtained with the baby lying on their back and most of the air collection is anterior, sometimes no rim or only a narrow rim of air may be seen at the edge of the lung. A lateral decubitus radiograph may be needed to confirm the presence of a pneumothorax.

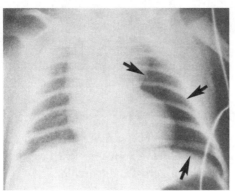

9. If you are not sure if a pneumothorax is present on the anteroposterior chest radiograph, obtain a lateral decubitus view.

10. Put the baby in the lateral decubitus position. The lung suspected of having the pneumothorax should be placed "up," and the unaffected side should be placed "down."

The baby's shoulders, back, and hips should be placed at right angles to the bed. The trapped air will "rise," shifting from the anterior chest to the lateral chest and outlining the lung.

11. Extend the superior arm over the baby's head.

12. Place the x-ray plate flat across the baby's back, also at right angles to the bed.

The x-ray beam will be positioned horizontally across the baby's bed. A lead apron should be worn by any personnel holding the x-ray plate or the baby in position.

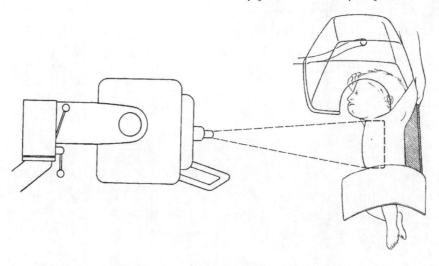

ACTIONS   **REMARKS**

Determining Chest Tube Position After Placement

13. Obtain a follow-up chest radiograph any time a chest tube is inserted. This is done to determine if the

    • Chest tube is positioned properly (see the radiograph below).

    • Pneumothorax has been completely evacuated.

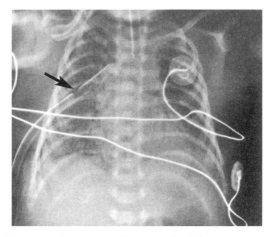

Correct placement of chest tube. There is a small residual pneumothorax at the superior aspect of the lung. The arrow points to one of the holes in the chest tube.

14. Assess the position of the chest tube. It should be directed toward the baby's head and then curved toward the midline.

The tip may touch but should not press against mediastinal structures.

15. Assess the position of the holes in the chest tube. These will appear as small, concave areas on the edge of the tube.

Because the holes are not outlined in radiopaque material, it may not be possible to assess the position of all of them. However, if the tube position is adjusted, be sure that all the holes stay within the baby's chest cavity.

ACTIONS   REMARKS

Determining Chest Tube Position After Placement (continued)

16. Determine if the pneumothorax has been
evacuated. If the pneumothorax is still present, several things should be considered.

• The chest tube is *positioned incorrectly*
(see the radiograph below).

— *Placed posteriorly:* The pneumotho-   On an anteroposterior radiograph, it is not
rax may be anterior to the lung,   possible to ascertain whether the chest tube
while the chest tube has been placed   is in front of or behind the lung. To differen-
behind the lung.   tiate this, you would need to obtain a cross-
table lateral view with the baby supine. The
— *Inserted too far:* On the radiograph,   x-ray plate is held vertically against the
measure the length the tube needs   baby's opposite chest wall, and the radio-
to be withdrawn. Withdraw the   graph is obtained horizontally across the
chest tube that amount by using the   baby's chest. Alternatively, the baby may be
black marks printed on the tube as   placed on their side on the x-ray plate with
reference points.   the radiograph obtained vertically.

— *Not inserted far enough:* The chest
tube must be withdrawn and a
new one inserted by using sterile
conditions.

• The chest tube *suction apparatus is not*   Recheck the system. See also Skill Unit:
functioning correctly.   Treating a Pneumothorax.

• The chest tube and system are working,   If you believe this to be the case and the baby's
but the *radiograph was obtained before*   clinical condition has improved, obtain a sec-
all the air could be withdrawn.   ond follow-up chest radiograph in 30 minutes.

• The tube is positioned correctly, but *not*   Change the baby's position to redistribute air
all of the air is accessible to the chest tube. pockets, allowing complete evacuation.

• One chest tube is not adequate.   While rare, a second chest tube may be
Note: A small residual pneumothorax   needed. Before a second chest tube is in-
may not need treatment if the   serted, thoroughly evaluate the position
baby's vital signs are stable and   and functioning of the first chest tube.
oxygenation is adequate.

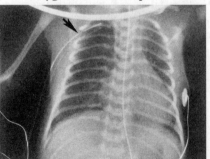

*Incorrect placement of a chest tube. Note the
tube has been placed very high and a hole
(arrow) is outside the chest cavity.*

ACTIONS	REMARKS

What Can Go Wrong?

ACTIONS	REMARKS
1. You misdiagnose a small pneumothorax.	Ask a second person to help you interpret the chest radiograph or obtain another radiograph 30 minutes later. If a pneumothorax is present, it will probably be larger and may have shifted location, making it easier to detect.
2. One pneumothorax is diagnosed and treated, but the baby's condition again deteriorates suddenly.	Transilluminate the baby's chest again or obtain another chest radiograph. A pneumothorax may have developed in the other lung or the chest tube may not be working, allowing the original pneumothorax to recur. Be sure to assess other factors that could have caused a rapid deterioration, such as inadequate ventilation or a dislodged endotracheal tube.

95

SKILL UNIT

Treating a Pneumothorax

These skill units will teach you how to aspirate a pneumothorax in an emergency and how to insert and secure a chest tube. You also will learn how to maintain a chest tube and how to manage chest tube suction. Not everyone will be required to learn how to relieve a pneumothorax. However, all staff members should read this unit and attend a skill practice session to learn the equipment and the sequence of steps so they can assist with needle aspiration and chest tube insertion.

- A video of needle aspiration may be viewed at https://neoreviews.aappublications.org/content/15/4/e163.
- A video of chest tube insertion may be viewed at https://www.youtube.com/watch?v=b1retCUzF38.
- A video of pigtail catheter placement for pneumothorax evacuation may be viewed at https://neoreviews.aappublications.org/content/15/6/e257.

It is critical that a time-out be taken prior to the procedure. The side of the pneumothorax should be carefully confirmed by the operator and the individual assisting.

Everyone will be required to know how to maintain a chest tube safely.

Study these skill units; then attend a skill practice and demonstration session. To master the skills, you will need to demonstrate each of the following steps correctly:

Needle Aspiration
1. Collect the equipment and, wherever possible, connect the pieces together.
2. Position the "baby" (mannequin).
3. Restrain the baby, if necessary.
4. Locate the fourth intercostal space in the midaxillary line to ensure the nipple area is avoided.
5. Cleanse this area with povidone-iodine and alcohol or with your institution's recommended technique.

Chest Tube Insertion
Set up suction
1. Collect the equipment.
2. Assemble the pieces.
   - Add water to the suction control and water seal chambers or set up the preset valve system.
   - Connect the tubing to the universal adapter and suction source.

Prepare the baby
1. Collect the equipment and prepare the "sterile" tray.
2. Position the baby.
3. Continue therapy and maintain support systems, such as oxygen delivery, thermal environment, and intravenous (IV) infusions.
4. Monitor the baby with a cardiac monitor and an oximeter.
5. Reposition tubes or wires, as necessary and appropriate.

6. Locate the fourth intercostal space at the anterior-axillary area.
7. Cleanse this area with povidone-iodine and alcohol.
8. Tape the chest tube in place.
9. Turn on and adjust the suction.
10. Identify whether air is being evacuated from the baby's chest.
11. Demonstrate how to check for leaks in the system.

Note: While successful relief of a pneumothorax depends on performing these skills correctly, actual insertion of a needle or chest tube is not included in these checklists. Physicians and selected nurses may be asked to participate in a demonstration and practice workshop for needle aspiration and chest tube insertion on mannequins or animal models, such as Cornish game hens from the grocery store.

Needle Aspiration

ACTIONS	REMARKS

Deciding When to Use Needle Aspiration

1. Is the baby's clinical condition deteriorating rapidly?

   Yes: Use needle aspiration to relieve the pneumothorax.

   No: Insert a chest tube to relieve the pneumothorax or wait for spontaneous resolution if the baby is not symptomatic.

Needle aspiration is used as an emergency procedure prior to placement of a chest tube.

Preparing the Baby and Equipment

2. Collect the following equipment:
   - 21- or 23-gauge butterfly needle

   or

   - 19- or 21-gauge percutaneous catheter
   - Short IV connecting tubing (T-connector) for use with a percutaneous catheter
   - 3-way stopcock
   - 10- or 12-mL syringe
   - Povidone-iodine or equivalent antiseptic solution
   - Sterile gloves, mask, cap
   - Antiseptic swabs
   - Sterile water swabs

3. Position the baby supine.

4. If necessary, restrain the baby or have someone hold the baby still.

5. Perform a time-out to confirm the baby's identification and side to be evacuated.

6. Determine the location of the fourth intercostal space at the anterior axillary line

Be certain to avoid insertion at or near the nipple area or surrounding breast tissue. Inappropriate placement of chest tubes can interfere with later breast development.

98

ACTIONS   **REMARKS**

Preparing the Baby and Equipment (continued)

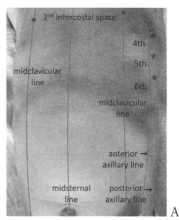

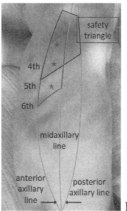

Figure 2.2. Locating the Fourth Intercostal Space
From Strutt J, Kharbanda A. Pediatric chest tubes and pigtails: an evidence-based approach to the management of pleural space diseases. *Pediatr Emerg Med Practice.* 2015:15(11).

7. Prep this area with antiseptic solution.

Allow the antiseptic solution to dry, and then remove it *completely* from the baby's skin by wiping it with sterile water swabs. If left in place, antiseptics can cause marked skin irritation. Many chlorhexidine solutions do not need to be removed. Follow your institution's policy on antiseptic solution use for neonates.

ACTIONS   **REMARKS**

Preparing the Baby and Equipment (continued)

8. Attach the butterfly needle to the 3-way stopcock and syringe.

Note: A percutaneous catheter (not shown) may also be used. With this, the short IV connecting tubing (T-connector) and stopcock should be connected but cannot be attached to the catheter until after it is inserted and the needle introducer is removed.

9. Turn the stopcock so it is open between the butterfly needle and syringe (shown below).

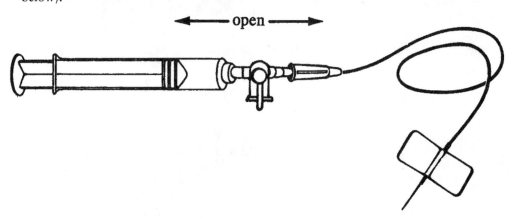

Evacuating the Air

10. Take the wings of the butterfly needle or percutaneous catheter between your thumb and forefinger.

ACTIONS   REMARKS

Evacuating the Air (continued)

11. Hold the needle or catheter perpendicular to the chest wall and insert it into either the fourth intercostal space, just above the fifth rib in the anterior axillary line or into the second intercostal space, just above the third rib in the midclavicular line (preferred insertion is anterior axillary, to avoid breast tissue).

Intercostal blood vessels run just below each rib. Avoid hitting these by inserting the needle just above the rib.

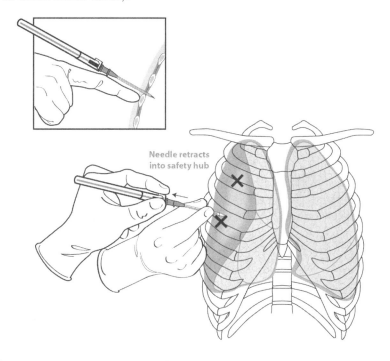

Locations for percutaneous aspiration of intrapleural air from the chest (either of the 2 Xs) or for placement of a chest tube (lower X)

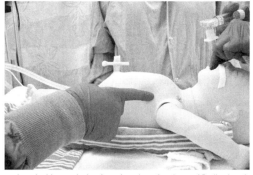
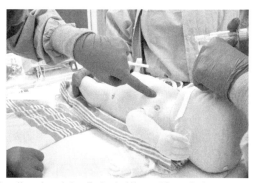

Reproduced with permission from American Academy of Pediatrics, American Heart Association. *Textbook of Neonatal Resuscitation.* Weiner GM, ed. 8th ed. American Academy of Pediatrics; 2021.

101

ACTIONS

REMARKS

Evacuating the Air (continued)

12. *If a butterfly needle is used,* as soon as the needle enters the skin, a second person should begin to "pull back" on the syringe plunger.

    Stop inserting the needle as soon as you get an air return. Hold it in this place.

    The air should come back easily with gentle pulling. Do not pull forcibly on the syringe plunger.

If a percutaneous catheter is used, stop inserting the catheter as soon as a "pop" is felt, indicating that the pleural space has been entered. Hold the catheter in place. A second person should remove the needle introducer and attach the IV connecting tubing (T-connector) and stopcock, and then begin to aspirate air by gently pulling back on the syringe plunger. Air withdrawal should come easily. Do not pull back forcibly.

Hold the needle or catheter still. Do not allow it to advance any farther into the chest cavity.

13. Continue to hold the butterfly needle (shown) or percutaneous catheter (not shown) in place while the second person gently pulls back on the syringe plunger to aspirate the air collection.

    You should begin to see a decrease in the baby's respiratory distress as air is withdrawn.

14. After the syringe has filled with air from the pneumothorax, close the stopcock to the needle or catheter and open it between the side port and syringe.

15. Empty the syringe of air by pushing the air out through the side port. (Note the direction of arrows in the illustrations.)

16. Continue to repeat this process until you can no longer aspirate air easily from the chest cavity.

17. As soon as you can no longer aspirate air easily from the chest cavity, withdraw the butterfly needle or percutaneous catheter.

This is done so that the re-expanded lung is not punctured by the needle. If using a blunt catheter, some clinicians will decide to tape the catheter in place until a radiograph has been obtained and reviewed.

18. A dressing is not needed over this site. The baby's skin and tissues will close tightly over the puncture point, preventing any air from entering from the outside.

19. Reassess the baby's condition and consider inserting a chest tube.

In many, but not all, cases, a chest tube will need to be inserted after needle aspiration of a pneumothorax.

PERINATAL PERFORMANCE GUIDE

Chest Tube Insertion

Note: The primary instruction is for a standard chest tube insertion, by using a surgical technique. A percutaneous technique is described in the Appendix at the end of this unit.

ACTIONS	REMARKS

Preparing the Equipment

1. Collect the following equipment:
   - 1% lidocaine
   - Small syringe with 26-gauge needle
   - Masks, caps, sterile gowns
   - Antiseptic swabs or povidone-iodine or equivalent solution
   - Sterile water swabs
   - Sterile 2-inch × 2-inch gauze
   - Sterile drapes
   - #15 knife blade
   - Knife handle
   - Small curved hemostat
   - Kelly clamp
   - Size 10F and 12F chest tubes with trocar
   - 3–0 suture on a curved needle
   - Needle holder
   - ½-inch adhesive tape
   - Clear adhesive dressing
   - Cotton-tipped swabs
   - Universal adapter (to fit between chest tube and suction tube)
   - Three-bottle suction apparatus
   - Suction source

Most of these items can be kept prepared on a sterile tray in the nursery. For wire-guided chest tube insertion, add a wire-guided apparatus kit; size 8F, 10F, or 12F wire-guided chest tubes; and sterile 5- to 10-mL syringe. (See the Appendix at the end of this unit.)

2. Set up the suction apparatus. This should be a 3-bottle water seal system or a system that works with preset valves.

Disposable units that incorporate all the principles of the 3-bottle system are commonly available. One example is shown in the diagram that appears with step 4.

3. Fill the section marked "suction control chamber" to between the 5- and 10-mL marks.

Usually, much lower suction levels are required for babies than are commonly used for adults. In almost all circumstances, chest tubes are placed in babies to evacuate air, not blood or fluid (which would require higher suction pressures).

4. Fill the section marked "water seal chamber" to the fill line.

Preparing the Equipment (continued)

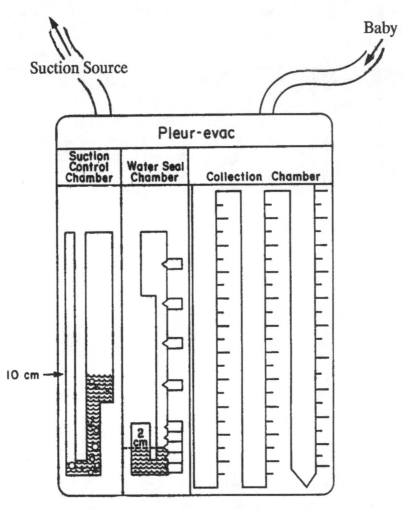

A Pleur-evac setup is shown in this illustration. Other 3-bottle commercially available products have chambers with similar function but may be labeled differently. Some of these products may regulate pressures with preset valves, rather than water seals.

5. Connect the suction tubing to the suction source.

   Do not, however, turn on the suction yet.

   (The illustration may be misleading because the water levels will not be different, and bubbles will not appear in the suction control chamber until the suction is turned on.)

6. Using aseptic technique, connect the universal adapter to the patient's drainage tube.

   Keep the patient end of the universal adapter covered with sterile gauze. Put this end near the baby so it can be connected to the chest tube as soon as it is inserted.

ACTIONS   **REMARKS**

Preparing the Baby

7. Perform a time-out to confirm the baby's identification and side to receive the tube.

8. Position the baby so the side with the pneumothorax is at a 60° upright angle.

   Place a blanket roll behind the baby's back.

   During the procedure, a second person will need to hold the baby's uppermost arm over the baby's head with the arm externally rotated.

This position is very important because it allows air to rise to the point of tube entry into the thoracic cavity.

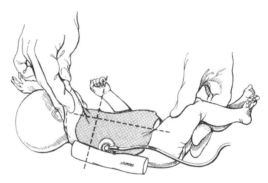

9. Maintain the baby's medical support. Be sure the oxygen therapy, IV infusions, and thermal environment are not interrupted.

   Heart rate and respiratory rate should be monitored throughout the procedure with an electronic cardiac monitor and oxygenation monitored with a pulse oximeter.

Increase the inspired oxygen concentration and provide additional supportive care if the baby's condition deteriorates.

10. Locate the baby's fourth intercostal space and sixth rib at the anterior-axillary area.

    This should be well away from the nipple area and surrounding breast tissue. Inappropriate placement of chest tubes can interfere with later breast development.

    Note: For illustration purposes, the ribs have been drawn larger than is anatomically correct.

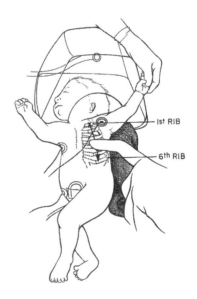

ACTIONS	REMARKS

Preparing the Baby (continued)

11. Draw up 1% lidocaine into a syringe. Clean the skin with antiseptic swab or solution and then inject the lidocaine to raise a small intradermal "button" over the sixth rib at the anterior-axillary point. Infiltrate the lidocaine into the subcutaneous tissue in a track up to the fourth intercostal space.

    To avoid overdose, do not use more than 0.5 mL of 1% lidocaine.

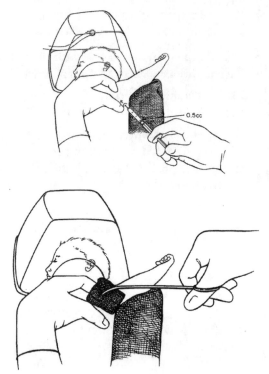

12. Put on the sterile gown, gloves, and a mask.

13. Scrub a generous area of the baby's skin from below the sixth rib to above the fourth intercostal space with antiseptic solution.

    Allow the antiseptic solution to dry, and then remove it *completely* from the baby's skin by wiping with alcohol or sterile water swabs. If left in place, antiseptics can cause marked skin irritation.

Some clinicians prefer to wait until after the tube is in place before cleaning the antiseptic solution off the skin.

Most commercial chlorhexidine solutions do not need to be removed.

14. Cover the area around the prepped skin with sterile drapes.

15. Attach the knife blade to the knife handle (if required) and make a 3- to 4-mm (¼-inch) full-thickness skin incision over the lidocaine "button" at the sixth rib.

    The incision in the skin should go completely through the skin but should be no longer than 3 to 4 mm (¼ inch).

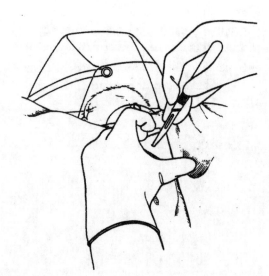

ACTIONS   REMARKS

Inserting the Chest Tube (Trocar Method)

16. Take the chest tube and slide the trocar up and down inside it to be sure it moves freely.

    If the trocar does not slide easily within the chest tube, "rinse" the chest tube with sterile saline.

17. Look at the baby's chest to estimate the length of chest tube to insert. The correct length is from the sixth rib to the fourth intercostal space and then across to the sternum. Note where this length falls in comparison with markings on the chest tube.

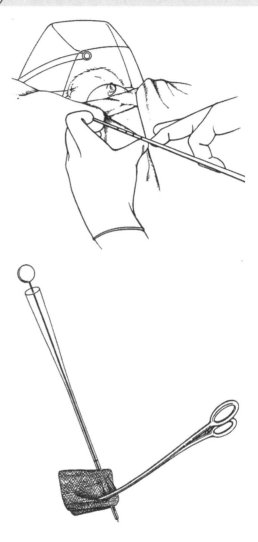

18. Take the chest tube and trocar and measure 2 cm (¾ inch) (or a shorter distance for tiny babies) from the tip of the chest tube.

19. Take a small piece of sterile gauze and wrap it once around the chest tube at this point.

20. Take the Kelly clamp and apply it firmly across the chest tube over the gauze 2 cm (¾ inch) (or shorter distance for tiny babies) from the tip of the tube.

    Note: After preparing the chest tube in this manner, set it aside (with clamp applied) until you create the skin tunnel (steps 21 through 24).

21. Take the small curved hemostat and insert the closed tip into the skin incision.

ACTIONS   **REMARKS**

Inserting the Chest Tube (Trocar Method) (continued)

22. By repeatedly spreading and closing the hemostat, create a tunnel from the sixth rib to the fourth intercostal space.

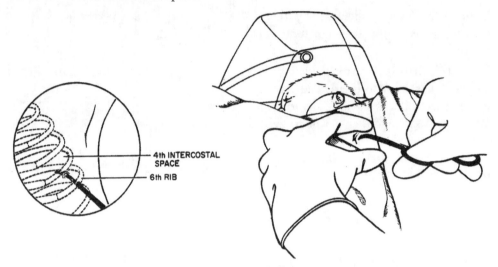

4th INTERCOSTAL SPACE

6th RIB

23. Slide the tip of the hemostat over the top of the fifth rib and into the fourth intercostal space.

    Do not insert the tip of the hemostat any deeper than necessary, or you may damage the lung tissue.

Slide the hemostat just over the top of the rib to avoid hitting the intercostal artery that runs along the lower edge of each rib.

Air collection of the pneumothorax provides a small space between the lung tissue and parietal pleura. This allows you to puncture the parietal pleura without touching the lung, unless you insert the hemostat too far. A rush of air may be heard as you enter the pneumothorax.

Note: Some clinicians prefer to use the point of the trocar, which remains in the tube, for puncturing through the pleura. If you choose to use this method, you must be very careful not to permit the trocar, with its tube, to enter too far into the chest. The Kelly clamp, described in step 20, will help to avoid this complication.

24. Remove the hemostat by again repeatedly spreading and closing the tips as you withdraw the hemostat through the tunnel.

ACTIONS   **REMARKS**

Inserting the Chest Tube (Trocar Method) (continued)

25. Place one hand on the baby's chest to steady it. Take the chest tube, with the Kelly clamp still applied, in the other hand and hold it firmly, as you would a pencil.

26. Place the tip of the trocar and chest tube through the skin incision.

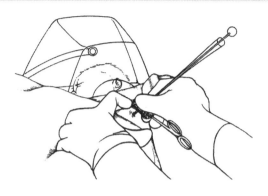

27. "Walk" the tip through the tunnel you previously made with the small hemostat.

    Continue to hold the chest tube perpendicular to the baby's chest. This will cause the skin to wrinkle above the chest tube as you walk it through the tunnel.

28. When you reach the fourth intercostal space, insert the chest tube until the baby's skin touches the Kelly clamp. You may feel the chest tube "pop" the parietal pleura. The Kelly clamp on the chest tube will prevent the tube and trocar from entering the chest too far.

    You will need to press firmly with the tube to insert it, but never apply insertion pressure higher up on the tube or on the knob of the trocar.

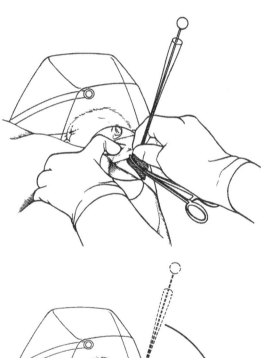

29. Hold the chest tube in this position as you remove the hemostat and gauze.

30. Hold the tube tip at that level as you swing the tube and trocar downward to an angle that is nearly parallel to the baby's body and pointed toward the baby's opposite shoulder.

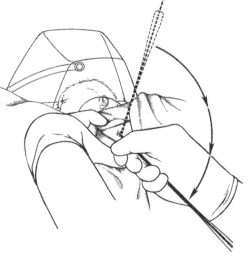

ACTIONS   **REMARKS**

Inserting the Chest Tube (Trocar Method) (continued)

When the tube is in the correct position, you should feel the tip press firmly against the underside of the fourth rib.

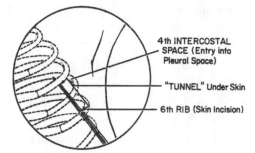

4th INTERCOSTAL SPACE (Entry into Pleural Space)

"TUNNEL" Under Skin

6th RIB (Skin Incision)

31. Hold on to the knob of the trocar and begin to advance the tube as it slips off the trocar.

    Be careful not to advance the trocar.

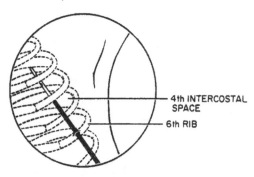

4th INTERCOSTAL SPACE

6th RIB

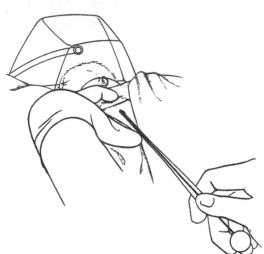

32. As the tube continues to slip off the trocar, remove the trocar completely.

33. You should see condensation develop within the lumen of the tube and may hear a rush of air.

You also may see a small amount of straw-colored or blood-tinged fluid in the tube. This is not uncommon in sick babies. More than a small amount of gross blood, however, is abnormal.

34. Advance the tube anteriorly toward the baby's opposite shoulder until you have inserted it the desired length determined earlier. Measure this according to the markings on the tube.

35. When the tube is inserted the desired distance, have someone promptly connect it to the universal adapter on the patient drainage tubing.

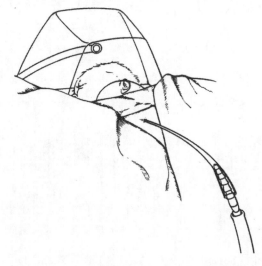

ACTIONS   REMARKS

Securing the Chest Tube

36. Be sure there is no tension on the tube while you suture and tape it in place. Maintain the tube in the same orientation, along the baby's side, pointed toward the opposite shoulder, to maintain it in proper position inside the chest.

Check the location of the chest tube markings frequently to be sure the tube has not slipped.

37. Place a full-thickness skin suture next to the skin incision. Then make several tight wraps around the tube. Avoid excessive suturing because it does not make the tube any more secure and may cause a constriction in the lumen of the tube if the sutures are too tight.

You may use the same suturing technique that is described in securing umbilical catheters (see Unit 3, Umbilical Catheters, in this book), except that you would omit the purse-string step.

38. Take 2 4-inch pieces of 1/2-inch adhesive tape.

39. Split each piece half the length of the tape.

40. Take one piece of tape and apply the base and half of the split section to the baby's skin. Wrap the other half of the split section in a spiral around the chest tube.

    Some people prefer to put clear adhesive dressing on the baby's skin and stick adhesive tape to that rather than directly to the baby's skin.

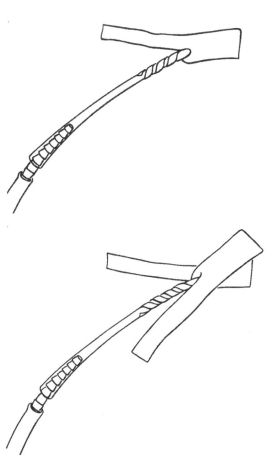

41. Take the other piece of tape and apply it in a similar manner to the chest tube, but from a different angle.

    Because the chest tube has been tunneled under the baby's skin, an occlusive dressing is not needed. The skin will close tightly over the chest tube and prevent any air from entering the chest cavity from the outside. Also, use of a petroleum substance will interfere with tape adherence to the skin.

    A transparent film adhesive dressing may be placed over the tube and entry site. Large occlusive dressings should be avoided because they can delay recognition of a slipped chest tube.

42. As soon as possible, return the baby to a supine position.

This is to avoid compromise of the baby's "good" lung, which is the one the baby has been lying on during the procedure.

ACTIONS

REMARKS

Maintaining Chest Tube Suction

43. Turn on the suction until minimal to moderate bubbling is seen in the **suction control chamber.**

Rapid, vigorous bubbling should be avoided.

44. Be sure all connections in the tubing are secure. Tape each connection with a *single* piece of tape wrapped in a spiral fashion (see illustration).

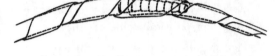

Do not over-tape the connections. An unreliable connection will be covered up but not secured by excessive tape.

Some people prefer, therefore, not to tape the connections at all, with the thought that, if they come loose, tape may mask the leak.

45. Bubbling in the **water seal chamber** indicates air is being evacuated from the baby's chest or there is a leak in the system.

Check for leaks in the system.

- Disconnect suction tubing from the suction source.

- Observe the water seal chamber for fluctuations that occur with the baby's respiration.

- If fluctuations occur with respirations, there are no leaks in the system. Bubbling in the water seal chamber indicates air is being evacuated from the baby's chest.

- If fluctuations do not occur with respiration, there is a leak in the system (check all connections) or the chest tube is blocked.

ACTIONS   **REMARKS**

Checking Chest Tube Placement

46. Obtain anteroposterior and lateral chest radiographs to locate the position of the tube within the chest accurately. Reposition the tube as indicated.

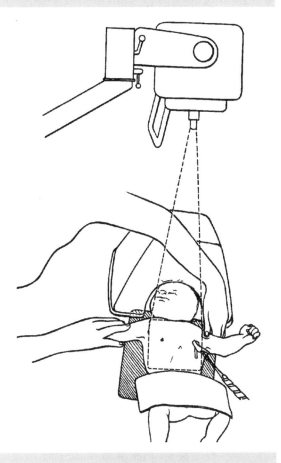

Removing the Chest Tube

47. Periodically change the baby's position to facilitate relocation of any air that might be trapped. This allows evacuation through the chest tube.

48. A baby with a pneumothorax generally requires a chest tube for several days.

    During this time, make frequent, regular observations of the baby and chest tube system.

49. When bubbling is no longer seen in the **water seal chamber,** turn the suction off but keep the 3-bottle system intact.

Discontinuing the suction simply converts the system to a 3-bottle water seal system. This allows passive evacuation of air from the chest, rather than active evacuation that occurs when suction is used.

ACTIONS	REMARKS

Removing the Chest Tube (continued)

50. When you are confident there is no further bubbling in the **water seal chamber,** clamp the chest tube while you watch the baby carefully for signs of deterioration as you wait for another chest radiograph to be obtained.

If you have been mistaken and the baby still has an active pneumothorax, clamping the chest tube will cause reaccumulation of the pneumothorax and collapse of the lung again. If this were to happen, you could simply remove the clamp as you look for bubbling again in the **water seal chamber.**

Note: If fluid is visible in the tube and there is no movement of the fluid with ventilatory efforts, it is likely the tube is no longer functional and is ready to be removed.

51. If you are confident the chest radiograph shows no evidence of a pneumothorax and the baby has remained stable while the tube has been clamped for 1 to 2 hours, remove the tape, cut the sutures, and slip the chest tube out.

Occasionally, removal of the tube will cause another pneumothorax to appear. Be prepared to transilluminate the baby's chest and insert another tube, if needed.

52. Dress the wound by covering it with a piece of occlusive film.

If the tube has been in for longer than 24 to 48 hours, a track may have formed. If so, a small occlusive dressing will prevent air from entering the chest through the incision.

53. Continue to observe the baby carefully and be alert for the possibility of the development of another pneumothorax.

APPENDIX

One type of percutaneous chest tube is used for the following skill. It is recommended that you also consult the manufacturer's website at www.cookmedical.com.

Wire-Guided Chest Tube Insertion

The following skill presents an alternative to the surgically placed chest tube skill, replacing steps 15 to 35. It is recommended that there are 2 sterile providers working together for appropriate and safe placement.

15. Open the chest tube insertion kit and identify the components.

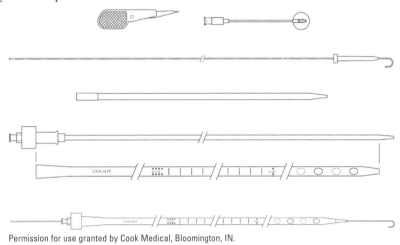

Permission for use granted by Cook Medical, Bloomington, IN.

16. Attach a sterile, empty 5- or 10-mL syringe to the 18-guage introducer needle from the chest tube set.

This syringe serves as a "handle" for the needle and allows aspiration of some of the air from the pneumothorax, thus confirming the needle tip is in the pleural space before inserting the guide wire.

Wire-Guided Chest Tube Insertion (continued)

17. Look at the baby's chest to estimate the length of chest tube to insert. The correct length will extend from the sixth rib to the fourth intercostal space laterally and then medially to the upper sternum (see the black line on the diagram to the right). Note where this length falls in relation to the black marks on the chest tube. By comparing the tube and its holes to the size of the baby's chest, you can insert the tube far enough down the chest wall to accommodate the tube.

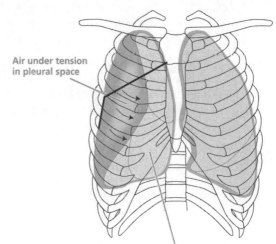

Air under tension in pleural space

Right lung compressed by pneumothorax

Reproduced with permission from American Academy of Pediatrics, American Heart Association. *Textbook of Neonatal Resuscitation.* Kattwinkel, ed. 6th ed. American Academy of Pediatrics; 2011.

In general, the tube will enter the skin around the sixth rib and will enter the chest in the fourth interspace (above the fifth rib). These landmarks can be difficult to discern. In extremely small babies, these entry points (and the need to place all of the tube's side holes *inside* the chest) can result in the relatively long tube reaching the apex of the chest cavity and curving behind the lung or pressing on mediastinal structures. In this situation, select a lower insertion point, taking care to avoid the diaphragm, liver, and spleen.

18. Using the included scalpel, make a full-thickness nick slightly larger than the diameter of the chest tube over the anesthetized skin at roughly the sixth rib.

19. Insert the introducer needle through the nick and under the skin at the anterior axillary line at the sixth interspace or lower, as described in the previous text. Direct the needle somewhat anteriorly (perpendicular to the ribs).

The goal is to direct the needle, wire, and, ultimately, chest tube anterior to the lung and toward the upper sternum. This is facilitated by the rolled position of the baby and introducing the needle from posterior to anterior of the baby's chest. Chest tubes that go posterior to the lung typically drain air poorly and may fail to control the pneumothorax.

Wire-Guided Chest Tube Insertion (continued)

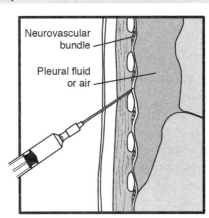

Neurovascular bundle

Pleural fluid or air

20. Tunnel under the skin toward the upper sternum, reaching to the upper aspect of the next higher rib (usually the fifth).

    Then raise the syringe and needle hub to a 45° angle and enter the chest over the upper (cephalad) edge of this rib to avoid the intercostal vessels and nerve.

    WARNING: Over-insertion of the needle or (subsequently) the dilators may result in serious harm.

    Aspirate with the syringe as you advance, to detect the pneumothorax and avoid advancing the needle beyond air collection. It is easy to inadvertently penetrate the lung with this sharp needle. Use great care to position the tip in the air pocket (pleural space).

21. Once the needle tip is inside the air collection, lower the syringe and needle hub toward the chest wall. The tip *must* be directed toward the upper sternum. If a free flow of air is not obtained, do not proceed with the next steps. Advance (a few millimeters) or withdraw the needle until air is encountered. If no air is found, discontinue the procedure and reevaluate.

22. While stabilizing the needle to avoid lung injury, remove the syringe.

    Air can enter (with spontaneous inspirations) or leave (under positive-pressure ventilation) the chest through this needle. Proceed promptly to the next steps or obstruct the needle with a sterile fingertip.

23. Using the plastic guide to straighten the wire, promptly insert the wire through the introducer needle. Advance until the mark on the wire approaches the needle hub. Once inside the chest, the tip of the wire will curve to present a blunt leading point.

    Advance in the direction of the upper sternum. The wire should advance without resistance. Do not force the wire into the chest.

Hold the needle in a hand resting on the chest or fingers directly against the skin. An instrument (clamp) can help disconnect a recalcitrant syringe. Take care not to dislodge or damage the needle. Because it will not be used again, the syringe can be removed by a second person without sterile gloves.

Ensure that the wire is advanced with the "curved" blunt leading end into the chest. Inserting the wire incorrectly can cause serious harm.

Wire-Guided Chest Tube Insertion (continued)

24. Remove the needle from the chest while stabilizing the wire in place. The needle is withdrawn along the stationary wire.

25. Remove the plastic guide and introducer needle from the wire entirely. The tip of the wire remains within the baby's chest.

26. Thread the dilator onto the wire and advance it through the chest wall along the wire, without moving the wire. Advance in line with the stationary wire to avoid kinking.

    Direct the dilator toward the upper sternum. Take care to avoid bending or kinking the wire. Do not force the dilator. Rotation of the dilator around the wire can assist in this step.

27. Remove the dilator from the wire and replace it with the chest tube on its inserter cannula. Advance the chest tube along the wire and through the chest wall in the direction of the upper sternum. Advance in line with the wire to avoid kinking.

    Again, rotate the tube around the wire and avoid bending or kinking the wire.

28. When all the side holes of the chest tube are inside the chest by 1 to 2 cm (0.4–0.75 inch), stabilize the tube and remove the guide wire from the chest and tube.

    Take care, when pulling on the wire, not to withdraw the chest tube from the pleural space.

29. Remove the internal inserter cannula from the lumen of the chest tube.

Wire-Guided Chest Tube Insertion (continued)

30. Attach the chest tube to the patient drainage tubing by using a universal adapter. Suction at 15 to 20 cm H_2O is typically applied when using this tube. A one-way Heimlich valve is sometimes used for transport, but a water seal system is more secure in the nursery.

Observe for fogging inside the tube, bubbles in the water seal chamber, and clinical improvement. Full recovery of respiratory function may take some time, but it should begin immediately.

You also may see a small amount of straw-colored or blood-tinged fluid in the tube. This is not uncommon in sick babies. More than a small amount of gross blood, however, is abnormal.

31. Secure the tube by using suture and tape and a clear plastic film, as described in step 36 in the main skill. No sutures are required to close an incision, but one stitch through the full thickness of the skin provides a good anchor for the tube.

32. Confirm the position and effectiveness of the tube by obtaining anteroposterior and lateral chest radiographs, as described in step 46 of the main skill.

GO TO STEP 36 in the main skill.

Unit 3: Umbilical Catheters

Objectives

In this unit you will learn

A. The definition of an umbilical catheter

B. The difference between venous and arterial catheters

C. When and how to use an umbilical *venous* catheter

D. When and how to use an umbilical *arterial* catheter

E. Where to position the tip of a venous or an arterial umbilical catheter

F. How to maintain umbilical catheters

G. Complications associated with umbilical catheters

Unit 3 Pretest

Before **reading the unit, please answer the following questions. Select the *one best* answer to each question (unless otherwise instructed). Record your answers on the test and check them against the answers at the end of the book.**

1. Below is an illustration of an umbilical cord. What is the structure labeled X?
   A. Umbilical artery
   B. Umbilical vein

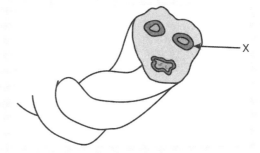

2. If a baby needed emergency medication in the delivery room, you would give the medication through an
   A. Umbilical venous catheter
   B. Umbilical arterial catheter

3. If a baby needed monitoring of blood oxygen, carbon dioxide, and pH levels, you would obtain blood samples from an
   A. Umbilical venous catheter
   B. Umbilical arterial catheter

4. Which of these dangers are possible with an umbilical venous catheter?

Yes	No	
____	____	Thrombosis
____	____	Blood infection
____	____	Brain damage
____	____	Kidney damage
____	____	Loss of toe from embolus

5. **True False** An umbilical venous catheter should be left in place until a baby is well.

6. **True False** If a constant infusion is to be given through an umbilical arterial catheter, an infusion pump must be used.

7. Umbilical venous catheters are most appropriately used for
   A. Administration of emergency medications
   B. Routine intravenous fluid therapy
   C. Obtaining blood samples for blood gas analyses
   D. Measuring central blood pressure

8. You are inserting an umbilical arterial catheter in a baby. The baby's toes on his right foot suddenly turn white. What should be done?
   A. Apply a warm compress to the right foot.
   B. Increase the amount of oxygen the baby is receiving.
   C. Remove the catheter.
   D. Observe the baby to see how long the toes stay white.

1. What is an umbilical catheter?

Immediately after birth, or within the next few days, a low-gauge catheter may be inserted into an umbilical artery or the umbilical vein of a newborn. Typically, there are 2 umbilical arteries and 1 vein (Figure 3.1)

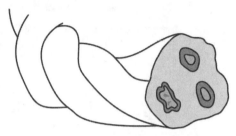

Figure 3.1. Drawing of a Cut Umbilical Cord

An umbilical catheter should have a rounded tip with a single hole in the center. This is to avoid formation of tiny clots that are associated with catheters that have multiple side holes. (Note: There are catheters available that have more than one lumen to permit administration of more than one type of fluid, but these will not be considered in this program.)

This catheter should also be radiopaque (visible on a radiograph) to allow determination of the exact position of the catheter after it has been inserted.

Umbilical arteries have relatively thick, muscular walls with pinpoint-sized lumens. In an umbilical cord cut close to the stump, the arteries can generally be found toward the baby's feet. The presence of only 1 artery is uncommon. A single artery is sometimes (not always) associated with certain anomalies, particularly renal malformations.

An *umbilical vein* is a relatively thin-walled vessel, larger than an artery, usually located toward the baby's head.

2. Where should the tip of an umbilical catheter be positioned?

An *umbilical venous catheter* (UVC) is inserted into the umbilical vein and then advanced through the ductus venosus into the inferior vena cava. The catheter tip should be located at or just above the level of the diaphragm, preferably as seen on a lateral, rather than an anteroposterior, chest radiograph, and ideally located at the junction of the inferior vena cava and the right atrium.

An *umbilical arterial catheter* (UAC) is inserted into either of the 2 umbilical arteries and then advanced into the abdominal aorta. The catheter tip should be located at a level between the sixth and ninth thoracic vertebrae (T6-T9; "high") or between the third and fourth lumbar vertebrae (L3-L4; "low").

The lower location, L3-L4, can be expected to be below the point where the intestinal and renal arteries branch from the aorta, while the higher location (T6-T9) is above these major vessels but is an area of high flow and thus less likely to allow clot formation.

Locating the tip in the region *between* these 2 optimal levels (between L4 and T6) should be avoided because this would place the tip at the level of the main arteries that feed the baby's vital abdominal organs. Therefore, any solutions injected into the catheter, or clots forming on the end of the catheter, would be more likely to enter the arterial beds of these organs.

Note: While some studies have shown fewer clinically evident short-term complications with catheters placed in high locations (T6-T9), some experts argue that more serious long-term complications may not have been detected with the techniques used in the studies. The position chosen should be defined by local standards.

3. When is an umbilical catheter used?

A. Umbilical venous catheter (Table 3.1)
- Emergency administration of medication or blood
- Exchange transfusions
- Emergency measurement of Pco_2 and pH (not Po_2)
- Fluid administration during the first several days after birth in preterm or sick babies

UVCs generally are not used for routine fluids except in extremely preterm or sick new-borns, unless another intravenous (IV) route is not available. If a peripheral IV (PIV) line is not available, however, many experts feel it is preferable to give fluids and medications through a UVC positioned above the liver (tip located at or just above the level of the diaphragm), rather than through a UAC.

B. Umbilical arterial catheter (Table 3.1)
- Drawing blood for blood gas analyses (the most common use for UAC)
- Obtaining central arterial blood pressure measurements

Infusion of blood, medications, or maintenance fluid solutions through a UAC is contro-versial. Insertion of a UAC *solely* for infusion of routine IV fluids is not recommended. However, if a UAC is in place for the purpose of arterial blood sampling or central blood pressure monitoring and another IV route is not available, routine IV fluids may be administered through a UAC.

Table 3.1. Uses for Umbilical Catheters		
Use	**UVC**	**UAC**
Emergency medications or blood	Yes, especially during first few days after birth	Not recommended
Exchange transfusions	Yes	Not recommended Note: UAC may be used to *withdraw* blood during exchange transfusion by using the con-tinuous technique, where a UVC or PIV route is used to infuse blood, although it will be prone to clotting unless frequently flushed or infused with IV fluid or heparinized flush solution. (See Book 4: Specialized Newborn Care, Unit 2, Ex-change, Reduction, and Direct Transfusions.)
Central arterial blood pressure measurements	Not applicable	Yes
Blood gas sampling • Emergency pH level and Pco_2 estimation • Routine Pao_2, $Paco_2$, pH level checks	• Yes, especially soon after delivery • Not applicable	• Not practical, longer procedure for placement, best to use UVC for emergency • Yes, especially if a high level of supplemental oxygen is needed for a prolonged period
Routine fluids • Extremely preterm or sick babies • Other babies Note: See Unit 5, Intrave-nous Therapy, in this book.	• Yes, especially soon after birth • Not recommended, unless a PIV or percutaneous catheter is not available	Not recommended, unless UAC is needed for arterial blood gases or central blood pressure, and a PIV or percutaneous catheter is not obtainable

Abbreviations: IV, intravenous; PIV, peripheral intravenous; UAC, umbilical arterial catheter; UVC, umbilical venous catheter.

Self-test A

Now answer these questions to test yourself on the information in the last section.

A1. Label the 3 blood vessels in the diagram below.

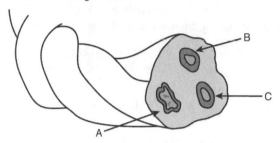

A2. Which of these features should an umbilical catheter have?

Yes	No	
____	____	Radiopaque
____	____	Beveled tip
____	____	Rounded tip
____	____	Single hole in tip center
____	____	Multiple tiny side holes near catheter tip

A3. Name at least 2 uses of umbilical venous catheters.

_____

_____

A4. What are 2 uses that are not recommended for umbilical arterial catheters?

_____

_____

A5. What is the most common use of an umbilical arterial catheter?

_____

A6. What is the recommended location for the tip of an umbilical

Arterial catheter: _____

Venous catheter: _____

Check your answers with the list that follows the Recommended Routines. Correct any incorrect answers and review the appropriate section in the unit.

4. How should umbilical catheters be maintained?

A. Umbilical venous catheter

A UVC may be required for medication administration during a resuscitation in the delivery room or for an exchange transfusion. Occasionally, a UVC may be placed for a longer period of use, such as when another route for administration of fluids is impractical. In such cases, one of the following procedures should be used to ensure the catheter does not become clotted:

1. Heparin lock
   - *Heparin concentration:* Large doses of heparin or an excessive number of flushes can result in systemic blood clotting problems in newborns, particularly very small

babies. The dosage of heparin that is hazardous is not well defined, but 1 to 2 units of heparin per milliliter of fluid is considered safe if amounts and frequency of flushes are kept to a minimum.

- *Flush volume:* Depending on catheter size, 0.5 to 1.0 mL of heparin solution is flushed through the UVC and the stopcock is turned off to the catheter. After a blood sample is drawn or any other solution is given through the catheter, the catheter should be flushed again with heparin-containing solution and the stopcock turned off to the catheter.
- *Record fluid given:* Care must be taken to avoid using more flush solution than necessary, or the baby may receive too much heparin or IV fluid. Each time the catheter is flushed, record the amount of flush solution used on the baby's "intake" record.

2. Continuous infusion – Preferred method

- Heparin should be added to a continuous infusion solution but in a concentration lower than that used for a heparin lock. For a continuous infusion, a heparin infusion rate of 0.12 U/kg/h is recommended.
- An infusion pump should be used to ensure that a constant, correct volume is infused. The use of an infusion pump will prevent backup of blood into the catheter and possible obstruction of the line with a thrombus.
- If heparin is not available immediately, a continuous infusion without heparin may be initiated until heparinized solution becomes available.
- After any blood sample is withdrawn, the catheter is flushed with 0.5 to 1.0 mL of the IV fluid or the 1 to 2 U/mL heparin solution and then reconnected to the constant infusion. Be sure to record the amount of flush solution used.

B. Umbilical arterial catheter

If a UAC is to be left in place to obtain frequent arterial blood samples for blood gas analyses, either one of the techniques described previously for UVCs may be used to prevent clotting.

Note: Some experts believe only a continuous infusion, *not* a heparin lock, should be used with a UAC.

If the continuous infusion method is used for a UAC, an infusion pump must be used, or blood will back up into the catheter because of the higher blood pressure in an artery.

C. Either type of catheter (venous or arterial)

- *Air bubbles:* Care must be taken to remove all air bubbles from the infusion tubing or an umbilical catheter. If present in an IV line or catheter, air bubbles will enter the bloodstream and can cause severe tissue damage. This can be a particularly severe complication of a UAC.
- *Clotted catheter:* You should always be able to get an *instantaneous* blood return from a UAC or UVC. If blood does not return easily, do not push fluid into the catheter. There may be a clot in the catheter, or the catheter tip may be wedged against the side of the vessel.

After the sterile field used during catheter insertion has been removed, do not advance the catheter farther because that would push an unsterile section of the catheter into the umbilical cord. You may withdraw the catheter about 1 cm and try to withdraw blood again. If blood still does not return, remove or replace the catheter.

127

- *Disconnected catheter:* If either type of catheter becomes disconnected or gets pulled out, massive blood loss can occur within a few seconds (particularly with a UAC). Catheter connections must be secure.

  Use Luer-Lok connections or another system for locking stopcock, tubing, and catheter connections.

  If blood loss occurs, immediately take the baby's blood pressure. If necessary, administer an appropriate volume of physiological (normal) saline solution to support the baby's circulation while you are waiting for compatible blood to be obtained. (See Unit 4, Low Blood Pressure [Hypotension], in this book.)

- *Excess fluid:* The volume and type of all constant infusion and flush solutions administered to the baby should be recorded, so that the amount of fluid a baby receives will be known. The following volumes of flush solution are all that are needed to flush Luer-Lok connection catheters of different sizes:

Catheter Size	Recommended Flush Volume
3.5F	0.4 mL
5F	0.6 mL
8F	1.0 mL

  The Infusion Nurses Society recommends flushing catheters with twice the dead-space volume. The flush volume recommended previously may not be the appropriate volume for your catheter. Check the volume of the catheter and the stopcock stated by the manufacturer.

- *Rapid fluid infusion:* Relatively large amounts of fluid can be infused quickly through a UVC or a UAC. This should be avoided. Rapid infusions of fluid can cause sudden, dangerous shifts in blood pressure and temporarily alter normal blood flow. All infusions and flush solutions through umbilical catheters should be administered slowly and steadily, generally at a rate no faster than 1 to 2 mL/kg/min.

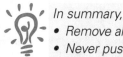

In summary,
- *Remove all air bubbles from the infusion tubing and the umbilical catheter.*
- *Never push fluid into a catheter that does not have an immediate blood return.*
- *Never advance a catheter when it is no longer sterile.*
- *Use a Luer-Lok or other system of locking connections.*
- *Record the volume of all flush solutions administered.*
- *Administer infusions and flush solutions through an umbilical venous or arterial catheter slowly and steadily. A rate no faster than 1 to 2 mL/kg/min is recommended.*

5. What complications are associated with umbilical catheters?

Umbilical arterial and venous catheters are extremely valuable tools that are often required for the care of sick babies. As with any medical treatment, complications are possible. With care, these complications can almost always be avoided.

A. Flow pathways determine many possible complications
   1. Umbilical venous catheter
      Solutions infused through a UVC placed at or just above the level of the diaphragm flow into the inferior vena cava. Solutions infused through a UVC placed below the

level of the diaphragm may flow through the venous circulation of the liver. Alternatively, when a UVC tip is too high above the level of the diaphragm, infusions may flow directly into the heart, quite possibly into the *left* atrium, which leads to arterial circulation, thus creating a risk of arterial emboli.

2. Umbilical arterial catheter

Solutions infused through catheters placed at L3-L4 flow to the legs. Solutions infused through a UAC placed at T6-T9 may flow to the liver, spleen, pancreas, kidneys, intestines, spinal cord, and legs.

B. Possible complications

1. Umbilical venous catheter
   - *Blood loss* from loose connections between, for example, the catheter and stopcock.
   - *Liver damage* from the infusion of hypertonic solution into the venous circulation of the liver.
   - *Perforation of the vein* if a catheter is inserted too vigorously.
   - *Pericardial tamponade* if the UVC is inserted too far into the heart.
   - *Thromboses (clots)* when blood backs up into the catheter. The clot that forms may then extend beyond the tip and into the vessel. Thromboses are more likely to occur when catheters with side holes, instead of a single hole in the center of a rounded tip, are used.
   - *Sepsis* (blood infection).
   - *Air embolus* with accidental infusion of air bubbles with fluid or medication. Air embolus also may be formed by air drawn into the circulatory system, if a baby inhales when an intrathoracic UVC is accidentally opened to the atmosphere.

2. Umbilical arterial catheter
   - *Massive blood loss* from a loose connection between catheter and stopcock.
   - *Blocked blood flow* during or after catheter insertion, as shown by blanching of a leg (turning white). The catheter must be withdrawn immediately to prevent permanent damage. After catheter removal, warming of the *opposite* leg may cause reflex improvement of blood flow to the compromised leg.
   - *Thrombi or emboli,* which may form from small blood clots on the catheter tip that may break off to embolize to one of the legs or vital organs located downstream from the catheter tip. Air bubbles pushed through the catheter will also form emboli.

     An embolus to a leg will cause one or more toes or the foot on the affected side to become cyanotic or blanched (white). The foot, leg, or buttock may be involved, and these areas should be carefully inspected for this complication after catheter insertion and frequently while the catheter is indwelling. Permanent damage may occur. Emboli to one of the abdominal organs will not cause visible changes but can cause permanent damage, often to the kidneys or intestines. Great care must be taken with all infusions through a UAC.
   - *Sepsis.*
   - *Hypoglycemia* can occur with catheters located above the third lumbar vertebra, located near the 10th thoracic vertebra, and used for continuous infusion. The pancreas may respond to glucose concentration in an IV fluid, rather than the baby's true blood glucose level, and produce additional amounts of insulin. This increased insulin secretion results in hypoglycemia.
   - *Hemorrhagic shock* secondary to a perforation of the umbilical artery as a complication of insertion of the catheter leading to massive blood loss into the abdomen.

129

6. How long can umbilical catheters be left in place?

While extremely valuable, UVCs and UACs are associated with possible complications and should be removed as soon as possible.

A. Umbilical venous catheters

UVCs should be removed as soon as the emergency is over, the exchange transfusion is completed, or another route of IV therapy is established. UVCs should not be in place longer than 7 to 10 days because of an increased risk of catheter-associated bloodstream infections and other complications.

B. Umbilical arterial catheters

UACs should be removed as soon as frequent sampling of arterial blood gases or central arterial blood pressure monitoring is no longer required. UACs should not be in place longer than 7 days because of an increased risk of catheter-associated bloodstream infections and other complications.

Because the risks associated with umbilical catheters are greater than those associated with PIVs, umbilical catheters should not be used as merely convenient routes for long-term fluid administration. Whenever possible, routine fluids should be infused through PIVs or, in babies in whom long-term venous access is required, percutaneously or surgically placed central venous catheters (not discussed here).

Self-test B

Now answer these questions to test yourself on the information in the last section.

B1. Identify the following complications as being associated with an umbilical venous catheter (UVC), an umbilical arterial catheter (UAC), or both.

UVC	UAC	
____	____	Blood loss from loose connections
____	____	Liver damage from infusion of hypertonic solutions
____	____	Sepsis
____	____	Blanching of a leg
____	____	Thrombosis

B2. **True** **False** It is generally recommended to leave an umbilical catheter in place once it has been inserted because it may be needed for long-term fluid therapy.

B3. What are 2 methods for maintaining an umbilical catheter?

_____

_____

B4. What equipment is required for continuous infusion through a UAC?

_____

B5. Medications, flush solutions, and all infusions through a UVC or UAC should be administered
  A. As quickly as possible
  B. Slowly and steadily

B6. A 1,600-g (3 lb 8 oz) preterm baby will require intravenous fluids for several days. What is the best route to use for this baby?

_____

Check your answers with the list that follows the Recommended Routines. Correct any incorrect answers and review the appropriate section in the unit.

UMBILICAL CATHETERS

Recommended Routines

All the routines listed below are based on the principles of perinatal care presented in the unit you have just finished. They are recommended as part of routine perinatal care.

Read each routine carefully and decide whether it is standard operating procedure in your hospital. Check the appropriate blank next to each routine.

Procedure Standard in My Hospital	Needs Discussion by Our Staff	Recommended Routine
_____	_____	1. Establish a policy to ensure the presence of a sterile umbilical catheter tray in each delivery room and in the nursery at all times.
_____	_____	2. Establish a policy of inserting an umbilical venous catheter during delivery room resuscitation when emergency medications are required.
_____	_____	3. Establish a routine to consider insertion of an umbilical arterial catheter in any newborn anticipated to require significant amounts of supplemental oxygen for longer than a short period.

Self-test Answers

These are the answers to the Self-test questions. Please check them with the answers you gave and review the information in the unit wherever necessary.

Self-test A

A1. A. Umbilical vein
    B. Umbilical artery
    C. Umbilical artery

A2.
Yes	No	
_X_	___	Radiopaque
___	_X_	Beveled tip
_X_	___	Rounded tip
_X_	___	Single hole in tip center
___	_X_	Multiple tiny side holes near catheter tip

A3. Any 2 of the following uses:
    • Administration of emergency medications, especially in the delivery room
    • Exchange transfusions
    • Emergency estimation of Pco_2 and pH level (not Po_2)
    • Fluid administration during the first few days in extremely preterm babies

A4. Not used for exchange transfusions (unless an umbilical arterial catheter used for withdrawal of blood with an umbilical venous catheter, or peripheral intravenous line used for infusion)
    Not used for medications or fluids, unless an umbilical arterial catheter is already in place (for blood gas sampling or central blood pressure monitoring) and another intravenous route is not available

A5. Drawing blood for arterial blood gas tests

A6. Arterial catheter: at a level between the third and fourth lumbar vertebrae (some experts prefer T6-T9).
    Venous catheter: at or just above the level of the diaphragm as seen on the lateral chest radiograph.

Self-test B

B1.
UVC	UAC	
_X_	_X_	Blood loss from loose connections
_X_	___	Liver damage from infusion of hypertonic solutions
_X_	_X_	Sepsis
___	_X_	Blanching of a leg
_X_	_X_	Thrombosis

B2. False   *Reason:* Except in special circumstances, routine fluid administration through an umbilical arterial or venous catheter should be avoided.

B3. Heparin lock
    Continuous infusion

B4. An infusion pump

B5. B. Slowly and steadily

B6. Peripheral intravenous line

Unit 3 Posttest

After completion of each unit there is a free online posttest available at www.cmevillage.com to test your understanding. Navigate to the PCEP pages on www.cmevillage.com and register to take the free posttests.

Once registered on the website and after completing all the unit posttests, pay the book exam fee ($15) and pass the test at 80% or greater to earn continuing education credits. Only start the PCEP book exam if you have time to complete it. If you take the book exam and are not connected to a printer, either print your certificate to a .pdf file and save it to print later or come back to www.cmevillage.com at any time and print a copy of your educational transcript.

Credits are only available by book, not by individual unit within the books. Available credits for completion of each book exam are as follows: Book 1: 14.5 credits; Book 2: 16 credits; Book 3: 17 credits; Book 4: 9 credits.

For more details, navigate to the PCEP webpages at www.cmevillage.com.

SKILL UNIT

Inserting and Managing Umbilical Catheters

This skill unit will teach you how to insert umbilical arterial catheters and umbilical venous catheters. Not everyone will be required to learn and practice umbilical catheterization. However, all staff members should read this unit and attend a skill session to learn the equipment and sequence of steps to assist effectively with umbilical catheterization. A video of umbilical catheter insertion may be viewed at https://www.youtube.com/watch?v=_eun4dq2BEY.

Staff members who will be asked to master all aspects of this skill will need to demonstrate each of the following steps correctly:

1. Restrain and measure the "baby" (mannequin) for catheter insertion.
2. Collect the equipment and prepare the "sterile" tray.
3. Prepare catheter, stopcock, and heparin solution.
4. Cleanse the umbilical cord and the surrounding skin; loosely cinch the umbilical tape around the stump. In the event of excessive bleeding from around the catheters after placement, the tie can be tightened.
5. Cut the cord to an appropriate length.
6. Identify the umbilical vessels.
7. Dilate the umbilical artery and insert the catheter. (You also may be asked to demonstrate venous catheterization.)
8. Check for blood return and flush the catheter with heparinized solution; turn the stopcock off to the catheter.
9. Suture the catheter in place (or temporarily tape it in place until the location is confirmed on a radiograph).
10. Tape the catheter in place after the radiograph has been obtained, the catheter location has been confirmed, and the catheter has been sutured in place.
11. Begin infusion or maintain the catheter with heparin lock.
12. Use sterile technique and standard precautions throughout the procedure.
13. Illustrate the techniques to stop bleeding from an umbilical artery and the umbilical vein.

Staff members who will be asked to master the assistant components of this skill will need to demonstrate each of the following steps correctly:

1. Restrain baby for catheter insertion.
2. Collect the equipment and prepare the "sterile" tray.
3. Hold the distal section of cord in an elevated position until it is cut off.
4. Hold the instruments to stabilize the umbilical cord or expose the artery or vein for catheterization, as needed by the person inserting the catheter.
5. Tape the catheter temporarily until placement is confirmed on a radiograph (unless the catheter was initially sutured in place).
6. Tape the catheter in place after the radiograph is obtained, the catheter location is confirmed, and the catheter is sutured in place.
7. Begin infusion or maintain the catheter with heparin lock.
8. Use sterile technique and standard precautions.
9. Illustrate the techniques to stop bleeding from an umbilical artery and the umbilical vein.

In addition to the practice session(s) scheduled by your coordinators, a special joint physician-nurse practice session may be arranged for nurses and perinatal care physicians in your hospital.

Note: The graph that accompanies step 10 for umbilical arterial catheters in this skill unit was adapted with permission from Klaus MH, Fanaroff AA. *Care of the High-Risk Neonate.* 6th ed. Philadelphia, PA: WB Saunders; 2013:592.

PERINATAL PERFORMANCE GUIDE

Inserting and Managing Umbilical Catheters

Note: The information presented in this skill unit pertains to the insertion of umbilical arterial catheters (UACs), as well as umbilical venous catheters (UVCs), to be used for exchange transfusions or prolonged intravenous (IV) fluid requirement.

UVCs, which are needed in the delivery room for administration of emergency medications, may be inserted with minimal preparation by one member of the resuscitation team (Box 3.1).

This guide uses one method for determining correct umbilical catheter placement (the Dunn method). Several studies have been conducted to determine the best method for calculating the appropriate umbilical catheter insertion depth. No method is perfect, and insertion should be confirmed with radiography or ultrasonography. Procedural videos can be found at https://www.youtube.com/watch?v=_eun4dq2BEY and https://www.nejm.org/doi/full/10.1056/NEJMvcm0800666?query=RES.

Box 3.1. Quick Steps for UVC/UAC Insertion

Position, restrain, and measure the baby for proper depth of insertion. Determine the catheter insertion distance.

Don a cap and mask, scrub, and put on a sterile gown and gloves. Use sterile technique throughout the procedure.

Prepare the equipment by maintaining sterile technique.

Clean the umbilical cord, stump, and the surrounding skin by using your institution's approved antiseptic solution, and place sterile drapes around the umbilicus.

Tie umbilical tape around the base of the umbilicus and cut the cord.

Identify the umbilical arteries and the umbilical vein.

Prepare the vessels. Dilate the umbilical artery if applicable.

Insert the venous and/or arterial catheter to the proper distance, check for blood return, and flush with heparinized solution.

Secure the catheter(s) and obtain a radiograph to confirm placement.

Step-by-Step Procedure

ACTIONS   **REMARKS**

Preparing the Equipment and Baby for Umbilical Catheterization (Inserter and assistant roles defined)

1. Perform a time-out per your institution's protocol.

2. Assign roles for inserter, assistant, and monitoring.

Two people, working together, make the job of inserting an umbilical catheter much easier. A third person should be present to monitor the insertion process to ensure all steps are done in a sterile fashion. With patience and careful preparation, insertion of an umbilical catheter can be accomplished quite easily. Failure occurs most often when there is inadequate preparation. The procedure will generally take about 30 minutes.

3. Maintain a properly heated and oxygenated environment. The baby should also be attached to a cardiac monitor or a pulse oximeter.

Temperature control can be best maintained during catheterization if the baby is placed under a radiant warmer.

4. Restrain the baby gently, but firmly.

Double half-hitch knots (shown at right), tied with gauze bandage around the baby's arms and legs and taped to the edges of the bed, work well. These knots will secure a baby's hand or foot but will not tighten further or constrict blood supply to the extremity.

Prefabricated restraints, typically with Velcro closure, may also be used. The use of circumcision "boards" or "trays" may interfere with maintaining sterility while obtaining a radiograph and are therefore not recommended.

After the procedure has been completed and a radiograph has been obtained to confirm the location of the catheter tip, return the baby to a more comfortable position.

Restraint is necessary because any movement by a baby will interfere with the procedure and lengthen the time needed to accomplish the catheterization.

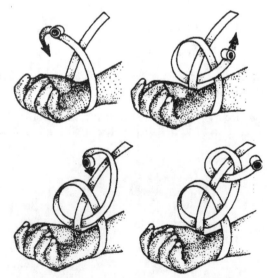

ACTIONS   REMARKS

Preparing the Equipment and Baby for Umbilical Catheterization (Inserter and assistant roles defined) (continued)

5. When the restraints have been tied and taped in place, the baby should be in a "spread eagle" position.

   Even the tiniest babies generally need some form of restraint.

   To accomplish umbilical catheterization quickly and easily, there must be

   • Excellent view of and access to the umbilicus

   • Good lighting

   • No risk of interference by movement of the baby during isolation of an umbilical vessel and delicate insertion of a catheter

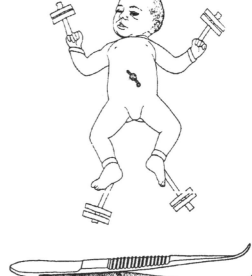

6. Certain instruments are especially helpful for umbilical catheterization. These are

   • One or 2 pairs of curved iris forceps

   • A pair of straight iris forceps

   Note: Forceps used should have smooth or serrated tips to grip the vessel firmly, but *not* toothed tips. Toothed tips will shred the edges of a vessel.

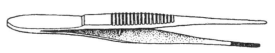

Curved and straight iris forceps
(shown actual size)

7. Other instruments for umbilical catheterization include

   • One pair iris scissors

   • One pair surgical scissors

   • One needle holder

   • Two curved mosquito clamps

   • Two straight mosquito clamps

   • One knife handle and blade

   • 2–0 silk suture

   • Umbilical tape

   • Three-way Luer-Lok (or similar) stopcock

ACTIONS   **REMARKS**

Preparing the Equipment and Baby for Umbilical Catheterization (Inserter and assistant roles defined) (continued)

8. The catheter should be sterile and radiopaque.

   The size of the catheter used depends on the size of the baby and the purpose of the catheter.

   Catheter Size for Umbilical Arterial Catheter

   - 3.5F for tiny babies (< 1,000 g [<2 lb 3 oz])
   - 5F for all other babies

   Some experts prefer size 3.5F in the aorta for most babies if the smaller catheter will feed into the correct position.

   Catheter Size for Umbilical Venous Catheter

   - 5F for all babies when UVC is used for emergency medications.
   - 3.5F for exchange transfusion for small babies.
   - Double-lumen catheters are often useful for administering several different solutions.

Determining Catheter Insertion Distance

9. Using a tape measure marked in centimeters, measure from the shoulder to a point equal to the level of the umbilicus (shown by the dashed line).

   Do *not* measure from the shoulder on a diagonal to the umbilicus (not shown, but a common mistake).

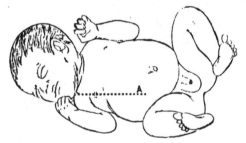

To determine shoulder-umbilicus length, measure along line A.

10. This measurement, when plotted on the graph to the right, will indicate the proper distance to insert a catheter.

    - The **dashed** line is for **venous** catheters.
    - The **solid** line is for **arterial** catheters, with the tip placed in the low position, at L3-L4.

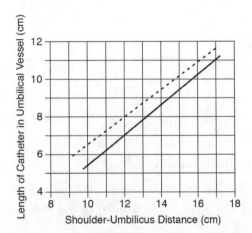

- - - - - - umbilical vein to junction of inferior vena cava and right atrium

——— umbilical artery to bifurcation of aorta

ACTIONS   REMARKS

Determining Catheter Insertion Distance (continued)

Example: A baby's shoulder-to-umbilicus distance is 13 cm.

Step 1 Find this shoulder-umbilicus distance on the horizontal scale (marked with the vertical arrow).

Step 2 Find where this distance intersects each of the black lines on the graph.

Step 3 Read where this point falls on the chart's vertical scale.

For the sample baby, this point is at 8 cm for an arterial catheter in the low (tip at L3-L4) position and at 8¾ cm for a venous catheter.

Another method for estimating appropriate length of catheter to insert is

- UVC length (cm) = umbilical-to-nipple length minus 1 cm

- UAC length (cm) = 9 plus 3 times baby's weight (kg) for a high location (T6-T9)

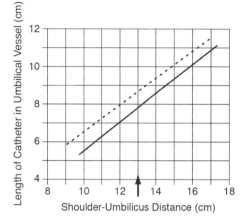

- - - - - umbilical vein to junction of inferior vena cava and right atrium

——— umbilical artery to bifurcation of aorta

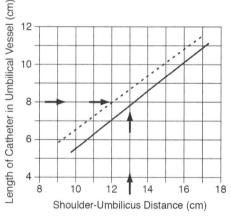

- - - - - umbilical vein to junction of inferior vena cava and right atrium

——— umbilical artery to bifurcation of aorta

11. A radiograph should be obtained to confirm catheter position prior to suturing the catheter in place and while the inserter remains sterile. The inserter can advance or retract the catheter after acquisition of an initial radiograph, if sterility has been maintained.

A catheter should *never* be inserted further after sterile drapes have been removed or after the exposed part of the catheter has been contaminated. If a catheter was not inserted a sufficient distance and the drapes have been removed or the catheter has been contaminated, it should be removed and a new catheter inserted under sterile conditions.

If a catheter must be repositioned, a repeat radiograph should be obtained to confirm correct positioning of the catheter.

ACTIONS	REMARKS

Preparing a Catheter

12. The first operator and assistant (second operator) should each put on a cap and mask, scrub, and put on a sterile gown and gloves.

13. Check the heparin solution.

A solution of 1 to 2 units of heparin per 1 mL of fluid is an appropriate concentration during catheter insertion or if the catheter is maintained as a heparin lock.

A lower concentration of heparin, such as 0.12 U/kg/h, is recommended if a slow continuous infusion will be given through the catheter, such as when it is used for central blood pressure monitoring.

14. Prepare the catheter, by using sterile technique.

   • Connect the catheter to a 3-way stopcock, which has been connected to a syringe containing heparinized solution, taking care to expel all air bubbles.

   • Fill the catheter, and the stopcock, with the heparinized solution.

   • Turn the stopcock *off* to the catheter.

Different stopcocks indicate the "off" direction in different ways.

You must be thoroughly familiar with the type of stopcock used in your hospital.

To avoid possible confusion, it is recommended that only one type of stopcock be used in all newborn care areas in your hospital.

15. Umbilical catheters are marked in various ways, depending on the manufacturer.

   Be sure to note the number and spacing of marks before inserting a catheter. Use these marks to help determine when the catheter has been inserted the appropriate distance.

   For the sample baby, the catheter should be inserted approximately 10 cm to place the tip at L3-L4.

ACTIONS   REMARKS

Preparing the Umbilical Cord

16. Clean the baby's umbilical cord, stump, and surrounding skin by using a surgical prep solution, such as povidone-iodine.

    The second operator should hold up the umbilical cord by using a straight mosquito clamp to secure the cord clamp.

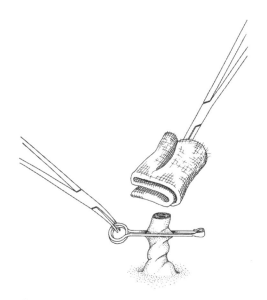

17. Place sterile drapes around the umbilicus.

    Two circumcision drapes folded in half work well for this, or an adhesive drape designed for eye surgery can secure the cloth drapes and "seal" the sterile field.

    Cloth drapes should extend over the sides and foot of the bed to allow the operator and equipment to touch those areas without contamination.

18. Loosely tie umbilical tape around the base of the umbilicus. The umbilical tape should *not* be knotted. Rather, it should be wrapped just once on itself (see illustration).

    This is done so the umbilical tape can be pulled tight very quickly in the event that one of the vessels bleeds when the cord is cut below the umbilical clamp.

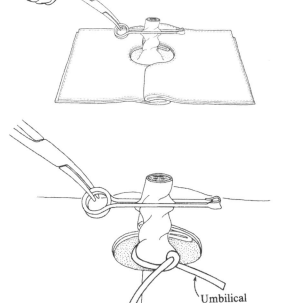

Umbilical Tape

ACTIONS

REMARKS

Preparing the Umbilical Cord (continued)

19. While the second operator continues to hold up the baby's umbilical cord with the mosquito clamp, cut the cord as evenly as possible with a knife blade. To do this, press the knife blade firmly against the side of the cord and use just 1 or 2 passes of the knife blade to cut cleanly across the cord. A stump of approximately 0.5 cm should be left.

    To avoid contamination of the sterile instruments and drapes, discard the cord remnant and clamp clear of the sterile field.

Avoid multiple back-and-forth sawing motions with the knife blade because these will lead to a ragged cord stump. If the stump is ragged, it will be more difficult to identify the vessels.

Cutting across the cord with scissors is also not recommended because doing so can crush the vessels.

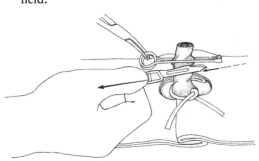

 Be careful! When you cut the cord, the vessels may bleed, sometimes profusely if from an umbilical artery. The second operator, with sterile gloves on, should be prepared to tighten the umbilical tape to stop the bleeding. If the cord has been cut too short, so that the tape comes off at this point, bleeding may be stopped by using techniques described at the end of this skill unit. Read these sections before proceeding with this step.

20. Now identify the umbilical vessels.

    There should be one vein, usually located toward the baby's head, and 2 arteries, usually located toward the baby's feet.

The vein is thin walled and larger than the arteries. The arteries are thick walled and the lumen is pin sized.

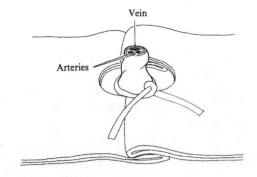

ACTIONS   REMARKS

Preparing the Umbilical Cord (continued)

21. If you cannot determine the vessels with visual inspection, rub the flat side of an instrument gently across the top of the cord stump.

    The resistance offered by the muscular tips of the arteries can be felt. The vein cannot be felt in this manner.

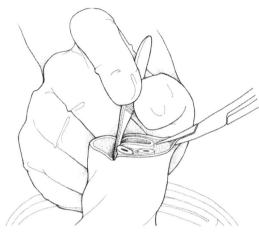

22. The second operator holds the edges of the cord stump with the mosquito clamps. One experienced operator can achieve placement of umbilical catheters by placing curved mosquito clamps in a "nose-up" position and allowing them to rest on the baby's abdomen to provide reasonable traction and positioning.

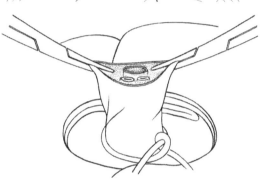

Inserting an Umbilical Arterial Catheter [Steps 23 (UAC) to 33 (UAC)]

23 (UAC). Select one artery for catheterization. The first operator should pick up the edge of the selected artery with the straight iris forceps.

    Note: The artery is fragile, so some clinicians prefer not to grasp the artery itself, but just the surrounding tissue, to achieve stability during insertion.

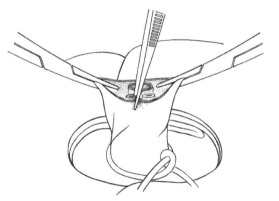

143

ACTIONS   **REMARKS**

Inserting an Umbilical Arterial Catheter [Steps 23 (UAC) to 33 (UAC)] (continued)

24 (UAC). The first operator then inserts one tip of the curved iris forceps into the lumen of the artery.

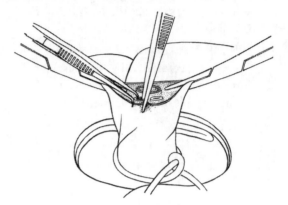

25 (UAC). Repeat step 24 several times. When the vessel has begun to dilate, insert both tips of the curved iris forceps.

Insert only the tips of the forceps. Do *not* attempt to probe deeply into the artery.

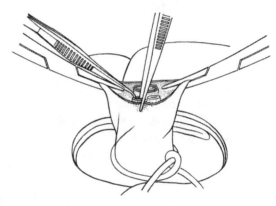

26 (UAC). Repeat step 25 several times, *slowly and patiently,* to dilate the entrance to the artery. Each time, spread the forceps a bit wider inside the artery, and hold the forceps open while sliding them out of the artery.

Use the instruments firmly but gently. *Never tug on the vessels,* but once you have the proper grip on an artery, hold it tightly.

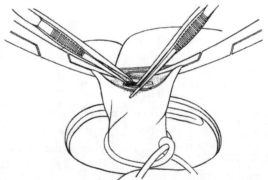

144

ACTIONS   REMARKS

Inserting an Umbilical Arterial Catheter [Steps 23 (UAC) to 33 (UAC)] (continued)

27 (UAC). Now, with one iris forceps holding one edge of the artery (or the surrounding tissue) and the curved iris forceps dilating the inside of the artery, the second operator should lay down one of the mosquito clamps, holding the edge of the cord, and use that hand to insert the catheter (using gloved fingers as shown or with a pair of non-serrated forceps).

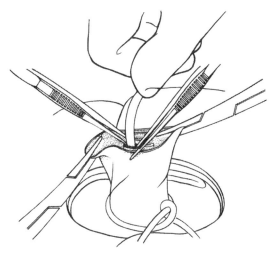

Grip the catheter near the tip. If held too far from the tip, the catheter will buckle and not enter the artery easily. If held too close to the tip, it will fall out of the artery when released in an attempt to advance it.

28 (UAC). Umbilical arteries curve toward the feet before curving upward toward the head. Therefore, it may be helpful to aim the tip slightly toward the baby's feet when first inserting a catheter.

29 (UAC). After 2 or 3 cm of the catheter has passed into the vessel, the curved iris forceps may be removed from the opening of the artery. Continue to grip the edge of the artery with the other iris forceps and the edge of the cord with the mosquito clamps.

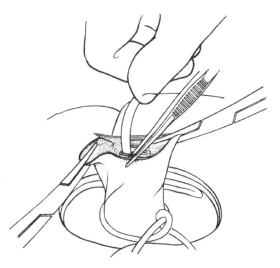

30 (UAC). Keep a *constant grip* on the catheter (with an instrument or your fingers) and continue to insert the catheter.

Be sure the cord stump is not pulled toward the left or right side of the baby because that may make it more difficult to insert the catheter.

- UAC insertion is sometimes aided by pulling the stump slightly toward the baby's head.

Never let go of the catheter until you have inserted it at least 2 cm into the vessel.

Once the catheter has been inserted the desired distance, it will stay there while it is being sutured and taped in place. However, if you let go of it after it has been inserted only a few centimeters, the pressure of the muscular artery may push the catheter out, forcing you to locate the artery once more, dilate it, and reinsert the catheter.

ACTIONS   REMARKS

Inserting an Umbilical Arterial Catheter [Steps 23 (UAC) to 33 (UAC)] (continued)

31 (UAC). As you insert the catheter, resistance may be met at 2 points:

- At the level of the abdominal wall, after the catheter has been inserted approximately 2 cm
- At the level of the bladder, after the catheter has been inserted approximately 5 to 7 cm

32 (UAC). If resistance does occur, apply only gentle, steady pressure to the catheter. With gentle, steady pressure, the artery will often relax enough to allow passage of the catheter.

Do not probe, pry, or repeatedly or forcefully push with the catheter.

If gentle, steady pressure on the catheter does not work, you may do 2 things:

- Remove the catheter and try a smaller size (3.5F is the smallest size).
- Attempt catheterization of the other umbilical artery.

33 (UAC). Insert the catheter the predetermined distance.

Use the marks on the catheter to estimate the proper depth of insertion.

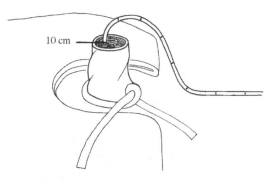

10 cm

For the sample baby, it was determined that the catheter should be inserted 10 cm. The type of catheter illustrated has black marks spaced in centimeters from the tip.

Continue to Step 34 after insertion of an umbilical catheter

ACTIONS

REMARKS

Inserting an Umbilical Venous Catheter [Steps 23 (UVC) to 33 (UVC)]

23 (UVC). The first operator should pick up the edge of the vein and the side of the umbilical cord with straight iris forceps.

The vein is thin walled and easily torn. To avoid this, pinch the side of the vein *and* the side of the umbilical cord together in the forceps.

- UVC insertion is sometimes helped by pulling the cord stump slightly toward the baby's feet.

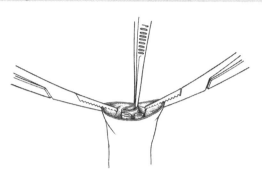

24 (UVC). The first operator now gently grasps the opposite side of the vein with another pair of iris forceps.

Because the vein is not a muscular vessel, it is not necessary to dilate it. Simply hold it open with the iris forceps.

The vein may bleed when first opened. If this happens, apply firm pressure on the baby's abdomen, just above the umbilicus.

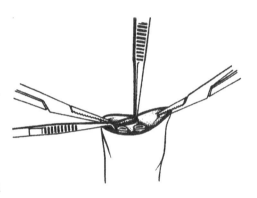

25 (UVC). The second operator should now lay down one of the mosquito clamps holding the edge of the cord and use that hand or forceps to insert the catheter.

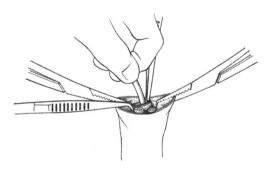

26 (UVC). The umbilical vein curves toward the baby's head and runs superficially under the skin several centimeters before curving downward toward the baby's spine. Therefore, it will be helpful, once inside the vein, to aim the tip of the catheter toward the baby's head.

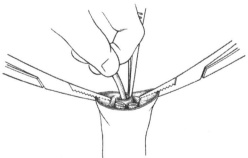

ACTIONS   **REMARKS**

Inserting an Umbilical Venous Catheter [Steps 23 (UVC) to 33 (UVC)] (continued)

27 (UVC). Continue to insert the catheter while always keeping a grip on it with forceps or your fingers.

28 (UVC). Insert the catheter the desired distance, as measured on the graph (see step 10 earlier in this skill), but use the *dashed* line to determine the distance for a *venous* catheter.

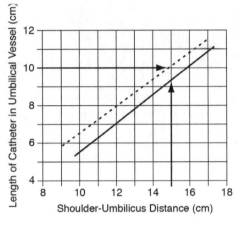

- - - - - umbilical vein to junction of inferior vena cava and right atrium

———— umbilical artery to bifurcation of aorta

Example: If the shoulder-umbilicus length for a specific baby is 15 cm, you would insert the catheter 12 cm (10 cm from the chart, plus 2 cm in case catheter withdrawal for repositioning is needed).

Another method for estimating appropriate length of catheter to insert is

Length of UVC (cm) to insert = umbilical to nipple length minus 1 cm

29 (UVC). If resistance is met, do *not* try to insert the catheter further.

Resistance indicates that the tip of the catheter has entered one of the small veins in the circulation of the liver.

30 (UVC). Withdraw the catheter 1 or 2 cm and twist it slightly in an attempt to aim the tip in a different direction. Gently attempt to insert the catheter in the desired distance.

Sometimes it is necessary to undertake this maneuver several times before the catheter will pass through the ductus venosus so that the tip can be placed above the diaphragm.

31 (UVC). *If repeated attempts to insert the catheter fail, seek another skilled person to attempt the procedure.*

In some cases, either upsizing or downsizing the catheter may be helpful.

32 (UVC). If the catheter still cannot be inserted so that the tip is above the level of the diaphragm, remove the catheter or withdraw it until 2 to 3 cm of it remains within the umbilical vein.

Check to be sure that an instantaneous blood return can be obtained with the catheter tip in this location.

ACTIONS REMARKS

Inserting an Umbilical Venous Catheter [Steps 23 (UVC) to 33 (UVC)] (continued)

33 (UVC). You may decide to leave the catheter in this position, but be aware that hypertonic solutions infused through the catheter will enter the circulation of the liver and may cause irritation or thrombosis.

While you should avoid locating the catheter tip below the level of the diaphragm, the exception to this is an emergency situation, when there is insufficient time to obtain a radiograph. In an emergency, insert a UVC just far enough to obtain a blood return (2–3 cm), before infusing medication or fluid.

Continue to Step 34 after insertion of an umbilical catheter

34. Turn the stopcock so that it is open between the catheter and the syringe containing the heparinized flush solution.

35. Pull back on the syringe. You should obtain an *immediate* blood return in the catheter.

If you do not obtain an immediate blood return, the catheter is placed incorrectly.

Do not push fluid into a catheter that does not have an instantaneous blood return.

36. After obtaining blood return in the catheter, pull any air bubbles into the syringe. Pull back only enough for air bubbles to enter the syringe. Generally, this can be done with little or no blood getting into the syringe.

Be careful not to infuse any air bubbles. Keep the syringe upright (with the barrel above the stopcock and catheter) so air bubbles will not enter the catheter.

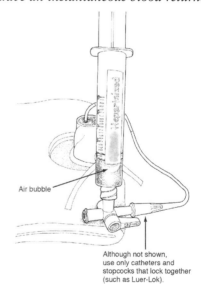

Air bubble

Although not shown, use only catheters and stopcocks that lock together (such as Luer-Lok).

37. Refill the catheter with the heparinized flush solution. Turn off the stopcock to the catheter.

Note: If a significant amount of blood entered the syringe, hold it upright so that the blood will stay near the stopcock and can be given back to the baby without also infusing the full amount of flush solution.

149

ACTIONS

REMARKS

Securing the catheter in place

38. The catheter is sutured in place (see step 45), and a sterile drape is placed over the sterile field and catheter while a radiograph is obtained. This is the preferred method.

    Or

    One operator and instrument tray remain sterile. The second operator removes the sterile drapes and tapes the catheter in place.

    A small rectangle of clear adhesive film may be used to protect the baby's skin (depicted as a faint gray line around the tape) before taping with adhesive tape, particularly if the baby is extremely preterm.

    Whether tape or suture is used, the catheter must be firmly secured in place before the radiograph is obtained.

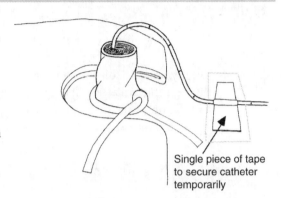

Single piece of tape to secure catheter temporarily

If the sterile drapes have been removed, the catheter may only be *withdrawn* if it is malpositioned. If the sterile drapes remain in place, then catheter may be inserted further.

If the catheter is taped, this is not the final taping. This temporary taping is done so the catheter will not become dislodged while catheter placement is checked with a radiograph.

Checking Catheter Placement

39. Obtain a portable radiograph of the baby's abdomen and chest.

The baby should be kept in the same heated and oxygenated environment throughout the entire radiography procedure.

40. The radiograph may be an anteroposterior or a lateral view. The anteroposterior view is obtained more easily than a lateral view, but a venous catheter is more precisely localized on the lateral view.

ACTIONS   REMARKS

Checking Catheter Placement (continued)

41. Umbilical *arterial* catheters

    When a catheter has been inserted the measured distance, the tip of the catheter should be in the aorta, above or below the major arteries that are feeding the abdominal organs.

    See the main section of this unit for a discussion of the relative risks associated with high versus low placement.

    On a radiograph, the catheter tip of a UAC should be between the level of the third and fourth lumbar vertebrae (L3-L4) for low placement, which is shown in the radiograph to the right.

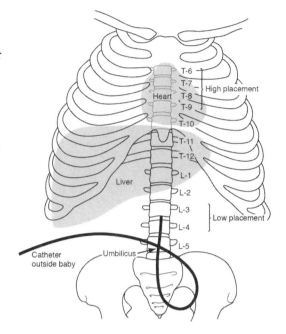

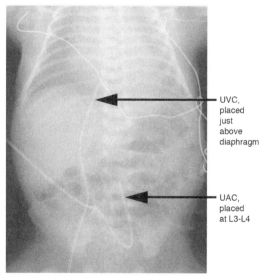

ACTIONS   REMARKS

Checking Catheter Placement (continued)

For high placement, the catheter should
be between the sixth and ninth thoracic
vertebrae (T6-T9) (shown on the radiograph to the right).

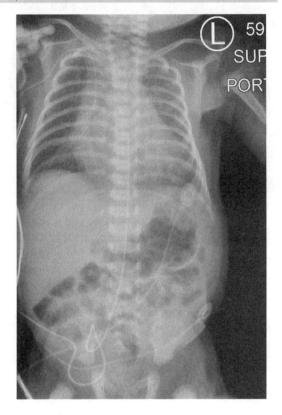

ACTIONS   REMARKS

Checking Catheter Placement (continued)

42. Umbilical *venous* catheters

    When the catheter has been inserted the proper distance, the tip of the catheter should be at the junction of the inferior vena cava and right atrium.

    This location is used because infusions of hypertonic solutions through a catheter in a lower position may go into the circulation of the liver and cause liver damage.

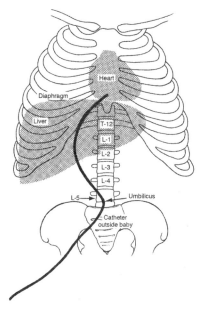

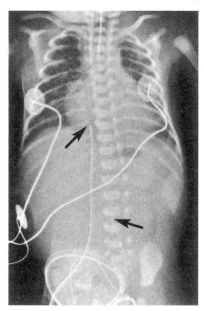

Correct placement of a UVC (upper arrow) and a UAC at L3-L4 (lower arrow).

The tip of the UVC is just above the level of the diaphragm.

On a radiograph, the catheter tip of a UVC should be at or just above the level of the diaphragm. The lateral view, shown below, is preferred because the diaphragm slants downward behind the heart and the catheter parallels the plane of the lateral radiograph, making measurements more accurate.

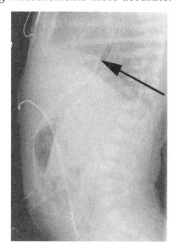

Lateral radiograph of correct UVC placement. The arrow tip points to the UVC at the level of the diaphragm. There is also a large-bore orogastric tube in the stomach.

ACTIONS   REMARKS

Checking Catheter Placement (continued)

43. When the radiographic results are known, reposition the catheter (if necessary).

44. To determine how far to withdraw or insert a catheter that needs to be repositioned, measure on the radiograph

    UVC: From the catheter tip to the diaphragm, preferably on the lateral view

    UAC: From the catheter tip to the third lumbar or sixth thoracic vertebra

    Using the marks on the catheter as a guide, reposition the catheter the distance you determine with the radiograph.

    If the catheter is repositioned, obtain another radiograph to check the location of the catheter tip.

*If you **removed the sterile drapes** and temporarily taped the catheter in place (see step 38), you may **only withdraw** a catheter to reposition it. If it needs to be inserted further, the catheter in place should be removed and a new catheter should be inserted, using the same procedure and sterile technique used with the first catheter.*

*If you **kept the sterile field intact** and sutured the catheter to secure it while the radiograph was obtained (see steps 38 and 44), you may cut the suture and **withdraw** or **insert** the catheter further to reposition it, and then secure the catheter with a new suture. When you cut the first suture, take great care not to nick the catheter.*

Securing a Catheter

45. Now suture and tape the catheter in place.

    A. Tie the suture to the catheter.

       1. Place a stitch through the umbilical cord stump by entering through the side of the cord and exiting from the cut surface. Tie this in place.

Be sure not to sew through any of the vessels.

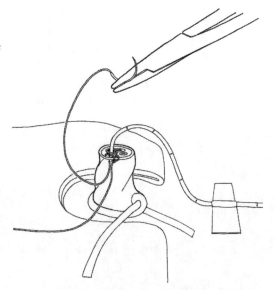

       2. Cut off the needle and tie the suture to the original.

ACTIONS   **REMARKS**

Securing a Catheter (continued)

3. Tie a knot to keep the suture tight.

4. Lace the tails of this knot around the catheter to form a "Chinese finger trap" and tie them in place. (See the series of drawings to the right.)

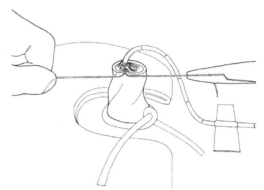

5. Wrap one end of the suture around the needle holder.

6. Put the needle holder on one side of the catheter and the end of this *same* piece of suture around the other side of the catheter. Pick up the free end of this suture with the needle holder and draw the suture down tight on the catheter.

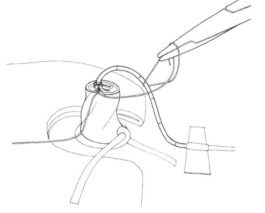

7. Repeat this with the other end of the knot from step 3.

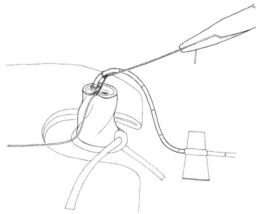

ACTIONS   REMARKS

Securing a Catheter (continued)

8. Finally, tie together both ends of
   the suture that have been knotted
   around the catheter.

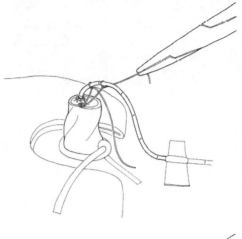

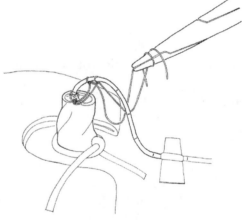

9. Cut off the loose ends of the suture, just beyond the knot.

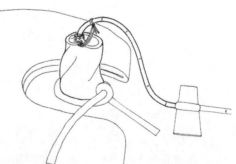

B. Completely remove the povidone-   If left in place, antiseptics can cause marked
   iodine used to prep the umbilical   skin irritation.
   area by wiping the baby's skin with
   alcohol or sterile water swabs.

C. The catheter can be pulled gently back
   through the suture by pushing the suture toward the baby with sterile iris
   forceps.

ACTIONS

REMARKS

Securing a Catheter (continued)

D. When the catheter is in its correct position, secure it to the baby with a "tape bridge."

Note: Some clinicians believe that if the suture has been secured well, a single piece of tape or adhesive dressing over the area where the catheter is sutured will be sufficient.

Also, commercial devices are available to replace tape bridges. Follow the manufacturer's application instructions.

1. Cut 2 strips of clear adhesive dressing, 2 to 3 inches long by ¾ inch wide.

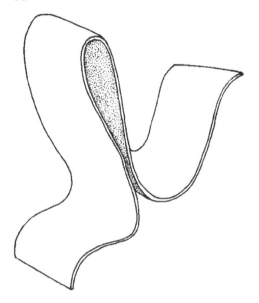

2. Place these strips on either side of the umbilicus.

   In the tape bridge illustration, clear adhesive film (indicated by the faint lines around the perimeter of the tape) is put on the baby's skin, under the adhesive tape.

3. Take a 4-inch strip of ½-inch adhesive tape and fold the center section on itself.

4. Tape this strip to one of the clear adhesive strips.

5. Repeat this with another piece of ½-inch adhesive tape and the other clear adhesive strip.

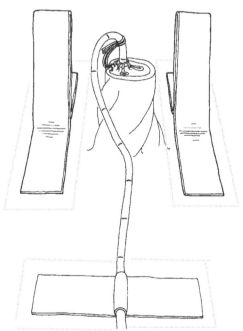

ACTIONS   REMARKS

Securing a Catheter (continued)

6. Next, wrap another piece of
   ½-inch adhesive tape from one side
   of the bridge to the other side,
   catching the catheter in the center.

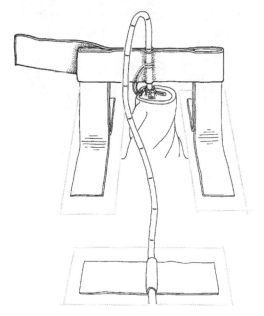

7. Loop the catheter over and catch a
   second section of the catheter with
   the adhesive tape.

   With the catheter secured in
   2 places in this manner, any traction exerted on the catheter will
   not pull directly on the suture.

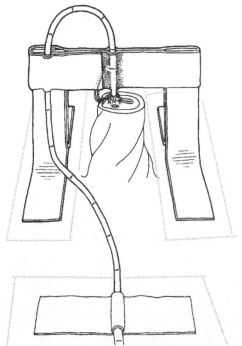

ACTIONS

REMARKS

Securing a Catheter (continued)

E. Some experts use clear adhesive film dressings to hold the catheter flat against the skin, thus facilitating prone positioning and kangaroo mother care.

In almost all cases, the loop of umbilical tape (shown in the figures from steps 18 to 44) can be removed after the catheter is secured in place. This is desirable because umbilical tape left around the cord for a prolonged period can become an area for bacterial growth or—if left on tightly—skin necrosis.

Only in rare situations will one of the umbilical vessels continue to ooze blood and require umbilical tape to be kept tightly pulled around the cord stump. In such cases, be sure the circulation to the skin at the base of the stump is not compromised.

F. Use a Luer-Lok or other system of locking connections between the tubing, stopcock, and catheter.

This is done to minimize the risk of disconnection, which could result in massive loss of blood from the baby.

G. Attach only locking syringes to the stopcock. These are syringes that twist into place and provide a more secure connection than syringes that fasten by simply being inserted into a stopcock.

Take this extra precaution because a loose connection may result in the baby losing a large amount of blood very quickly.

EMERGENCY VS NON-EMERGENCY PLACEMENT OF A UVC

When a UVC is inserted in an emergency for the administration of medications, it may be done with minimal preparation. In such situations, there is generally only enough time to put on a pair of sterile gloves, insert the catheter 3 to 5 cm, check for blood return, and then begin administration of emergency drugs.

When the insertion of a UVC is *not* for emergency purposes, a procedure similar to the one outlined for UACs should be followed. In fact, steps 1 through 22 and steps 34 through 45 are the same. The differences occur in steps 23 through 33 of the arterial catheterization skill. The corresponding steps for venous catheterization follow.

Unit 4: Low Blood Pressure (Hypotension)

Objectives

In this unit you will learn to

A. Identify babies at risk for low blood pressure, including which babies are at risk for blood loss.

B. Recognize the complications of hypotension.

C. Identify blood pressure measurements within and outside the normal (reference) range for babies of different birth weight and age categories.

D. Recognize and treat a newborn in shock.

E. Take accurate blood pressure measurements.

Note: Blood pressure graphs in this unit were derived from data published in *J Perinatol.* 1995;15(6):470–479.

Unit 4 Pretest

Before reading the unit, please answer the following questions. Select the *one best* answer to each question (unless otherwise instructed). Record your answers on the test and check them with the answers at the end of the book.

1. Blood pressure occurs as a result of
   A. Pumping action of the heart
   B. Volume of blood
   C. Tone of the blood vessels
   D. All of the above

2. A palpation blood pressure most closely approximates the
   A. Mean blood pressure
   B. Diastolic blood pressure
   C. Systolic blood pressure
   D. Pulse blood pressure

3. What is the recommended initial dosage of fluids to increase the blood volume of a 2,000-g (4 lb 6½ oz) baby who is in shock?
   A. 10 mL
   B. 20 mL
   C. 50 mL
   D. 100 mL

4. Which of the following amounts is the best estimate of the total blood volume of a 2,000-g (4 lb 6½ oz) baby?
   A. 180 mL (6 oz)
   B. 250 mL (8⅓ oz)
   C. 300 mL (10 oz)
   D. 420 mL (14 oz)

5. What minimum amount of blood loss would put a 2,000-g (4 lb 6½ oz) baby into shock?
   A. 15 mL (½ oz)
   B. 25 mL (⅚ oz)
   C. 45 mL (1½ oz)
   D. 75 mL (2½ oz)

6. Which of the following fluids is the best fluid to use to restore a baby's blood volume?
   A. 5% dextrose in water
   B. Sodium bicarbonate
   C. 10% dextrose in water
   D. Physiological (normal) saline solution

7. What can happen to babies with low blood pressure?
   A. Acidosis can develop.
   B. Vital organs can be damaged.
   C. Rapid respirations can develop.
   D. B and C
   E. A, B, and C

(continued)

Unit 4 Pretest (*continued*)

8. **True   False**   If a term baby is born with a blood pressure of 26 mm Hg, the first action should be to crossmatch the baby's blood and administer compatible blood.

9. Low blood pressure in newborns is associated with all of the following conditions, except
   A. Poor oxygenation
   B. Polycythemia
   C. Sepsis
   D. Central nervous system insult

10. A baby weighing 1,800 g (4 lb) has a blood pressure of 32/12 mm Hg at 30 minutes of age. How would this baby's blood pressure be described?
   A. Hypertensive
   B. Within reference range
   C. Hypotensive

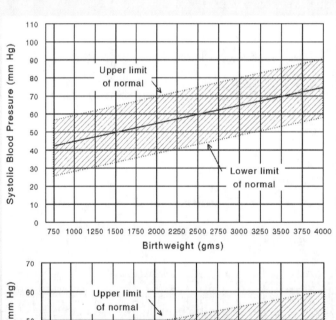

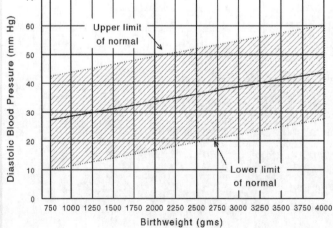

1. What is blood pressure?

Blood pressure is the amount of force pushing blood through the circulatory system. This force is determined by 3 factors: pumping action of the heart, tone of the blood vessels, and amount of blood or blood volume.

- *Systolic* pressure occurs at the end of each heart contraction. It is the higher number in a blood pressure measurement.
- *Diastolic* pressure occurs immediately before each contraction (resting period). It is the lower number in a blood pressure measurement.
- *Mean* pressure is about halfway between systolic and diastolic pressure.

Hypotension means low blood pressure. *Hypovolemia* means low blood volume, which is one cause of hypotension.

2. How do you check a baby's blood pressure?

Multiple methods are used to measure blood pressure. The oscillometric method is the primary means of measuring blood pressure noninvasively in babies. Palpation is acceptable but rarely used. The *auscultation* (listening with a stethoscope) method used for adults is not appropriate for babies. Other methods for measuring a baby's blood pressure are also available (eg, Doppler, central arterial), but they require equipment that is more specialized and are therefore not discussed in this unit. (See Book 4, Specialized Newborn Care, Unit 1, Direct Blood Pressure Measurement.)

With *oscillometric measurement,* oscillations in the arterial wall caused by pressure changes within the artery are detected. This method provides accurate readings, although it may give a slightly higher reading than that registered from an indwelling arterial catheter. Separate machines may be used, or some cardiac monitors have a blood pressure channel and cable that connects between the blood pressure cuff and monitor. In either case, oscillometric measurements are displayed as systolic, diastolic, and mean blood pressure values. The oscillometric device is the most common device used if an indwelling arterial catheter is not available.

Palpation measurement provides a single value that is slightly lower than systolic pressure, but this method is not as accurate as most other instrumentation methods and is now generally used only when there is an electronic equipment failure. Measurement is obtained by using a blood pressure cuff, manometer, and the care provider's index finger. The palpation method may provide a reasonably reliable mean pressure reading if the true systolic pressure is greater than 20 mm Hg.

3. Which babies should have their blood pressure checked?

All babies should have their blood pressure checked as a routine vital sign. Some babies will require more frequent blood pressure readings because they are at risk for hypotension. At-risk babies include

A. Babies suspected of having hypotension
   Babies in whom hypotension should be suspected are those with

   - Rapid respirations
   - Paleness or mottled coloring of the skin

- Weak pulses and rapid heart rate
- Prolonged capillary refill time

    Note: To test *capillary refill time*, press firmly for 5 seconds centrally over the mid-point of the sternum, forehead, or one of the long bones in a baby's arm or leg. After pressure is released, the blanched fingerprint area should disappear in 1 to 2 seconds as the skin capillaries refill with blood. If the fingerprint remains longer than 2 to 3 seconds, the baby has slow capillary refill time—although this is a relatively insensitive test.

B. Babies suspected of having blood loss (hypovolemia)
- Due to a tear in an umbilical vein or artery (inspect the cord closely because a tear may not be obvious)
- Due to a cord clamped incompletely, allowing blood loss from the baby
- Due to accidental cutting of the placenta during cesarean delivery
- Due to the presence of placenta previa or placental abruption (the risk of fetal blood loss is significantly higher with placenta previa than with placental abruption, but it can occur with either condition)
- Due to accumulation of blood in the placenta, secondary to cord compression
- Due to internal bleeding caused by trauma (difficult delivery)

C. Babies suspected of having congenital heart disease
For these babies, blood pressure measurements should be obtained in all 4 extremities. Differences in pressures among the extremities may suggest specific cardiac defects. For example, if the mean blood pressure in the legs is lower than that measured in the right upper extremity, one might suspect a coarctation of the aorta. Further interpretation of these blood pressure differences is not discussed in this program.

D. Babies born from a multifetal pregnancy
In identical (monozygotic) multifetal pregnancies, sometimes an abnormal connection exists between placental circulations of the fetuses. Fetal-fetal transfusion may result, with one fetus becoming the "blood donor" to the other "recipient" fetus.

Usually, this is a chronic process that allows the donor fetus to compensate for loss in blood volume but not for loss of red blood cells. Therefore, a donor fetus is usually not hypovolemic but is often anemic. If the abnormal connection is long-standing, the donor fetus may become severely anemic, which may lead to development of *hydrops*, a generalized fetal edema that occurs as a result of extreme, chronic anemia. A recipient fetus is typically a ruddy red color from polycythemia.

Blood pressure and hematocrit values should be checked in multifetal pregnancies (eg, twins, triplets). (See Unit 9, Identifying and Caring for Sick and At-Risk Babies, in this book, for information about hematocrit values.)

E. Babies born after fetal-maternal transfusion
Sometimes, an abnormal connection occurs between fetal and maternal circulation in the placenta, which results in fetal-maternal transfusion. The reverse direction of maternal-fetal transfusion apparently does not occur, probably because the pressure gradient in the intervillous space in the placenta favors a flow direction from the fetus to the woman.

When fetal-maternal blood loss occurs, the newborn may present with findings similar to the donor fetus described in the previous paragraphs (section D) on fetal-fetal transfusion.

If fetal-maternal transfusion is suspected, the mother's blood can be tested for the presence of fetal cells by using the Kleihauer-Betke (acid elution) test.

F. At-risk and sick babies

All at-risk and sick babies, especially those suspected of having an infection, require more frequent blood pressure readings.

Self-test A

Now answer these questions to test yourself on the information in the last section.

A1. **True** **False** Blood pressure depends entirely on how hard the heart pumps blood through the circulatory system.

A2. **True** **False** A transfusion from the fetus to the pregnant woman can occur in utero.

A3. Which of the following methods is/are being recommended in this unit for checking a baby's blood pressure? (Select all that apply.)

   A. Oscillometric method
   B. Palpation
   C. Auscultation
   D. Doppler method

A4. Which babies should have their blood pressure checked?

_____

_____

_____

_____

_____

A5. Hypotension means low blood _____, while hypovolemia means low blood

_____.

A6. If a fetus-to-fetus transfusion develops in utero, it can cause _____ in the donor fetus and _____ in the recipient fetus.

Check your answers with the list that follows the Recommended Routines. Correct any incorrect answers and review the appropriate section in the unit.

---

4. What is the normal (reference) newborn blood pressure range?

The blood pressure of newborn babies is much lower than that of older children or adults. In addition, neonatal blood pressure varies according to a baby's birth weight and age. Blood pressure increases with increasing birth weight, advancing gestational age, and the number of days and weeks since birth.

At birth, a baby's blood pressure is closely related to the birth weight and gestational age. Figures 4.1, 4.2, and 4.3 show the reference (normal) range of systolic and diastolic pressures for babies of different birth weights during the first day after birth, as a function of gestational age at birth, and as a function of postmenstrual age, respectively.

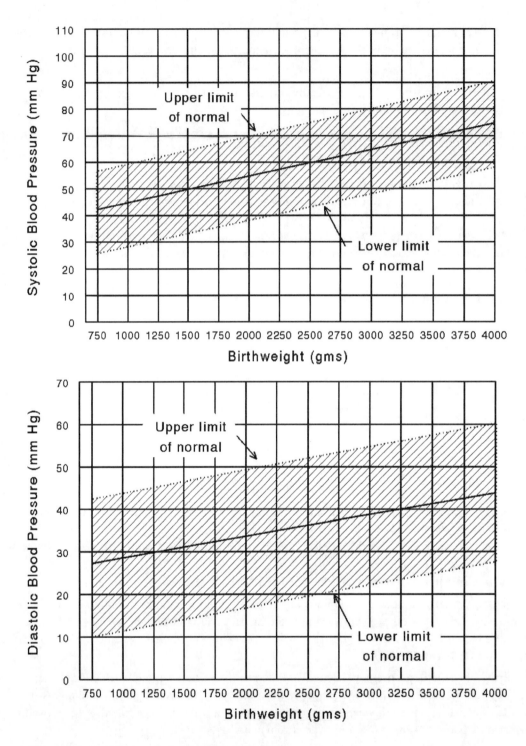

Figure 4.1. Blood Pressure During the First Day After Birth

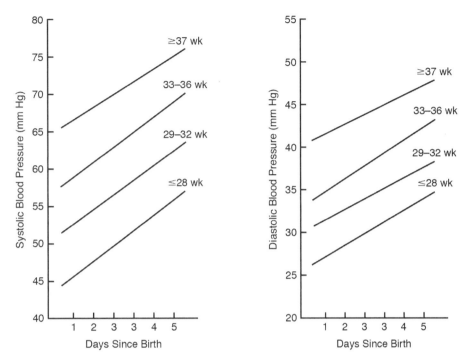

Figure 4.2. Blood Pressure for Babies of Different Gestational Ages During the First 5 Days After Birth

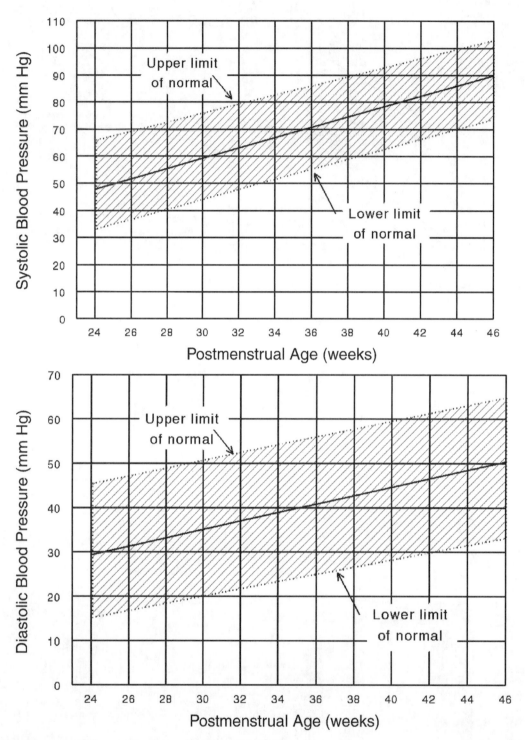

Figure 4.3. Blood Pressure for Babies of Different Postmenstrual Ages

During the first 5 days after birth, there is a predictable increase in blood pressure for babies of all birth weights and gestational ages. Figure 4.2 shows the increase in systolic and diastolic blood pressure during that time for babies of 4 different gestational age groups (≤ 28 weeks, 29–32 weeks, 33–36 weeks, and ≥ 37 weeks).

After 5 postnatal days, there is a much slower, but also predictable, increase in blood pressure for all babies.

Blood pressure for babies older than 5 days is closely related to postmenstrual age. Postmenstrual age is a baby's gestational age at birth, plus the number of weeks since birth. For example, a 2-week-old baby born at 32 weeks' gestational age has a postmenstrual age of 34 weeks. Figure 4.3 shows the reference (normal) range of systolic and diastolic pressures for babies of different postmenstrual ages.

5. What is the normal (reference) newborn blood volume range?

Babies have only about 90 mL of blood per kilogram of body weight (about 40 mL/lb).

Example: A 1,500-g (3 lb 5 oz) baby only has about 135 mL of blood.

   90 mL/kg $\times$ 1.5 kg = 135 mL (4.5 oz)

Example: A 7-lb (3,175-g) baby only has about 280 mL of blood.

   40 mL/lb $\times$ 7 lb = 280 mL (9.47 oz)

6. How much blood loss will cause shock?

If babies lose 25% or more of their blood volume, they will probably go into shock. *Shock* is a complex clinical syndrome involving inadequate perfusion of the body's vital organs, which is caused by an acute failure of circulatory function. When this occurs, inadequate amounts of oxygen and nutrient substrate are delivered to the body tissues, and removal of metabolic waste products is also inadequate.

Example: A baby is born weighing 2,000 g (4 lb 6½ oz).

- What is the baby's approximate blood volume? 90 mL/kg $\times$ 2 kg = 180 mL
- How much blood would this baby need to lose to go into shock?
  180 mL $\times$ 25% = 45 mL (about 3 Tbsp)

 Babies in shock require immediate treatment.

If this same baby is born to a woman with placenta previa or placental abruption, the woman may easily lose 1,000 mL of blood during delivery. If only 5% (50 mL) of this blood is the baby's, the baby most likely will go into shock.

Note: Babies also lose blood from blood sampling for laboratory tests. It is recommended to
- Take the minimum amount of blood required for the test(s).
- Keep a record of the amount withdrawn for each test and a tally of the total amount of blood withdrawn.

Self-test B

Now answer these questions to test yourself on the information in the last section. Refer to the graphs or charts in the unit, as necessary, to answer these questions.

B1. Of the following values, which value(s) is/are within normal limits for systolic blood pressure for a newborn with a birth weight of 3,000 g (6 lb 10 oz)? (Select all that apply.)
   A. 36 mm Hg
   B. 42 mm Hg
   C. 56 mm Hg
   D. 72 mm Hg

B2. A 2,100-g (4 lb 10 oz) baby is born at your hospital. The initial blood pressure is 60 mm Hg. How would this baby's blood pressure be described?
   A. Within normal range
   B. Hypertensive
   C. Hypotensive

B3. What is the normal blood volume range of a newborn?
   _____ mL/kg or _____ mL/lb

B4. What minimum blood loss would put a healthy 2,400-g (5 lb 4½ oz) baby into shock?
   A. 14 mL
   B. 54 mL
   C. 108 mL
   D. 216 mL

B5. Why is a baby at risk for low blood pressure if the mother loses a large volume of blood during delivery?
   _____
   _____

B6. What are the possible consequences of frequent sampling of blood for laboratory tests in babies?
   _____

B7. The normal diastolic blood pressure range for a 1-day-old, 1,750-g (3 lb 14 oz) baby is approximately _____ to _____ mm Hg. The normal systolic blood pressure range for the same baby is approximately _____ to _____ mm Hg.

Check your answers with the list that follows the Recommended Routines. Correct any incorrect answers and review the appropriate section in the unit.

7. What are the causes of hypotension in the newborn?

Hypovolemia is only one of many causes of low blood pressure. It is important to make every attempt to establish the cause of hypotension and treat it appropriately. For example, a baby may be hypotensive because of poor oxygenation, which will cause the heart to beat poorly and the blood vessels to dilate. Appropriate treatment would therefore be to administer oxygen or assist the baby's ventilation. The following causes of hypotension should be considered:

- Blood loss (hypovolemia)
- Poor oxygenation
- Severe acidosis
- Sepsis (blood infection)
- Poor cardiac output
- Severe central nervous system insult

Sick babies may be hypotensive from a combination of multiple factors. If not corrected, these factors may lead to a worsening cycle of acidosis and hypoxia.

8. What happens to babies with low blood pressure?

A baby's body will try to adjust so that vital organs receive adequate blood flow and oxygen from the available blood volume. As a result, the following complications may occur:

A. Inadequate oxygenation

Loss of blood volume also means a loss of red blood cells. Remaining red blood cells may not be able to carry sufficient oxygen to the brain and other vital organs. A baby may try to compensate for this by breathing fast. Babies may not, however, be able to take in enough oxygen to maintain adequate blood oxygen levels.

B. Poor perfusion leading to acidosis (low blood pH level)

Low blood pressure will result in the closing off or constriction of smaller blood vessels to less vital organs (skin, muscles) in an effort to preserve blood flow to more vital organs (brain, heart, lungs). Consequences of this restricted blood flow include

- *Increased production of lactic acid*: Restricted oxygen supply forces a less-efficient, more acid-producing form of metabolism to be used.
- *Reduced removal of lactic acid*: Restricted blood flow limits the amount of metabolic waste products that can be removed.

Lactic acid that accumulates in the tissues may result in lowering the pH level of the blood.

 In addition to the clinical appearance of rapid respirations, pale or mottled skin color, weak pulse, rapid heart rate, and slow capillary refill time, hypotensive babies are likely to be hypoxic and develop metabolic acidosis.

9. What do you do for babies with hypotension from blood loss (hypovolemia)?

As mentioned previously, babies may have low blood pressure from blood loss. If you suspect hypovolemia—particularly if there is a history of possible blood loss—treatment involves the administration of a blood volume expander to increase the baby's blood volume.

A. Check the baby's blood pressure to confirm it is low

If the blood pressure is low, consider leaving the deflated blood pressure cuff in place to be able to obtain more frequent measurements, or insert an indwelling arterial catheter (see Unit 3, Umbilical Catheters, in this book) if possible.

B. Choose an appropriate blood volume expander

An isotonic crystalloid solution (physiological [normal] saline [0.9% NaCl]) is recommended to improve blood volume in a symptomatic hypotensive, hypovolemic baby. If indicated, packed red blood cells may be administered. Theoretically, crossmatched whole blood is the best blood volume expander. Whole blood, however, is usually not immediately available and carries a higher risk than other volume expanders. **Do not wait. Ensure your center has a protocol in place for the quick administration of a blood volume expander.**

C. Administer 10 mL/kg (4 mL/lb) of blood volume expander intravenously
Although it is important to begin infusion of a blood volume expander immediately, the fluid should be administered *slowly and steadily*. Sudden shifts in blood volume place a baby at risk for an intraventricular hemorrhage (bleeding in the brain), particularly if the baby is significantly preterm. If blood is provided to a baby for any other reason (eg, anemia) in the presence of normal blood pressure, the rate of administration should be slower than the rate used for emergency blood volume expansion.

 Although acute hypotension from volume loss should be corrected relatively rapidly (steady intravenous infusion over 5–10 minutes), fluids administered for any reason other than emergency volume expansion should be delivered more slowly, especially in preterm babies.

D. Recheck the baby's blood pressure
- *If within normal range:* Continue checking the baby's blood pressure (every 10 minutes, and then at longer intervals) to ensure that it has stabilized.
- *If still low:* Consider administering another dose of volume expander and recheck the baby's blood pressure every 10 minutes until you achieve the desired response, and then recheck at longer intervals per your institution's policy. Discuss further interventions with the attending licensed independent practitioner if the blood pressure remains low without response to 2 rounds of volume expansion.

E. Investigate other possible causes of hypotension

10. What do you do for hypotensive babies if you do not suspect blood loss?

Always look for the cause of low blood pressure. (See Section 7, What are the causes of hypotension in the newborn?) In babies who have had significant perinatal compromise, the initial blood pressure reading may frequently be low because of severe hypoxia and acidosis. The most important treatment for these babies is to perform rapid and efficient resuscitative measures. These measures alone will usually restore a baby's blood pressure to the normal range. If they do not, medications, such as dopamine or dobutamine, may be required to increase cardiac output.

Babies with sepsis may also be hypotensive. If sepsis is suspected as the cause of low blood pressure, the baby's blood should be cultured, and antibiotics should be administered to the baby promptly.

Finally, babies with congenital heart disease, such as hypoplastic left heart syndrome or severe aortic stenosis, may also have low blood pressure. If such a condition is suspected, physicians from the nearest tertiary medical center should be contacted, and the baby should be urgently evaluated by a pediatric cardiologist. The baby may need to be treated with a prostaglandin E_1 infusion before and during transport to the tertiary hospital.

Self-test C

Now answer these questions to test yourself on the information in the last section.

C1. List the fluid(s) recommended as an emergency blood volume expander. _____

_____

C2. What is the recommended starting amount of volume expanders?

_____ mL/kg (_____ mL/lb)

C3. What is the recommended rate of administration of volume expanders? _____

_____

C4. How is low blood volume treated?

    A. Administer blood volume expander to increase blood volume.

    B. Administer caffeine to improve cardiac output.

    C. Administer epinephrine to increase the tone of the blood vessels.

C5. Physical examination and blood pressure measurement indicate that a baby is in shock. Blood loss is suspected. What should be done?

    A. Send blood for crossmatching and give blood as soon as it is available.

    B. Give physiological (normal) saline solution immediately.

C6. List 3 of the possible causes of hypotension in a baby.

_____

_____

_____

Check your answers with the list that follows the Recommended Routines. Correct any incorrect answers and review the appropriate section in the unit.

LOW BLOOD PRESSURE (HYPOTENSION)

Recommended Routines

All the routines listed below are based on the principles of perinatal care presented in the unit you have just finished. They are recommended as part of routine perinatal care.

Read each routine carefully and decide whether it is standard operating procedure in your hospital. Check the appropriate blank next to each routine.

Procedure Standard in My Hospital	Needs Discussion by Our Staff	Recommended Routine
_____	_____	1. Consider including blood pressure as a part of initial assessment for all newborns.
_____	_____	2. Require repeated blood pressure measurements for babies at risk for hypotension.
_____	_____	3. Be sure sterile physiological (normal) saline solution (0.9% NaCl) for intravenous use is always immediately available in each delivery room and nursery.
_____	_____	4. Check all blood pressure cuffs to ensure availability of appropriate-sized cuffs for newborns of all sizes.
_____	_____	5. Ensure a policy is in place for quick administration of blood volume expander.

Self-test Answers

These are the answers to the Self-test questions. Please check them with the answers you gave and review the information in the unit wherever necessary.

Self-test A

A1. False   *Reason:* In addition to the pumping action of the heart, blood pressure also depends on the tone of the blood vessels and volume of blood.

A2. True

A3. A and B

A4. Babies with suspected blood loss

Babies with signs of low blood pressure

Babies suspected of having heart disease

Babies born from multifetal pregnancies

All at-risk and sick babies

Note: A baby with fetal-maternal transfusion would fall into the "at-risk and sick" group of babies because such babies are likely to have signs similar to a donor fetus in fetal-fetal transfusion. After immediate treatment and stabilization of the baby, a Kleihauer-Betke (acid elution) test of the mother's blood might then be done to document or rule out fetal-maternal transfusion.

A5. Hypotension means low blood *pressure*, while hypovolemia means low blood *volume*.

A6. If a fetus-to-fetus transfusion develops in utero, it can cause *anemia* in the donor fetus and *polycythemia* in the recipient fetus.

Self-test B

B1. C and D

B2. A. Within normal range

B3. *90* mL/kg or *40* mL/lb

B4. B. *54* mL (2.4 kg × 90 mL/kg = 216 mL; 216 mL × 25% = 54 mL)

B5. If only a small fraction of the blood lost is the baby's blood, the baby can go into shock.

B6. Low blood volume and low blood pressure. A running total of the amount of blood withdrawn should be kept.

B7. The normal diastolic blood pressure range for a 1-day-old, 1,750-g (3 lb 14 oz) baby is approximately *16* to *48* mm Hg. The normal systolic blood pressure range for the same baby is approximately *36* to *68* mm Hg.

Self-test C

C1. Normal (physiological) saline solution; lactated Ringer injection also may be used.

C2. *10* mL/kg (*4* mL/lb)

C3. Over *5* to *10* minutes (volume expansion begun immediately, but fluid given slowly and steadily)

C4. A. Administer blood volume expander to increase blood volume.

C5. B. Give physiological (normal) saline solution immediately. (Start giving normal saline solution immediately, infusing steadily over 5–10 minutes. The baby should not be left in shock while waiting for blood to be crossmatched.)

C6. Any 3 of the following causes:

• Low blood volume or blood loss

• Poor oxygenation

• Severe acidosis

• Severe central nervous system insult

• Poor cardiac output

• Sepsis

Unit 4 Posttest

After completion of each unit there is a free online posttest available at www.cmevillage.com to test your understanding. Navigate to the PCEP pages on www.cmevillage.com and register to take the free posttests.

Once registered on the website and after completing all the unit posttests, pay the book exam fee ($15) and pass the test at 80% or greater to earn continuing education credits. Only start the PCEP book exam if you have time to complete it. If you take the book exam and are not connected to a printer, either print your certificate to a .pdf file and save it to print later or come back to www.cmevillage.com at any time and print a copy of your educational transcript.

Credits are only available by book, not by individual unit within the books. Available credits for completion of each book exam are as follows: Book 1: 14.5 credits; Book 2: 16 credits; Book 3: 17 credits; Book 4: 9 credits.

For more details, navigate to the PCEP webpages at www.cmevillage.com.

SKILL UNIT

Measuring Blood Pressure

This skill unit will teach you how to take oscillometric and palpation blood pressure measurements on a baby.

Study this skill unit; then attend a skill practice and demonstration session.

To master the skill, you will need to demonstrate each of the following steps correctly. At least one of the blood pressure measurement techniques needs to be demonstrated on 3 different babies.

Oscillometric Blood Pressure Measurement
1. Select cuff. Two different criteria for cuff size have been proposed. Either should result in approximately equal results.
   a. Cuff that is 75% or greater of the limb circumference, and the cuff length should be at least two-thirds of the length of the upper limb.
   b. A bladder width that measures approximately 40% of the upper arm circumference.

Note that these recommendations are referring to the inflatable bladder and not to the fabric that may be used to encase the bladder.

2. Set monitor to appropriate mode: manual mode or automatic with determined cycle time.
3. Position cuff around baby's arm or leg.
4. Activate operation of the machine or oscillometric blood pressure mode on the cardiac monitor.
5. Record baby's systolic, diastolic, and mean blood pressure.
6. Set alarm limits for a specific baby (when automatic mode used), as appropriate.
   Note: Automatic mode will not be used for all babies. It is most useful for babies who require frequent blood pressure measurements. You will need to know how to obtain oscillometric measurements in manual and automatic mode.

Palpation Blood Pressure Measurement
1. Select cuff.
2. Wrap cuff around the baby's arm or leg.
3. Connect gauge to cuff; check to see the gauge reads zero.
4. Palpate artery; inflate cuff.
5. Release cuff pressure at an appropriate rate.
6. Determine when arterial pulsation first occurs (this is the systolic reading); deflate cuff.
7. Record palpation blood pressure. A diastolic pressure reading cannot be measured when obtaining a manual blood pressure by palpation.

Measuring Blood Pressure

ACTIONS	REMARKS

Deciding to Take a Baby's Blood Pressure

1. Ask yourself, "Is there a reason why this baby's blood pressure might be low?" • Is/was there a cause for blood loss? • Was the baby born from a high-risk pregnancy? • Is the baby sick for any reason, such as perinatal compromise, acidosis, suspected sepsis, or other illness? • Does the baby have signs of shock? • Is a cardiac abnormality suspected? • Was the baby born from a multifetal pregnancy (eg, twin, triplet)? Yes: Take blood pressure as soon as possible. (This may be done in the delivery room.) No: Blood pressure measurement may be taken as a part of routine vital signs.	Neonatal blood loss can occur with • Umbilical cord tear • Incomplete clamping of umbilical cord • Placenta previa or placental abruption • Accidental cutting of the placenta during cesarean delivery • Trauma to the baby with internal bleeding • Accumulation of blood in the placenta secondary to cord compression Babies who are hypotensive (in shock) typically have • Rapid respirations • Rapid heart rate • Weak pulses • Pale or mottled appearance • Slow capillary refill time

Preparing to Obtain an Oscillometric Blood Pressure

2. Collect the appropriate equipment. • Oscillometric blood pressure machine or appropriate cable for the cardiac monitor. • If using a separate machine, plug the monitor into a grounded outlet and turn on the power. • Appropriate-sized blood pressure cuff. Cuffs may be sized according to the baby's weight; follow manufacturer's guidelines for selecting size.	Proper operation of an oscillometric device or the peripheral blood pressure mode on a cardiac monitor is specific to each brand of equipment. Detailed knowledge of equipment used in your hospital is essential. Cuffs are usually disposable and should be used once and then discarded or kept at the baby's bedside and used only for that baby. Size of the cuff is important. A cuff that is too large or too small will give inaccurate readings. (See Preparing to Take a Baby's Blood Pressure by Palpation, step 3.)

ACTIONS   REMARKS

Deciding Which Mode of Operation to Use

3. Ask yourself

- Is the baby's condition unstable, requiring frequent blood pressure measurements?

- Is the baby's blood pressure being taken as a part of routine vital signs?

If frequent measurements are needed, select the automatic mode. This means the monitor will automatically reinflate the blood pressure cuff and obtain a new measurement once every cycle period. Some monitors have preset cycle periods. For other monitors, you program the specific cycle time you want.

If blood pressure measurements are needed infrequently, select the manual mode. This means the monitor will measure the baby's blood pressure only when you activate it.

4. If the automatic mode is selected, determine the cycle period to be used.

Generally, an automatic cycle time of 3 minutes or less does not provide sufficient deflation time to allow adequate circulation to the extremity between cuff inflations.

Rotate cuff location.

When the cuff is inflated repeatedly on an arm or leg, over an extended period, the baby's extremity can be bruised, especially if the baby is significantly preterm.

Cycle periods of 5 to 10 minutes are usually appropriate for unstable babies. However, be sure to change cuff location periodically.

Obtaining an Oscillometric Blood Pressure Measurement

5. Wrap the cuff around the baby's extremity so it fits snugly but does not constrict blood flow.

   Some cuffs are designed to be positioned in a particular way.

The baby's upper arm or calf may be used. The arm is preferred unless you are evaluating for coarctation of the aorta, when upper and lower extremities are measured.

For example, an arrow may indicate the point that should be positioned over the artery.

6. Connect the blood pressure cuff to the machine or cardiac monitor channel and begin operation.

7. Read blood pressure values off the monitor. Systolic, diastolic, and mean arterial values are measured.

For example, if a baby's blood pressure is registered as 64 systolic, 40 diastolic, with a mean arterial pressure (MAP) of 52, record this as

64/40 mm Hg, MAP 52 mm Hg

Note: This is sometimes written as 64/40 (52) mm Hg

8. Set the upper and lower alarm limits 10 mm Hg higher and 10 mm Hg lower than the baby's initial systolic blood pressure reading. If a baby is hypotensive, re-adjust alarm limits as blood pressure is corrected.

181

ACTIONS	REMARKS

What Can Go Wrong?

1. The monitor is out of calibration and does not give accurate values.	Follow the manufacturer's recommendations regarding calibration and maintenance. Any time you are in doubt about values given by the monitor, double-check your findings with another monitor or a palpation blood pressure measurement. Remember, palpation gives a single value that is slightly lower than the baby's systolic pressure.
2. The baby wiggles while you are taking blood pressure. The values given are inaccurate or the machine does not register any blood pressure.	The baby needs to be quiet and still while the cuff is inflated and measurements are taken, or the extremity needs to be held still during this time.
3. Circulation in the baby's extremity is compromised or the skin is bruised.	Be sure the time between automatic cycles is 5 minutes or longer. Observe the baby's extremity for signs of circulatory compromise. Rotate location of cuff placement.
4. The monitor gives a blood pressure reading, but the simultaneous heart rate it records is significantly different than the baby's heart rate.	This almost surely is not an accurate blood pressure measurement. Take blood pressure again. If the baby is crying, calm the baby before rechecking the measurement.

ACTIONS   **REMARKS**

Preparing to Take a Baby's Blood Pressure by Palpation

1. Does the baby need a blood pressure measurement?

    See the beginning of this skill (oscillometric section).

2. Collect the proper equipment.

    • A standard mercury or aneroid manometer (blood pressure gauge) with bulb inflator

    • Appropriate-sized blood pressure cuff

    Blood pressure gauge, inflator, and cuff are the only items needed.

    The inflatable part of the cuff, called the *bladder,* should be long enough to wrap at least three-fourths of the way around the baby's arm or leg.

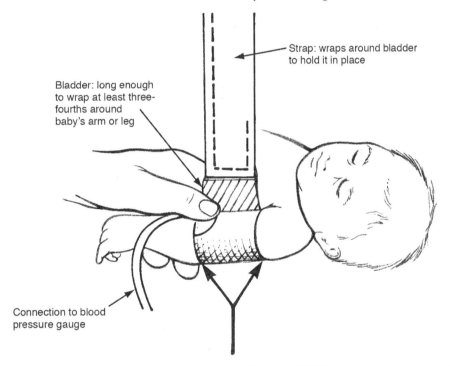

Strap: wraps around bladder to hold it in place

Bladder: long enough to wrap at least three-fourths around baby's arm or leg

Connection to blood pressure gauge

3. Do you have the correctly sized cuff?

    Yes: Go ahead with taking blood pressure.

    No: Get the correctly sized cuff.

    Cuffs with bladders that are too small (especially if it does not wrap at least three-fourths of the way around baby's arm or leg) may give extremely inaccurate readings, which are usually much higher than the true blood pressure. Cuffs with bladders that are too large will often give inaccurate low readings.

4. Wrap the blood pressure cuff around the baby's upper arm or thigh.

    The cuff should be neither loose nor tight. A too-tight cuff will give a falsely low blood pressure reading because it will restrict blood flow.

5. Connect the cuff to the blood pressure gauge.

6. Check to see that the gauge reads zero.

    If the gauge does not read zero, adjust it or get a different gauge.

183

ACTIONS   REMARKS

Obtaining a Palpation Blood Pressure Measurement

7. Hold the baby's arm straight, with
the palm and inner part of the arm
facing you.

8. Using your index finger of this same
hand, feel for the pulse in the baby's brachial artery.

9. When you feel the pulse well, keep your
index finger lightly pressed over this spot.

10. Using your other hand, pump up the cuff
until the mercury or needle reads approximately 100 mm Hg. You will no longer
be able to feel the pulse.

You can usually palpate the artery (feel the
pulse) just above the crease of the elbow and
slightly toward the inside of the arm.

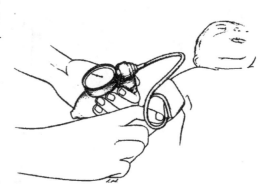

11. Release the screw clamp, let the mercury
or needle fall fairly quickly until it
reaches about 80 mm Hg, and then
slow the rate of fall to approximately
2 mm Hg per second.

12. Watch the top of the mercury column or
needle as it drops. Note the reading on
the blood pressure gauge when you first
begin to feel the artery pulsate beneath
your index finger.

13. After the arterial pulsation has been felt,
the cuff may be rapidly deflated.

14. Record the blood pressure reading and
the method used.

*It is important that the mercury or needle
falls slowly. If allowed to fall too quickly,
the blood pressure reading will be
falsely low.*

The blood pressure reading when you first
feel the baby's pulse is slightly less than the
systolic blood pressure.

For example, if the arterial pulsation was
first felt at 48 mm Hg, the blood pressure
reading may be abbreviated and recorded as
48 mm Hg/palpation (or 48 mm Hg/P).

ACTIONS	REMARKS

What Can Go Wrong

1. You press your index finger too firmly over the brachial artery.	You will restrict the blood flow through the artery and get a falsely low blood pressure reading.
2. You are not certain when you first feel the pulse.	A very sick baby may have a weak pulse, making it difficult to obtain an accurate palpation blood pressure reading.
3. You may perform the blood pressure measurement correctly but not take blood pressure often enough.	A sick and unstable baby needs frequent blood pressure determinations. One reading within reference range does not mean the baby's blood pressure will stay within the reference range.
4. The strap may be wrapped too tightly or the cuff may be left inflated.	This may restrict blood flow to the baby's limb for a long time and cause tissue damage.
5. The bladder of the cuff is too small.	Readings will be falsely high.
6. The bladder of the cuff is too large.	Readings will be falsely low.
7. You may release the pressure in the cuff too fast.	Readings will be falsely low.

Unit 5: Intravenous Therapy

Objectives

In this unit you will learn

A. The purpose of intravenous therapy

B. Routes and types of fluid therapy

C. What fluid losses within and outside of reference range may occur in a baby

D. How to tell if a baby is getting too much or too little fluid

E. When to stop an intravenous infusion

Note: In this unit you will *not* learn fluid management for complex situations (eg, a severely compromised baby, an extremely preterm baby, a baby requiring parenteral nutrition).

In any situation in which fluid management seems to be a problem, further consultation should be obtained.

Unit 5 Pretest

Before reading the unit, please answer the following questions. Select the *one best* answer to each question (unless otherwise instructed). Record your answers on the test and check them with the answers at the end of the book.

1. Which of the following babies should receive intravenous (IV) therapy?

   Yes   **No**

   ____   ____   A 1,590-g (3 lb 8 oz), vigorous baby on the first day after birth

   ____   ____   A 3,175-g (7 lb) baby with Apgar scores of 6 at 1 minute and 9 at 5 minutes

   ____   ____   A 3,620-g (8 lb) baby with suspected sepsis who has ingested 120 mL (4 oz) of formula during the past 24 hours

   ____   ____   A 2,720-g (6 lb), vigorous baby whose mother was hospitalized with bacterial pneumonia at 20 weeks of gestation

2. An umbilical venous catheter is appropriately inserted when a baby weighing 1,900 g (4 lb 3 oz) needs
   A. Frequent blood gas determinations
   B. An exchange transfusion
   C. 10 days of IV antibiotics
   D. IV fluids to supplement oral intake

3. Which IV fluid should be used during the first 24 hours after birth for a baby with no specific complications?
   A. 10% dextrose in water with 10% sodium bicarbonate added
   B. Lactated Ringer injection
   C. 10% dextrose in ¼ normal physiological (normal) saline with 20 mEq of potassium chloride (KCl) added to each 1,000 mL
   D. 10% dextrose in water

4. How much fluid does a term baby need after the first 48 hours of postnatal age?
   A. 80 mL/kg per 24 hours
   B. 100 mL/kg per 24 hours
   C. 120 mL/kg per 24 hours
   D. 180 mL/kg per 24 hours

5. **True**   **False**   At 2 days of age, a baby's sodium level is 150 mEq/L. This may indicate that the baby is receiving too much fluid.

6. A baby who is designated to receive nothing by mouth has been receiving IV therapy for 4 days. Which test(s) should this baby routinely receive?
   A. Blood electrolyte values
   B. Hemoglobin and hematocrit values
   C. Complete blood cell count
   D. Serum bilirubin level

(*continued*)

Unit 5 Pretest (*continued*)

7. A 6-day-old, 2,500-g (5 lb 8 oz) baby is receiving the targeted amount of IV and/or oral fluid. How much would you expect the baby's daily urine output to be?
   A. 40 mL
   B. 100 mL
   C. 140 mL
   D. 200 mL

8. Approximately how much IV fluid should a 2,700-g (5 lb 15 oz) baby receive during the third day after birth?
   A. 225 mL per 24 hours
   B. 275 mL per 24 hours
   C. 325 mL per 24 hours
   D. 375 mL per 24 hours

1. What is intravenous therapy?

Intravenous (IV) therapy means fluid, blood, or medication given through a needle or catheter that has been inserted into a vein.

2. What is the purpose of intravenous therapy?

IV therapy has several purposes, including

- Replacing or maintaining body stores of water and electrolytes
- Replenishing blood volume
- Administering medication
- Providing calories, in the form of glucose (calories in the form of protein and fat can also be delivered intravenously but are not discussed in this unit)

3. Which babies should receive intravenous fluids?

- All sick babies
- Babies with low blood glucose levels
- All babies who are designated to receive nothing by mouth or who cannot ingest an adequate amount of fluid via nipple or tube feedings
- Infants weighing less than 1,800 g (<4 lb) at birth

4. What routes are used for intravascular infusion in babies?

Different intravascular routes are used for different purposes.

- *Umbilical artery*
  - Used for arterial blood gas sampling or direct blood pressure monitoring.
  - May be used to withdraw blood during exchange transfusion.
  - Not used for blood, medications, or fluids unless another IV route is not available (and only on rare occasions; some institutions do not allow any infusions other than fluid, to keep the vessel open—check your institution's guidelines).
- *Umbilical vein*
  - Used for exchange transfusion, emergency medications, or fluids during the first few days after birth (usually up to 7 days) in preterm babies or babies who are small for gestational age.
  - May be used for IV fluids or parenteral nutrition.
  - Depending on the catheter placement within the umbilical vein (low lying or central), a higher concentration of glucose can be used. This may be useful in babies with refractory hypoglycemia or to optimize parenteral nutrition in preterm or growth-restricted infants.
- *Peripheral vein* (hand, foot, or scalp vein)
  - Used for maintenance fluids, medications, or blood transfusion.
- *Peripherally inserted or surgically placed central venous catheter*
  - Used for long-term maintenance fluids and parenteral nutrition in extremely preterm babies or babies with long-term nutritional needs.
  - These central venous lines are not covered in the Perinatal Continuing Education Program (PCEP) books.

Self-test A

Now answer these questions to test yourself on the information in the last section.

A1. Which of these babies should receive intravenous (IV) therapy? (Select all that apply.)

   A. A baby weighing 3,175 g (7 lb) with sepsis and unstable heart rate

   B. A baby weighing 3,620 g (8 lb) who is ingesting 30 mL of formula per day

   C. A baby weighing 1,500 g (3 lb 5 oz) on the first day after birth

A2. Describe the IV route you would use for these purposes.

   A. Administer blood to the baby with vital signs within reference range:_____

   B. Draw blood for blood gas analysis:_____

   C. Administer emergency medications during resuscitation:_____

   D. Administer antibiotics:_____

   E. Perform an exchange transfusion:_____

A3. Name 4 reasons why you might use IV therapy for a baby.

   _____

   _____

   _____

   _____

A4. A 2-hour-old baby weighing 1,800 g (4 lb) develops hypoglycemic seizures and is given a bolus of 10% dextrose in water by umbilical vein. What would you do next for this baby?

   _____

   _____

Check your answers with the list that follows the Recommended Routines. Correct any incorrect answers and review the appropriate section in the unit.

---

5. How does a baby lose fluid?

A. Losses within reference range

   A baby typically loses fluid from the *skin and respiratory passages*. This is called *insensible water loss*. In term babies, insensible loss usually amounts to about 35 to 40 mL/kg/d. Insensible water losses may be higher in preterm babies, especially extremely-low-birthweight babies.

   The remainder of a baby's typical fluid loss is in feces and urine.

B. Losses outside of reference range
   - Vomiting
   - Diarrhea
   - Bleeding
   - Excessive urine output
   - Frequent blood sampling
   - Increased insensible loss
     — *Phototherapy:* May increase insensible loss by as much as 40%.
     — *Radiant warmer:* May increase insensible loss by as much as 100%.
     — *Extremely preterm babies:* Insensible loss may increase by as much as 100% because of respiratory losses and losses through immature skin.

6. Which intravenous solutions are used for babies?

For simplicity of computation, electrolyte requirements are presented in this unit in terms of electrolyte *concentration* in the IV fluid (eg, ¼ physiological [normal] saline solution). Recommendations will result in delivery of the appropriate amount of electrolytes to babies with kidney and heart function within reference range. Babies with impaired kidney or cardiac function present complex management problems and require frequent adjustment of their IV electrolyte solutions.

While receiving IV therapy, a baby's blood electrolyte and glucose levels need to be checked. The composition of IV fluid is readjusted if values are not within reference ranges.

The following IV solutions are suggestions for short-term maintenance therapy. Individualized therapy is needed for babies that require long-term or complex management.

A. During the first 24 hours after birth
- Ten percent dextrose in water (D10W) for most babies.
- Some babies will require concentrations of dextrose higher or lower than 10%. Infants born to diabetic mothers (and requiring IV therapy) may benefit from calcium added to their electrolyte solution. However, caution should be used when administering calcium-containing solutions through a peripheral IV, because clinically significant tissue damage from extravasation of the fluid can occur.

B. After 24 hours of postnatal life
Ten percent dextrose in water (or other appropriate concentration of dextrose) in ¼ normal saline solution (which contains 38 mEq/L NaCl) with 20 mEq of potassium (as potassium chloride) per 1,000 mL of fluid. (This preparation is commercially available.)

C. Unusual circumstances
- *Sick babies:* These babies may need other solutions, such as blood or fluids with a higher or lower electrolyte concentration. Long-term fluid management may become complex and is not covered in the PCEP books.
- *Babies with low blood glucose levels* (see Book 1: Maternal and Fetal Evaluation and Immediate Newborn Care, Unit 8, Hypoglycemia): These babies may require more glucose than is supplied in D10W. Solutions of D12.5W, D15W, or even D20W are sometimes needed. However, if concentrations of glucose higher than D12.5 are needed, this solution will need to run through a centrally located catheter (ie, peripherally inserted central catheter, umbilical venous catheter).

  A dextrose delivery (ie, glucose infusion rate) of 4 to 6 mg/kg/min during the first few days after birth is usually required to achieve a blood glucose level of 45 to 80 mg/dL. However, some babies, such as babies of diabetic mothers, may require up to 12 to 14 mg/kg/min to achieve an acceptable blood glucose level. Dextrose delivery rate (DDR) can be calculated as follows:

  $$DDR = \frac{\% \text{ dextrose} \times \text{rate}}{6 \times \text{weight in kg}}$$

  or

  $$\text{Desired IV rate} = \frac{DDR \times 6 \times \text{weight in kg}}{\% \text{ dextrose}}$$

Examples

A 3,500-g (7 lb 11 oz) baby receiving D10W at 12 mL/kg/h would have a DDR of 5.7 mg/kg/min

or

To receive a DDR of 5 mg/kg/min by using D10W, a 3,500-g (7 lb 11 oz) baby receiving D10W would require an IV rate of 10.5 mL/h.

- *Extremely preterm babies:* Blood glucose levels should be closely monitored, and the dextrose concentration should be adjusted accordingly. In general, the goal should be to avoid a DDR or glucose infusion rate of less than 4 mg/kg/min. Fluids containing fat and protein will also be needed, but fluid therapy and nutrition for tiny babies are not covered in the PCEP books.

7. How much fluid does a baby need?

A. Preterm (see Section 7C, Extremely preterm babies), term, and post-term babies
- *During the first 24 hours after birth*: 80 mL/kg/24 h. During the first postnatal day, babies need less fluid than they do later in life. Over the next 2 days, fluid requirements gradually increase.
- *From 24 to 48 hours after birth*: 100 mL/kg/24 h
- *More than 48 hours after birth*: 120 mL/kg/24 h

Frequently, an at-risk baby may be able to manage nipple or tube feedings but may not ingest a sufficient amount to provide the volume of fluid the baby needs for a 24-hour period. The additional fluid the baby requires may be supplied via a peripheral IV.

B. Babies after resuscitation

Newborns who had low Apgar scores or required prolonged resuscitation may not have kidney or heart function within reference range. Fluids may need to be restricted to as little as 35 to 40 mL/kg/d (insensible losses) for term babies or somewhat higher for preterm babies.

C. Extremely preterm babies
- *During the first 24 hours after birth*, extremely preterm babies need more fluid. This is because of their proportionately larger surface area compared with their body weight, as well as the lack of keratinization of their skin, which results in greater insensible water losses through the skin. These babies should receive 100 mL of fluid or more for each kilogram (2 lb 3 oz) of body weight during the first 24 hours after birth (100 mL/kg/24 h).
- *After 24 hours of postnatal life*, fluid management for extremely preterm babies becomes very complex. Insensible water losses are variable and unpredictable. Complications such as patent ductus arteriosus, intraventricular hemorrhage, hyperglycemia, and electrolyte imbalance become much more likely. These conditions mandate special considerations for fluid management, which are not discussed in this program. Consult regional perinatal center staff.

Example: You are caring for a 3-day-old, 3,100-g (6 lb 13½ oz) term baby who is being evaluated for neurological depression.

1. How much fluid does the baby need per day?
- The baby needs 120 mL of fluid per kilogram of body weight per day.
- Therefore, 120 mL × 3.1 kg = 372 mL of fluid needed per day.

2. You find the baby will ingest only 30 mL every 3 hours by nipple. How much fluid is the baby getting by nipple per day?
   - $24 \div 3 = 8$ feedings per 24-hour period
   - 8 feedings $\times$ 30 mL = 240 mL per day by nipple

3. You should give the baby more fluids via IV. How much IV fluid does the baby need?
   372 mL needed per day $-$ 240 mL received via feedings = 132 mL needed via IV per day

4. What rate of flow per hour should you use to give the baby 132 mL in 24 hours?
   132 mL $\div$ 24 hours = 5.5 mL/h

Self-test B

Now answer these questions to test yourself on the information in the last section.

B1. What special action will you probably need to take for babies who are placed under radiant warmers or phototherapy lights?

_____

B2. When is 5% dextrose in water (D5W) or D10W (without saline or potassium chloride) usually used as the intravenous (IV) fluid for babies?

_____

B3. A newborn baby weighs 3,000 g (6 lb 10 oz). How much fluid does the baby need during the first 24 hours after birth?

_____

B4. How much fluid should a 2,500-g (5 lb 8 oz) baby take in each 24 hours after the first 48 hours of postnatal life?

_____

B5. The baby in question B4 ingests 150 mL/24 h by bottle feedings. How much IV fluid should the baby receive to supplement liquids received from feedings?

_____

B6. What is insensible water loss?

_____

B7. You are caring for a 3-day-old neonate who is being treated with antibiotics for suspected sepsis. The baby weighs 2,600 g (5 lb 12 oz). The baby is vigorous but ingests only 20 mL of formula every 3 hours. How much fluid should the baby be given intravenously?

_____ mL per day

_____ mL per hour

B8. Most babies who have experienced severe perinatal compromise will require _____ fluids during the first few days after birth.
   - **A.** Increased
   - **B.** Decreased

Check your answers with the list that follows the Recommended Routines. Correct any incorrect answers and review the appropriate section in the unit.

8. How do you know if a baby is getting too much or too little fluid?

A. Day-to-day changes in body weight

- *With the exception of some post-term babies or babies that are small for gestational age, babies typically lose weight during the first few days after birth.* After that, reference daily weight gain is approximately 20 to 30 g (0.7–1.0 oz) per day. (See Unit 6, Feeding, in this book for details on caloric requirements and expected weight gain.)

  Obtaining daily weights is not always practical with sick babies. If it is possible to weigh the baby, the most accurate weights are obtained when a baby is weighed on the same scale at the same time of day, before a feeding. It is also important to note if any equipment is weighed with the baby.

- *Excessive weight gain* may mean a baby is receiving more fluid than necessary, a baby's kidneys are not making urine as well as they should, or a baby is in congestive heart failure.

- *Excessive weight loss* may be due to an inadequate fluid or calorie intake, the kidneys making too much urine, or a baby losing extra fluid by some other route.

B. Volume of urine output

- *Reference volume of urine output* in a 24-hour period is approximately 40 mL/kg of body weight (1–2 mL/kg/h).

  1. Urine output may be estimated by weight
     - The dry weight of a diaper is calculated. (If commercial disposable diapers are used, an average dry weight may be determined, rather than weighing each separate diaper.)
     - After a baby voids, the wet diaper is weighed, and the difference between the dry and wet weight in grams is determined. This difference is a close estimate of the number of milliliters of urine voided by the baby.
     - If a baby is placed under a radiant warmer, it is important to weigh diapers frequently because urine in a diaper will evaporate quickly under a radiant warmer.

  2. Urine may be collected to measure output

     In cases of urinary retention or when it is critical to measure exact urine output, an indwelling urinary catheter may be placed by an experienced provider. This risk of infection with catheter placement and its prolonged usage must be balanced with the need to document exact urine output or treat urinary retention. In such situations, an ultrasound bladder scanner could help determine whether or not the bladder contains urine. Consider consulting your regional center.

     Although challenging to effect adequate securement and prevent leakage, a commercially available plastic bag placed over the baby's genitalia, with the edges sealed with adhesive, may be used to collect urine. To avoid frequent removal and reapplication of the bag and adhesive, a feeding tube may be inserted into the bag through a tiny slit. The tube is sealed in the insertion slit with plastic tape to prevent leaks around the tube. A syringe is attached to the feeding tube, and urine is aspirated from the bag for measurement and/or analysis.

- *Decrease in urine output* may occur when there is inadequate fluid intake or the kidneys are damaged and unable to make urine normally, especially after an episode of severe hypoxia. Babies with heart disease may have low urine output and retain fluid, as reflected by excessive weight gain.

- *Increase in urine output* may occur when a baby is getting too much fluid or the kidneys are damaged and unable to conserve fluid appropriately.

Self-test C

Now answer these questions to test yourself on the information in the last section.

C1. What is the expected weight gain per 24 hours of a baby who is appropriate size for gestational age, weighing 3,000 g (6 lb 10 oz) at 5 days of age?

_____
_____

C2. What is the expected urine output of a baby weighing 2,000 g (4 lb 6½ oz)?

_____ mL/24 h

_____ mL/h

C3. A baby is receiving intravenous therapy. What would you do to obtain the baby's daily weight?

Yes	No	
____	____	Obtain the baby's weight at the same time each day.
____	____	Remove all equipment attached to the baby.
____	____	Use the same scale for every weight.
____	____	Weigh the baby before a feeding.
____	____	Weigh the baby immediately after a feeding.

C4. What are 2 methods of measuring urine output?

_____
_____

C5. A 2,500-g (5 lb 8 oz) baby's daily urine output is 40 mL.

Is this in the reference range? ___ Yes ___ No

If not, what could have caused this?

_____

C6. A 2,000-g (4 lb 6½ oz) baby born at 35 weeks of gestation who is an appropriate size for gestational age gains 120 g (4 oz) in 24 hours. Is this the same, larger, or smaller than the expected weight gain?

_____

Check your answers with the list that follows the Recommended Routines. Correct any incorrect answers and review the appropriate section in the unit.

9. When are intravenous infusions stopped and restarted?

A. Infiltration of intravenous fluid into subcutaneous tissues
IV infiltration is detected by

- *Increase in the pressure registered by the IV pump:* Many IV pumps indicate the pressure required to infuse an IV solution. If the pump indicates a specific pressure, it should be recorded whenever a new IV is started and checked every hour throughout infusion. Whenever an increase in pressure is noted or a warning alarm of occlusion is activated, the IV site should be investigated carefully because an infusion pressure increase is often the first sign of an infiltration.

- *Puffiness around the insertion site:* When puffiness or swelling is present, un-tape and remove the IV catheter. Insert a new IV in a different site.

- *Fluid not pushed easily through the IV:* To check this, gently flush the IV catheter with IV fluid or normal saline. If this fluid flushes easily, with no sign of swelling, the IV almost surely is not infiltrated. Assess the administration set (IV tubing) for closed clamps or tubing kinks.

- *No blood return in the IV needle tubing when it is disconnected from the rest of the IV tubing:* A brisk, definite blood return is a good indication that the IV has not infiltrated. However, blood return is not an entirely reliable indicator. Occasionally, a non-infiltrated IV will not have a blood return, and sometimes a delayed or minimal blood return occurs with an infiltrated IV.
- *Persistent fussiness or irritability of the baby:* This may happen when the infiltrated skin is painful.

B. Thrombophlebitis and intravenous infiltration
Thrombophlebitis is detected by

- *Warmth over the insertion site*
- *Redness along the vein*
- *Tenderness around the insertion site*

The baby may become fussy and irritable or cry when the area near the IV is touched.

Thrombophlebitis is an inflammation of a vein associated with the formation of a clot, or thrombus, within the vein. Thrombophlebitis occurs much less often in babies than it does in adults. This is because peripheral IVs generally infiltrate more easily and more often in babies before thrombophlebitis has time to develop. If thrombophlebitis develops, treatment is to remove the IV catheter and insert another at a different site.

Some medications may cause severe tissue damage, despite prompt removal of an infiltrated IV catheter. In such cases, treatment with medication at the infiltration site (eg, hyaluronidase) or consultation by a plastic surgeon or wound care team may be warranted. If not addressed promptly or treated properly, IV infiltrates may result in infection, scarring, and even loss of mobility at the site. Follow your institution's policies on extravasation prior to removing the IV catheter.

 It is important to detect thrombophlebitis or infiltration early and discontinue intravenous (IV) infusion through that insertion site without delay.

Some medications and IV solutions are extremely irritating and may cause severe tissue damage if an infiltrated IV catheter is not removed immediately.

10. When are intravenous infusions discontinued?

When a baby meets all of the following requirements, infusion of IV fluid may be stopped:

- There is adequate intake of calories and fluid via nipple or tube feedings.
- The baby has recovered from an illness and is stable.
- IV infusion is no longer needed for glucose or medication administration.

11. What is an intravenous lock?

Occasionally, medically stable babies who are managing full feedings will continue to require IV medications (most commonly, antibiotics). These may be given through an IV lock. An IV lock does not require a continuous infusion of IV fluid. The catheter should be connected to a T-connecter and then a needleless access device, which can be accessed with a syringe of either normal saline or a dilute solution of heparin (0.25–0.5 U/mL). Heparin solutions are available in several concentrations, so it is good practice to standardize the type used in your hospital. Before each infusion of medication, assess for patency by flushing the IV with normal saline. After each medication administration, the IV should be flushed with normal saline to clear the dead space of the IV tubing (generally recommended flush volume is 0.5–1.0 mL). Additionally, the IV should be flushed periodically (every 4–6 hours) to assess for patency. Between uses, the IV lock should be clamped off to prevent blood from backing up into the catheter. Despite these precautions, sometimes a clot will develop in the tip of the catheter.

- If there is a clot in the tip, do not flush solution through the IV lock, because the clot could be dislodged and released into the baby's bloodstream.
- If the IV has become infiltrated, do not force fluid through the IV lock, because this would put the solution or medication into the baby's subcutaneous tissues.

If the IV lock cannot be flushed *easily*, do not force fluid through it. Remove the catheter and insert a new IV catheter in a different site.

12. What facts about intravenous therapy are important to remember?

1. Consider using IV fluids for babies weighing less than 1,800 g (<4 lb).

2. Obtain consultation for fluid management of babies with severe perinatal compromise and extremely preterm babies.

3. Usual IV solutions (except for extremely preterm babies) include the following:
   - *During the first 24 hours:* D10W
   - *After the first 24 hours:* D10W with ¼ normal saline solution and 20 mEq potassium chloride (KCl) per liter

   Adjust the IV dextrose concentration higher or lower than D10W according to a baby's blood glucose level.

4. Daily fluid requirements
   - *During the first 24 hours:* 80 mL/kg/24 h.
   - *After the first 24 hours:* Gradually increase to 120 mL/kg/24 h by 72 hours.
   - *Extremely preterm babies (younger than 28 weeks' gestational age) during the first 24 hours:* 100 mL (or more)/kg/24 h.

5. Daily reference weight gain (4–6 days or more after birth)
   About 20 to 30 g/d

6. Daily reference urine output
   About 40 mL/kg/24 h or 1 to 2 mL/kg/h

7. Reference insensible water loss
   About 35 to 40 mL/kg/24 h (increase dramatically when a baby is placed under phototherapy lights or a radiant warmer or is extremely preterm)

Self-test D

Now answer these questions to test yourself on the information in the last section.

D1. How can you determine whether an intravenous (IV) line is infiltrated?

_____
_____
_____

D2. When does a baby no longer need an IV infusion?

_____
_____
_____

D3. A baby receiving IV fluids begins to fuss and cry, and nothing you do will soothe the baby. What might be the cause of the baby's crying?

_____

Check your answers with the list that follows the Recommended Routines. Correct any incorrect answers and review the appropriate section in the unit.

INTRAVENOUS THERAPY
Recommended Routines

All the routines listed below are based on the principles of perinatal care presented in the unit you have just finished. They are recommended as part of routine perinatal care.

Read each routine carefully and decide whether it is standard operating procedure in your hospital. Check the appropriate blank next to each routine.

Procedure Standard in My Hospital	Needs Discussion by Our Staff	Recommended Routine
_____	_____	1. Arrange staffing patterns to ensure constant availability of personnel with the capability of starting and monitoring a peripheral intravenous (IV) line in a baby.
_____	_____	2a. Establish a policy of delivering IV fluids to all babies who • Are sick • Have inadequate intake from nipple or tube feedings
_____	_____	2b. Consider starting IV fluids in babies weighing less than 1,800 g (<4 lb) at birth.
_____	_____	3. Establish a routine of measuring urine volume and daily weights of all babies receiving IV fluids.
_____	_____	4. Establish a policy for managing IV lines regarding: • Appropriate IV fluids for the specific type of IV catheter being used • Maintaining patency

Self-test Answers

These are the answers to the Self-test questions. Please check them with the answers you gave and review the information in the unit wherever necessary.

Self-test A

A1. A, B, and C. (All the babies listed should receive intravenous therapy. A is a sick baby; B is receiving inadequate oral intake; and C weighs less than 1,800 g [<4 lb] and would not be managing full feedings by the first day after birth.)

A2. A. Administer blood to the baby with vital signs within reference range: *Peripheral intravenous line*

    B. Draw blood for blood gas analysis: *Umbilical arterial catheter or radial artery sampling*

    C. Administer emergency medications during resuscitation: *Umbilical venous catheter (low lying)*

    D. Administer antibiotics: *Peripheral intravenous line*

    E. Perform an exchange transfusion: *Umbilical venous catheter. If an umbilical artery catheter is in place, withdraw blood via an umbilical arterial catheter and infuse blood or saline via an umbilical venous catheter*

A3. Replace or maintain body stores of water and electrolytes.
Replenish blood volume.
Give medication.
Provide calories, in the form of glucose.

A4. Run a continuous infusion of D10 through the umbilical vein catheter.

Self-test B

B1. Increase the fluid intake to account for increased insensible water losses.

B2. During the first 24 hours after birth

B3. 240 mL (80 mL × 3.0 kg)

B4. 300 mL (120 mL × 2.5 kg)

B5. 150 mL (300 mL − 150 mL)

B6. Body fluid lost through the skin and respiratory passages

B7. *152 mL per day*
6.3 mL per hour
2.6 kg × 120 mL = 312 mL total fluid required per day
20 mL × 8 hours = 160 mL via nipple
312 mL − 160 mL = 152 mL intravenously
152 mL ÷ 24 hours = 6.3 mL per hour

B8. B. Decreased

Self-test C

C1. Approximately 20 to 30 g/24 h

C2. *Approximately 80 mL/24 h*
Approximately 2 to 4 mL/h (1–2 mL/kg/h)

C3.

Yes	No	
X	___	Obtain the baby's weight at the same time each day.
___	X	Remove all equipment attached to the baby.
X	___	Use the same scale for every weight.
X	___	Weigh the baby before a feeding.
___	X	Weigh the baby immediately after a feeding.

C4. Determine the weight (in grams) of the urine by weighing each wet diaper and subtracting the dry diaper weight. If an indwelling urinary catheter is in place, urine can be measured in the collection device attached to the catheter.

C5. No
The baby is getting too little fluid or the baby's kidneys and/or heart are not functioning properly.

C6. Larger

Self-test D

D1. If an intravenous line flushes easily with a syringe or has a brisk, definite blood return, it is probably not infiltrated. Difficulty in flushing an intravenous line, an increase in infusion pressure, or puffiness at the site are indications that an intravenous line is likely infiltrated.

D2. Adequate intake of calories and fluid via nipple or tube feedings
Recovered from an illness and is stable
No longer needs intravenous line for glucose or medications

D3. The intravenous line is infiltrated.

Unit 5 Posttest

After completion of each unit there is a free online posttest available at www.cmevillage.com to test your understanding. Navigate to the PCEP pages on www.cmevillage.com and register to take the free posttests.

Once registered on the website and after completing all the unit posttests, pay the book exam fee ($15) and pass the test at 80% or greater to earn continuing education credits. Only start the PCEP book exam if you have time to complete it. If you take the book exam and are not connected to a printer, either print your certificate to a .pdf file and save it to print later or come back to www.cmevillage.com at any time and print a copy of your educational transcript.

Credits are only available by book, not by individual unit within the books. Available credits for completion of each book exam are as follows: Book 1: 14.5 credits; Book 2: 16 credits; Book 3: 17 credits; Book 4: 9 credits.

For more details, navigate to the PCEP webpages at www.cmevillage.com.

SKILL UNIT

Peripheral Intravenous Infusions

This skill unit will teach you how to start a peripheral intravenous (PIV) line in a baby. Not everyone will be required to start PIV lines. Everyone should read this skill unit, however, to learn the equipment and sequence of steps to be able to assist with starting a PIV line.

You will need to demonstrate mastery of the skill by inserting and stabilizing an intravenous (IV) line for a baby in your nursery the next time a baby needs an IV catheter placed. Preliminary practice may be possible on certain mannequins.

To master the skill, you will need to demonstrate each of the following steps correctly:
1. Collect and prepare the proper equipment.

2. Demonstrate proper IV insertion technique.

3. Secure the IV catheter.

4. Monitor the IV site and the fluid intake.

Note: Illustrated in this skill unit are conventional IV equipment and insertion devices. Increasingly, shielded catheters for PIV insertion and IV tubing with needleless access ports are becoming available to protect the health professional from exposure to blood and needlesticks. *Shielded catheters* are ones in which the needle can be withdrawn into the insertion hub and locked within a cover once the catheter has been inserted.

Insertion and taping of these devices are essentially the same as shown in this unit, but each brand of IV insertion device requires its own insertion technique. These techniques are very similar to each other but also slightly—but importantly—different. You will need to become familiar with the specific insertion devices used in your hospital and master the specific technique to insert each device. See the video at https://www.youtube.com/watch?v=bu5zgfZFViY for demonstration of peripherally inserted central catheter technique.

PERINATAL PERFORMANCE GUIDE

Inserting and Managing Peripheral Intravenous Infusions

Note: Although the exact technique of peripheral intravenous infusion (PIV) insertion and taping may vary, the principles are always the same. The following method is just one of several that work well. Only PIV insertion into the hand or foot is discussed. Central, long-line catheter insertion and maintenance are not covered.

Whatever method is used, it is important to expect to succeed in starting an IV and, therefore, to have everything ready. A good IV placement can be ruined by delay in proper taping or by clotting of the line due to delay in starting infusion of IV fluid. It is always helpful to have another set of hands to assist with the insertion.

ACTION	REMARKS
Collecting Equipment for a PIV	

1. Gather all of these materials.

   • *Intravenous solution—check to ensure it is*

      — Prepared as ordered

      — Labeled with the following information:

         ▪ Solution

         ▪ Electrolytes or other medications, if any, added to the IV fluid

         ▪ Date and time it was prepared

         ▪ Patient name

It is recommended that an IV solution be changed every 24 hours, regardless of the amount of fluid left in the bottle or bag. This is to minimize the chance of an infection being transferred to the baby through IV fluid. The administration set (IV tubing) up to, but not including, the IV catheter should be routinely changed every 24–96 hours. Follow your hospital's (infection control) guidelines and the Infusion Nurses Society standards for changing IV fluids and administration sets.

   • *Intravenous pump*

To provide a consistently accurate IV delivery rate, a pump is essential.

   • *Intravenous tubing*

      — IV tubing needed for the specific IV pump being used

      — *Microbore bacterial filter* (optional for routine IV therapy)

      — Tubing with a measuring chamber (optional)

This will be specific to the pump you are using.

Tubing with a measuring chamber can also be used. Review your hospital's policy for the appropriate equipment to use.

   • *IV fluid solution*

      — IV bag

      or

      — Appropriately sized syringe, if using a syringe pump

The smallest-volume bag of fluids available should be used. Newer pumps also have the capability of using a syringe to administer fluids.

205

ACTION	REMARKS

Collecting Equipment for a PIV (continued)

- *IV dressing*
  — Adhesive transparent film dressing
- *Tape, precut*
  — ½-inch tape cut into one 1-inch strip
  — ½-inch tape cut into one 3-inch strip
  — Clear adhesive film dressing cut to fit over the insertion site

For infection prevention purposes, the IV insertion site should be covered with a clear adhesive film that allows visualization of the site.

- *Small tourniquet*

An elastic band is sometimes used as a tourniquet around an extremity.

- *Intravenous board* (optional, for an arm or leg site)

An extremity board is occasionally used to immobilize the limb of a large, vigorous baby.

- *Intravenous catheters*

A catheter size 24 is used for most babies; a size 22 is used for large veins.

- *Antimicrobial solution*

Follow your hospital's protocol for the appropriate selection and use of an antimicrobial solution. It is important to note that whichever is used, it is most effective when allowed to dry. The site should not be palpated after cleaning.

- *Sterile 2-inch x 2-inch gauze*

Gauze may be needed for positioning the catheter.

- *T-connector*

This is a short piece of tubing, with a medication port, that is inserted between the catheter and the main IV tubing.

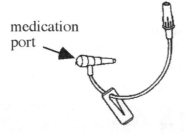

medication port

- *Needleless access device*

This is a cap that allows the IV tubing and/or syringes to be attached safely.

Preparing the Equipment

2. Run the IV solution through the tubing, taking care to eliminate all air bubbles.

If using a syringe pump, also draw a specific amount of IV solution into the syringe.

3. Insert the tubing into the pump according to the manufacturer's directions.

4. Set the IV rate but do not start the pump.

5. Draw up a syringe of flush solution.

Use either a pre-filled normal saline syringe or draw up a syringe with normal saline.

ACTION	REMARKS

Preparing the Equipment (continued)

6. Connect the syringe to the T-connector via the needleless access device and fill the connector with the flush solution, leaving 2 to 3 mL of flush solution in the syringe.

Keep the T-connector, needleless access device, and syringe connected.

7. Select an appropriate vein. Choose the largest vein in a convenient, relatively easy place to insert, stabilize, and protect the catheter.

It is prudent to avoid using a vein in the antecubital space (the bend of the elbow). Leave this vein available to obtain blood for laboratory tests or to obtain central access if needed in the future (ie, for peripherally inserted central catheter placement), unless no other IV site is available.

8. For an extremity vein, consider the use of an arm or leg board to stabilize the extremity.

    Note: In most situations, an extremity board is not needed. This information is provided in case a board is useful to protect an IV in a large or active baby.

    • Be sure the board is the appropriate length. If the selected vein is in a foot, for example, the board should be short enough not to rub in the popliteal space (the bend of the knee) but should be long enough to stabilize the ankle joint.

    • The extremity may be secured before or after the IV catheter is inserted and taped in place.

    • Check for capillary refill to make sure the tape is not too tight.

If an extremity board is used, secure the extremity above and below the insertion site. Use Velcro wraps or face a section of adhesive tape with another, shorter piece of tape long enough to go over the top of the extremity, leaving the ends of the longer piece sticky to secure to the underside of the board.

The important thing is to prepare the IV board at this point in the procedure. Actual taping of the arm or leg can be done later, in step 24.

Gently press and release the baby's toes or fingers. Note how quickly the blanched area turns pink again. There should be an almost instantaneous pink flush. If this does not happen, loosen the immobilization device slightly and check again.

9. Immobilize the baby.

This is always a safe practice, but immobilization may not be necessary with very small or sick babies. A mummy wrap, however, is often necessary for large or vigorous babies. Alternatively, ask for assistance.

If clinically appropriate, consider offering the baby a pacifier dipped in sucrose solution to comfort the baby during the procedure.

207

ACTION	REMARKS

Preparing the Equipment (continued)

10. Cleanse the intended insertion site with antimicrobial solution.

11. Allow the antimicrobial solution to dry.

This is necessary to provide appropriate antimicrobial benefit of cleansing the skin.

Inserting an IV Catheter

12. If starting an arm or leg IV catheter, consider using an elastic band for a tourniquet (shown in the illustration below).

If using an elastic band, be certain it is removed after the IV catheter is inserted.

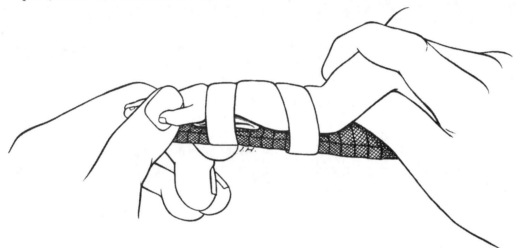

13. The person holding the baby or the person inserting the IV catheter may use their (gloved) fingers to spread the skin over the insertion site to keep it taut.

With the skin taut, the vein will roll less as the catheter and needle are inserted.

Be careful not to contaminate the area that was just cleansed.

14. Take the catheter and hold the hub between your thumb and index finger with the bevel (slanted part) of the needle facing upward.

15. **Insert the catheter directly into the vein.** Do not try to thread it through the skin.

Proceed slowly, because there is normally a slight delay in the backflow of blood into the catheter hub that indicates the vein has been entered.

ACTION	REMARKS

Inserting an IV Catheter (continued)

16. When the backflow of blood is first seen, *stop*.

17. Remove the needle from the catheter.

18. Release the elastic band.

Care must be taken to avoid puncturing the opposite side of the vein.

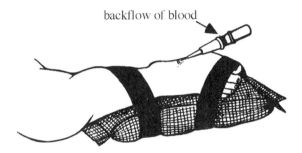

backflow of blood

19. *Thread* the catheter into the vein as far as it will go *easily.*

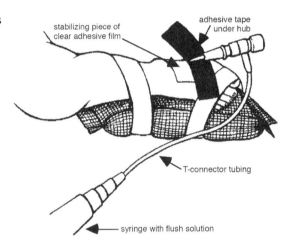

stabilizing piece of clear adhesive film

adhesive tape under hub

T-connector tubing

syringe with flush solution

20. Stabilize the catheter with an adhesive transparent film dressing, covering the insertion site and two-thirds of the catheter hub.

21. Connect the T-connector, needleless access device, and syringe with the flush solution to the catheter. Flush a small amount of solution through the catheter.

22. Observe the insertion site and the ease or difficulty of pushing the flush solution.

If the area in the skin near the tip of the catheter becomes swollen, the catheter is in the subcutaneous tissue and not in the vein. It should be removed immediately.

ACTION

REMARKS

Securing an IV Catheter

23. When the catheter flushes easily, tape it in that position with the 3-inch piece of adhesive tape. Adhesive skin closures (eg, Steri-Strip) may be used instead of tape.

    - Slide the tape under the catheter hub, with the sticky side facing up.

    - Crisscross the ends over the hub and tape the ends to the clear adhesive dressing that covers the insertion site.

    - A 2 × 2 piece of gauze under the hub (not shown) may be useful to protect the baby's skin from the hard hub pressing into it.

    Do not over-tape!

    Additional tape will not make the catheter any more secure, but it will make early detection of an infiltration more difficult.

Do not cover the site with tape. The insertion site and the inserted catheter should remain visible for observation.

adhesive tape crisscrossed over hub

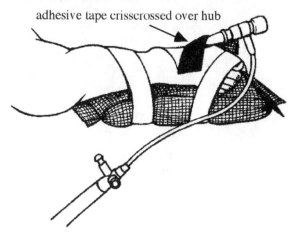

24. Recheck the ease with which the catheter can be flushed after it is taped in place. If it continues to flush easily, connect the IV tubing and begin the infusion.

In most cases, an arm or leg immobilization device is not needed with IV catheters. If one is indicated and it was not taped in place earlier (step 8), secure the baby's arm or leg to the IV board now, as shown in previous illustrations.

25. Be sure to include the T-connector tubing under the tape (not shown).

This is extremely important so that any pull on the IV tubing will pull against the tape and not the catheter.

Monitoring an IV Line

26. Record the amount of IV fluid infused during the insertion procedure and the time at which continuous IV infusion was started.

27. Record the amount of IV fluid infused each hour. Compare this with the ordered amount of IV fluid and the readout on the pump. Adjust the flow rate as necessary.

    Total the amount of IV fluids administered every 8 hours, or at least every 24 hours, per your institution's policy.

ACTION	REMARKS

Monitoring an IV Line (continued)

28. If the pump you are using measures the infusion pressure, record the pressure when the IV fluid is started.

29. Inspect the insertion site at least every hour for signs of infiltration.

To minimize possible tissue damage from infiltrated IV fluid, it is important to detect an infiltration as early as possible.

Unit 6: Feeding

Unit 6 Pretest

***Before* reading the unit, please answer the following questions. Select the *one best* answer to each question (unless otherwise instructed). Record your answers on the test and check them with the answers at the end of the book.**

1. In which of the following situations is a newborn most at risk for feeding intolerance?
    A. When the baby's mother has ulcers
    B. When there was excess amniotic fluid
    C. When the baby's mother has hypoglycemia
    D. When there was minimal amniotic fluid

2. Which of the following babies is most likely to develop feeding problems?
    A. A 3-day-old, term baby who has not produced stool
    B. A 3,200-g (7 lb 1 oz) baby
    C. A baby with a myelomeningocele
    D. A baby with an estimated gestational age of 43 weeks

3. How does formula for preterm newborns differ from that for term newborns?
    A. Higher protein concentration
    B. Higher caloric density
    C. Higher concentrations of vitamins and minerals
    D. All of the above

4. A 2-hour-old, term baby that is appropriate for gestational age has rapid, shallow respirations at a rate of 80 breaths per minute. The baby is requiring only 30% oxygen. How would you provide fluids/nutrition for this baby?
    A. Nipple feedings
    B. Nasogastric or orogastric tube feedings
    C. Peripheral intravenous fluids
    D. Delay fluids/feedings until the baby is 24 hours old.

5. **True   False**   A 2,000-g (4 lb 6½ oz) baby who is small for gestational age will require more calories to grow than a 2,000-g baby who is appropriate for gestational age.

6. **True   False**   Most preterm newborns initially lose weight and then slowly regain weight to arrive at their birth weight by approximately 2 weeks of age.

7. **True   False**   Preterm newborns born prior to 34 weeks of gestation have higher protein, vitamin, and mineral needs and often require fortified human (breast) milk until they are ingesting more liberal volumes.

8. Which of the following babies require tube feedings instead of nipple feedings?
    A. Babies born at 30 weeks' gestational age who are appropriate for gestational age with a strong suck reflex
    B. Babies born at 36 weeks' gestational age who are small for gestational age with polycythemia
    C. Babies born at 40 weeks' gestational age with hyperbilirubinemia who require phototherapy
    D. Babies born at 43 weeks' gestational age who are small for gestational age with a strong suck reflex

(*continued*)

Unit 6 Pretest (*continued*)

9. Which of the following procedures should usually be performed before each tube feeding?

    A. Aspirate the baby's stomach contents, record the amount, and discard the aspirated fluid.

    B. Check for a soft, nondistended abdomen.

10. **True**   **False**   The placement of a feeding tube should be checked before every feeding.

11. **True**   **False**   Term babies with increased work of breathing and supplemental oxygen requirement may be fed orally.

12. **True**   **False**   A combination of nipple and tube feedings may be appropriate for some babies.

Part 1: Feeding Principles

Objectives

In Part 1 of this unit you will learn

A. The goals of feeding

B. The importance of human (breast) milk and evidence-based strategies to support breastfeeding

C. To recognize the risks associated with feedings

D. To identify babies who are at risk for feeding problems

E. To determine how much and how often a baby should be fed

F. To determine if a baby should be fed via feeding tube or nipple

G. To determine if multivitamin or iron supplements are needed

Note: • Throughout this unit, the general term *milk* is used to indicate human (breast) milk or formula.

　　　• *Kilocalories* is often shortened to *calories* in everyday usage.

　　　• Nutritional management of extremely-low-birth-weight babies (<1,000 g [<2 lb 3 oz]) is not discussed.

1. What are the goals of feeding?

- To achieve optimal growth
- To promote optimal brain development
- To nourish the gut
- To promote a healthy immune system

2. What is the importance of human (breast) milk and evidence-based strategies to support exclusive breastfeeding?

- Human (breast) milk from the baby's own mother is the optimal source of nutrition for all babies—term and preterm—with rare exceptions.
- Advantages of breastfeeding and breast milk are greater for the preterm baby who has an immature gastrointestinal tract, although certain supplements may be indicated (described herein).
- A review of current American Academy of Pediatrics (AAP) recommendations for breastfeeding may be found in American Academy of Pediatrics Section on Breastfeeding. Breastfeeding and the use of human milk. *Pediatrics*. 2012;129(3):e827–e841. Updated guidelines are anticipated in 2021.
- Certain hospital practices, such as providing immediate skin-to-skin care, rooming-in, and feeding on cue, have been shown to increase the rates of breast milk feeding and help more mothers achieve their breastfeeding goals.
- The World Health Organization Ten Steps to Successful Breastfeeding (Box 6.1) have been endorsed by the AAP. They highlight the importance of signaling a mother's body within the first hour after delivery and include helping mothers establish and maintain their milk supply, even if they are separated from their newborn.

Box 6.1. Ten Steps to Successful Breastfeeding

Critical management procedures

1a. Comply fully with the *International Code of Marketing of Breast-milk Substitutes* and relevant World Health Assembly resolutions.

1b. Have a written infant feeding policy that is routinely communicated to staff and parents.

1c. Establish ongoing monitoring and data management systems.

2. Ensure that staff have sufficient knowledge, competence, and skills to support breastfeeding.

Key clinical practices

3. Discuss the importance and management of breastfeeding with pregnant women and their families.

4. Facilitate immediate and uninterrupted skin-to-skin contact and support mothers to initiate breastfeeding as soon as possible after birth.

5. Support mothers to initiate and maintain breastfeeding and manage common difficulties.

6. Do not provide breastfed newborns any food or fluids other than breast milk, unless medically indicated.

(continued)

> **Box 6.1. Ten Steps to Successful Breastfeeding (*continued*)**
>
> 7. Enable mothers and their infants to remain together and to practice rooming-in 24 hours a day.
> 8. Support mothers in recognizing and responding to their infants' cues for feeding.
> 9. Counsel mothers on the use and risks of feeding bottles, teats, and pacifiers.
> 10. Coordinate discharge so that parents and their infants have timely access to ongoing support and care.

Adapted from World Health Organization, United Nations Children's Fund. *Implementation Guidance: Protecting, Promoting, and Supporting Breastfeeding in Facilities Providing Maternity and Newborn Services: The Revised Baby-Friendly Hospital Initiative.* Geneva, Switzerland: World Health Organization, 2018. https://apps.who.int/iris/bitstream/handle/10665/272943/9789241513807-eng.pdf?ua=1. Accessed January 21, 2020.

- Hospital physicians and nursing staff play an important role in helping a mother feed her baby at the breast, if mother and baby are stable, or initiate pumping within the first hour or as soon as possible after delivery. The subsequent capacity to establish a full milk supply has been shown to depend somewhat on the timing of the first milk expression, preferably no later than 6 hours after delivery.
- After the initiation of milk expression and if the mother is stable, hospital staff caring for the mother who is separated from her newborn should have a system in place that ensures she is able to express her milk by using hand expression and breast pumping combined with breast compression at least 8 times every 24 hours and there is a way to safely store and deliver to baby any colostrum or milk that is expressed.

Breast milk is the preferred nutrition source for babies born at all gestational ages. There are rare contraindications to feeding a baby breast milk (Box 6.2). Any contraindications to breastfeeding should be documented in the medical record and conveyed to the team caring for the newborn.

> **Box 6.2. Contraindications to Breastfeeding**
>
> - Babies with classic galactosemia
> - Mothers with active, untreated tuberculosis, HIV-1, or HIV-2
> - Mothers receiving antimetabolites or chemotherapeutic agents, until these substances are cleared from her milk
> - Mothers using drugs such as cocaine
> - Mothers with herpes simplex lesions on the breast or active varicella

A. Babies born at 37 weeks' gestational age or later
- Babies born at $37^{0/7}$ to $38^{6/7}$ weeks' gestational age are *early term,* as defined by the American College of Obstetricians and Gynecologists. These babies are more vulnerable to complications, such as feeding or respiratory problems.
- *Term* is defined as $39^{0/7}$ to $41^{6/7}$ weeks.
- Breast milk is the preferred source of nutrition, unless there is a contraindication.
- All mothers should be given current, evidence-based information about the importance of breast milk and the physiology and management of breastfeeding so that they may make an informed choice for themselves.

- Pasteurized donor milk is an option for breastfeeding babies who have a short-term medical need for supplementation (eg, hypoglycemia that is not responsive to breastfeeding), while the mother's breast milk production is "ramping up."
- If, after receiving educational information, commercial formula is the mother's preferred choice, any one of several standard commercial formulas, all of which have a caloric density of 20 kcal/oz, are appropriate for babies born at 37 weeks' gestational age or later, without complications.

B. Preterm babies born at less than 37 completed weeks of gestation
- Preterm babies' immature gastrointestinal tracts can easily be injured if given anything other than breast milk, if feedings are advanced too quickly, or if given formula that is too concentrated. The more preterm the baby, the greater the risk of intestinal damage.
- Preterm babies also have greater nutritional requirements than babies born at term and require supplemental calories, protein, and various additional nutrients, whether they are receiving breast milk or commercial formula.
- Milks for providing enteral nutrition to the preterm baby include
  — *Breast milk:* If a baby is too preterm or too sick to feed at the breast, the mother can collect milk that can then be fed via nasogastric or orogastric tube, as described later in this unit. Fresh milk that is collected with clean equipment by using an approved protocol may be given directly to the baby. Because mothers usually cannot be available to their hospitalized baby for every feeding, the milk can be frozen and thawed for later use. Another option is the implementation of a protocol for the use of donor breast milk for babies who do not have mother's milk available. Babies born at less than approximately 35 weeks' gestational age who are fed breast milk may need commercially available breast milk fortifiers added to their feedings. Manufacturers' instructions should be followed when adding these fortifiers.
  — *Commercial formulas for preterm babies:* Most commercial formulas for preterm newborns are derived from cow's milk. These formulas also have a higher caloric density and more vitamins, minerals, and protein than standard baby formulas. While breast milk and commercial formulas for term newborns have a caloric density of approximately 20 kcal/oz, formulas designed for preterm babies contain 22 or 24 kcal/oz. Infants born prior to 34 weeks of gestation, if not receiving breast milk, will require a preterm formula to meet their nutritional needs.
  Note: Meeting protein goals for a preterm newborn weighing less than 1,500 g (<3 lb 5 oz) in the first 5 days of age is associated with improved developmental outcomes. Feedings should be initiated in small volumes, with a protein goal of 3 to 4 g/kg/d in the first 7 to 10 days after birth. This will require the use of either a breast milk–based fortifier or a cow's milk—based fortifier to reach a minimum of 24 kcal/oz or by using a commercially prepared preterm infant formula. Consult a regional center for babies weighing less than 1,500 g.

 Preterm babies have immature intestines that are easily injured. Use only breast milk, usually fortified with an appropriate supplement, whenever possible.

C. Late preterm babies ($34^{0/7}$ to $36^{6/7}$ weeks' gestational age) or preterm babies approaching discharge

As babies born significantly preterm approach discharge weight, they still have unique, but changing, nutritional requirements.

1. Breastfeeding babies

Breastfeeding babies who were born preterm and are now breastfeeding may need additional calories, protein, iron, and other minerals than can be provided with nonfortified breast milk until they reach 36 to 37 weeks' postmenstrual age. The baby's growth patterns and/or laboratory results will help determine when fortification is no longer necessary.

2. Non-breastfeeding babies

Non-breastfeeding babies may be switched to a formula intended to meet the special needs of the growing preterm baby after hospital discharge. These formulas contain 22 kcal/oz, plus the additional minerals, vitamins, and iron required for a baby who has not had a full intrauterine gestation. If more than 22 kcal/oz is needed to support adequate growth, recipes for 24 kcal/oz or more can be provided at discharge. (*J Pediatr Gastroenterol Nutr.* 2008;46[1]:99–110.)

D. Babies with certain digestive problems

There are many special formulas that contain less or no lactose, hydrolyzed or elemental proteins, and/or a blend of long-chain and medium-chain fats for easier digestion or intolerance. Although these formulas differ considerably in their composition, nearly all contain 20 kcal/oz. Discussion of these formulas is beyond the scope of this educational unit.

3. What are the associated risks of oral and/or gastric tube feedings?

- Babies may aspirate (inhale) milk into their lungs as they eat.
- Babies may vomit and aspirate the vomitus into their lungs.
- Aspiration of breast milk or formula into the lungs can lead to pneumonia.
- Babies with respiratory distress cannot breathe as easily with a full stomach.
- Babies with respiratory distress or other acute illness may not have the energy or coordination to orally feed and effectively breathe at the same time.

4. Which babies are at risk for developing feeding problems? (Table 6.1)

Table 6.1. Feeding Risk Factors and Recommended Responses	
Risk Factor	**Response**
Excessive mucus	• Do *not* feed the baby until a tube is passed into the baby's stomach to rule out tracheoesophageal fistula and esophageal atresia.[a]
History of maternal polyhydramnios (often associated with GI anomalies)	• Monitor the baby's feeding tolerance carefully. If abdominal distension or vomiting develops, give the baby nothing by mouth,[a] insert an NG or OG tube, and obtain an abdominal radiograph.

(continued)

Table 6.1. Feeding Risk Factors and Recommended Responses (*continued*)	
Risk Factor	**Response**
Distended abdomen	• Insert an NG or OG tube and withdraw air/fluid to decompress the baby's stomach. • Do *not* feed the baby until obstruction and ileus have been ruled out.[a]
Respiratory distress, rapid breathing, or depressed activity	• Do *not* feed the baby by bottle or allow the baby to breast-feed until the respiratory rate is less than approximately 60 breaths per minute, with no increased work of breathing, and the baby can coordinate sucking, swallowing, and breathing.[a,b]
Babies younger than 32 to 34 weeks' gestational age may be able to suck, swallow, and breathe adequately but *may not be able to coordinate* these activities.	• Feed the baby by NG or OG tube or administer IV fluids until oral feedings can be attempted. • Preterm babies, depending on gestational age and health status, may also have special nutritional needs, which may require breast milk fortifier or preterm infant formula. • During feeding, allow skin-to-skin time. Kangaroo care provides benefits to the baby and parents, such as increased mean daily weight gain and increase in successful breastfeeding. • After 2 days of age, initiate oral care with colostrum and breast milk when the baby is hemodynamically stable or per your institution's protocol. (*Oral care* refers to the practice of keeping a baby's mouth clean, which can prevent or reduce tooth decay. Oral care is performed with a swipe of a piece of gauze or a washcloth dampened with colostrum, breast milk, or water.) • Provide oral stimulation with a pacifier during NG or OG feedings.
Vomiting of green material or persistent vomiting or spitting	• Stop feedings.[a] • Obtain an abdominal radiograph to evaluate for possible intestinal obstruction. Give the baby nothing by mouth. • Place an NG or OG tube to decompress the baby's stomach. • Consult a regional perinatal center for immediate evaluation and perform an upper GI examination to rule out malrotation or volvulus, if resources are available.
No stool by 48 hours of age	• Obtain a careful history to ensure that there was not meconium passage at delivery or a diaper with stool that had been changed and not recorded. • Evaluate the baby for adequate oral intake. • Perform a clinical assessment for abdominal distension and anal-rectal patency. • Stop feedings. • Evaluate the baby for obstruction or ileus. • Consult a regional perinatal center and evaluate the baby for congenital megacolon (Hirschsprung disease).

(continued)

Table 6.1. Feeding Risk Factors and Recommended Responses (*continued*)	
Risk Factor	**Response**
Prolonged resuscitation (perinatal compromise increases the risk for developing an ileus or necrotizing enterocolitis)	• Give the baby nothing by mouth until stable. • Consider giving the baby nothing by mouth for at least 24 to 48 hours or until bowel sounds are heard. • Provide oral care with colostrum or breast milk as long as the baby is hemodynamically stable.[a]
Sepsis (increases the risk for developing an ileus)	• Give the baby nothing by mouth until stable.[a] • Provide oral care with colostrum or breast milk as long as the baby is hemodynamically stable.

Abbreviations: GI, gastrointestinal; IV, intravenous; NG, nasogastric; OG, orogastric.

[a] Maintain hydration and blood glucose levels by administering IV fluids.

[b] Tube feedings may be appropriate for some babies. See Part 2, Tube Feeding, in this unit.

5. How do you know how much milk is needed by a baby who is appropriate for gestational age?

A. Determine total daily volume of milk needed
- Initially, the stomachs of healthy early term and term babies are small.
  — Physiological volumes for newborns in the first 0 to 4 days after birth are significantly lower than they are on day 5 and beyond, coinciding with lactogenesis stage II, or the making of ounces of milk, in the mother (Figure 6.1).

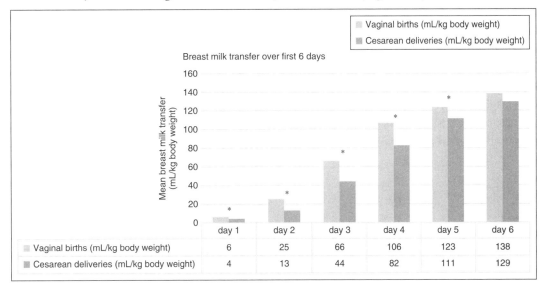

Breast milk transfer over first 6 days

	day 1	day 2	day 3	day 4	day 5	day 6
Vaginal births (mL/kg body weight)	6	25	66	106	123	138
Cesarean deliveries (mL/kg body weight)	4	13	44	82	111	129

Figure 6.1. Milk Volume Estimated by Breast Milk Transfer Over the First 6 Days in Vaginal and Cesarean Births
*= Adjusted difference $P < .05$.
From Feldman-Winter L, Kellams A, Peter-Wohl S, et al. Evidence-based updates on the first week of exclusive breastfeeding among infants ≥35 weeks. *Pediatrics.* 2020;145(4):e20183696.
Derived in part from Evans KC, Evans RG, Royal R, Esterman AJ, James SL. Effect of caesarean section on breast milk transfer to the normal term newborn over the first week of life. *Arch Dis Child Fetal Neonatal Ed.* 2003;88(5):F382.

- Appropriate feeding should allow weight gain of 15 to 20 g/kg/d for a newborn weighing less than 2,000 g (<4 lb 6½ oz) and 20 to 40 g/d for a newborn weighing more than 2,000 g.
- Volume requirements should increase each day after birth. Babies who are appropriate for gestational age (AGA) will generally require a minimum of 100 to 120 kcal/kg of body weight by day 4 to 5 to maintain metabolic functions, gain weight, and allow for some losses in the stool.
  — In general, for newborns fed breast milk or commercial infant formula, aim for more than 150 mL/kg/d once the baby is older than 5 to 6 days of age.
  — If a newborn can ingest only 130 mL/kg/d, calories should be increased* to 24 kcal/oz.
  — If a newborn ingests less than 130 mL/kg/d but is meeting hydration needs, consider increasing* the caloric density to 27 kcal/oz or consulting a regional center.
  *If the baby's weight pattern is not consistently meeting expectations, the growth pattern is more important than maintaining specific volumes. If the baby is growing well, baby is getting what baby needs from a caloric standpoint.

B. Determine feeding frequency

Newborns need to eat 8 to 12 times a day, preferably spaced throughout the day in response to feeding cues. However, the time lapse between feedings should not be longer than 4 hours for preterm newborns. Babies weighing less than 1,500 g (<3 lb 5 oz) usually do not display periods of arousal frequently enough for nutritional needs to be met and require a more scheduled feeding regimen. Table 6.2 provides *general guidelines* for AGA babies. For all newborns, regardless of gestational age, it is optimal to try as much as possible to time feedings with the baby's sleep-wake cycles by feeding the baby when the baby begins to stir, awaken, or be in a lighter sleep pattern, rather than feeding on a set schedule. Oral feeding practice is most effective when the baby self-awakens. Changing the baby's diaper or placing the baby skin-to-skin with the mother are ways to gently coax the baby into a more awake state prior to feeding.

Table 6.2. Feeding Guidelines for Babies Who Are Appropriate for Gestational Age		
Baby's Weight and EGA	**Feeding Frequency**	**Feeding Method**
1,000–1,499 g (2 lb 3 oz to 3 lb 5 oz) EGA <32–34 wk	The baby should be fed 8 to 12 times in 24 hours, preferably spaced throughout the day. When the baby begins to feed by mouth, initiate oral feedings when the baby shows feeding cues.	Feed by NG or OG tube. Continue providing oral care with breast milk. The baby may snuggle and root at the breast during a feeding.
1,500–1,800 g (3 lb 5 oz to 4 lb 6½ oz) EGA >32–34⁶/⁷ wk	Watch for awake/alert periods or feeding cues for oral feedings, 8 to 12 times in 24 hours. The time between feedings should not exceed 4 hours.	Feed the baby orally (unless contraindicated), followed by NG or OG tube feedings for the remainder of the feeding, if the baby is not ingesting the full amount.

(continued)

Table 6.2. Feeding Guidelines for Babies Who Are Appropriate for Gestational Age (*continued*)		
Baby's Weight and EGA	**Feeding Frequency**	**Feeding Method**
>1,800 g EGA 35$^{0/7}$–36$^{6/7}$ wk	Feed the baby on demand or with every feeding cue, 8 to 12 times in 24 hours. The time between feedings should not exceed 4 hours.	Feed the baby orally (unless contraindicated), followed by NG or OG tube feedings for the remainder of the feeding, if objective data support the finding that the baby is not ingesting enough volume (ie, output and weight pattern are suboptimal). If breastfeeding, the baby should be allowed to go to the breast with every feeding cue, and mothers should be taught to use breast massage and compression to maximize their milk transfer and hand express their breasts after each feeding to maximize milk production signaling to the mother's body and intake of the infant. A feeding should be observed and assessed by using an objective tool, such as LATCH (*l*atch, *a*udible swallowing, *t*ype of nipple, *c*omfort [breast/nipple], *h*old [positioning]), and consideration should be given to having the mother pump to ensure adequate milk production signaling and milk removal. (*J Obstet Gynecol Neonatal Nurs.* 1994;23[1]:27–32.) The baby should be evaluated at least every 12 hours for adequacy of intake, output, and fluid status, with a low threshold for supplementation if medically necessary.
Healthy, early term and term babies >2,500 g (>5 lb 8 oz) EGA >37 wk	Feed the baby on demand or with every feeding cue at least 8 to 12 times in 24 hours.	Feed orally (unless contraindicated). If breastfeeding, the baby should be allowed to go to the breast with every feeding cue, and mothers should be taught to use breast massage and compression to maximize their milk transfer and to hand express after each feeding. A feeding should be observed and assessed by using an objective tool, such as LATCH. Any breast milk expressed should be fed to the baby by using a method other than an artificial nipple, such as a syringe, cup, or spoon.

Abbreviations: EGA, estimated gestational age; NG, nasogastric; OG, orogastric.

C. Determine the target volume per feeding for newborns that are requiring supplementation or ingesting commercial infant formula
Example: A 1,600-g (3 lb 8 oz) AGA baby born at 33 weeks' gestational age who is feeding approximately every 3 hours, for a total of approximately 8 feedings per day.

Therefore, if the feeding goal is 240 mL/d (1.6 kg × 150 mL/kg), each feeding volume would be 30 mL (240 mL/d ÷ 8 feedings/d).

D. Gradually increase the feeding volume to reach the target amount
If a baby is preterm or has been sick, work up slowly to the calculated volume of feedings. This may take several days.

 To maintain hydration and prevent hypoglycemia, babies who are not receiving full feedings should receive intravenous (IV) fluids until adequate milk intake has been established. As the volume of enteral milk feeding increases, the volume of IV fluids should be reduced. Babies weighing less than 1,800 g (<4 lb 6½ oz) require IV parenteral nutrition while receiving a slow advance of feedings.

The speed with which full feedings can be achieved depends on the baby's degree of illness or prematurity. General guidelines for preterm babies are shown in Table 6.3.

- *Example:* The 1,600-g (3 lb 8 oz) baby described earlier might first be given a feeding of 5 mL. If that is managed well, consider increasing the feeding volume by 1.5 to 3.0 mL every third feeding until the baby is receiving the full targeted amount of an average of 30 mL every 3 hours, or 240 mL/d. Alternatively, advancing feedings by 20 to 30 mL/kg/d to a goal of 150 mL/kg/d is commonly done in many NICUs.

Table 6.3. Suggested Guidelines for Increasing Feedings for Preterm Babies		
Baby's Weight	**Starting Volume**	**Progression**
<1,200 g	2 mL/kg at each feeding	1 mL/kg approximately every 12 h or 10–20 mL/kg/d
1,200–1,800 g	2–3 mL/kg at each feeding	1–2 mL/kg approximately every 9 h or 20–30 mL/kg/d
>1,800 g	5 mL/kg at each feeding	5–10 mL approximately every other feeding or 30 mL/kg/d

6. How do you know how much milk is needed by a baby who is small for gestational age?

Most preterm babies and babies who are born small for gestational age (SGA) need additional kilocalories per kilogram of body weight for achievement of catch-up growth. For babies who are SGA and born at a later gestational age, the amount of volume and calories they need will be determined on the basis of their clinical course (eg, do they have an appropriate amount of output, have they started gaining weight at an appropriate rate).

When starting feedings, work up slowly to the calculated volume.

- In general, for an SGA newborn feeding on breast milk or standard infant formula, aim for more than 150 mL/kg/d, and increase the caloric intake to 24 kcal/oz once the baby is more than 4 to 5 days old.
- Powdered infant formula can be mixed to a higher caloric density if needed, to ensure a steady weight gain pattern.

- There are also commercially prepared preterm infant 24 kcal/oz formulas available for infants born preterm. Note: These are not recommended for term infants or infants who have reached 3.5 kg (7 lb 11 oz), due to excessive minerals and protein in the formula.
- If a newborn receives adequate oral intake for hydration but consistently less than 130 mL/kg/d, consider increasing to 27 kcal/oz fortified breast milk or formula or consulting a regional perinatal center, depending on how the baby is growing.

Self-test A

Now answer these questions to test yourself on the information in the last section. Refer to the graphs or charts in the unit, as necessary, to answer these questions.

A1. What can happen if a baby of 30 weeks' estimated gestational age is fed by mouth?

_____

A2. A woman with polyhydramnios delivered a full-term, vigorous baby. Thirty minutes after birth, the baby is noted to have excessive mucus. What would you do before the first feeding?
  A. Suction the baby's mouth and nose with a bulb syringe, and then feed the baby.
  B. Insert an orogastric or nasogastric tube and feed the baby with the tube in place.
  C. Insert an orogastric or nasogastric tube and evaluate for obstruction before feeding.

A3. **True   False**   Formulas with high osmolarity are preferred for preterm babies.

A4. A baby weighs 1,800 g (3 lb 15½ oz) and is appropriate size for gestational age. The baby is in no distress. How often would you feed this baby?

_____

A5. A baby weighs 2,300 g (5 lb 1 oz) at 40 weeks' gestational age.
  A. How often would you feed this baby?

  _____

  B. Is this baby small, large, or appropriate size for gestational age?

  _____

  C. How much would you eventually give the baby at each feeding?

  _____

A6. A 2-day-old baby is requiring 50% oxygen and breathing at a rate of 70 breaths per minute. The baby's estimated gestational age is 36 weeks. This baby should be fed via
  A. Intravenous fluids only
  B. Oral feedings while oxygen is being delivered to the baby's face
  C. Nasogastric or orogastric tube feedings

Check your answers with the list that follows the Recommended Routines. Correct any incorrect answers and review the appropriate section in the unit.

---

7. How can you tell if a baby is growing satisfactorily?

Very-low-birth-weight (ie, <1,500 g [<3 lb 5 oz]) babies will lose weight for more than the few days exhibited by babies born closer to term. Additionally, the more preterm babies are, the longer they will take to regain birth weight.

Fenton growth curves are appropriate tools to follow the growth of newborns during hospitalization, after discharge from the hospital, and up to 52 weeks' postmenstrual age-corrected gestational age (Figure 6.2). However, World Health Organization growth curves can also be used once a baby reaches approximately 40 weeks' corrected gestational age.

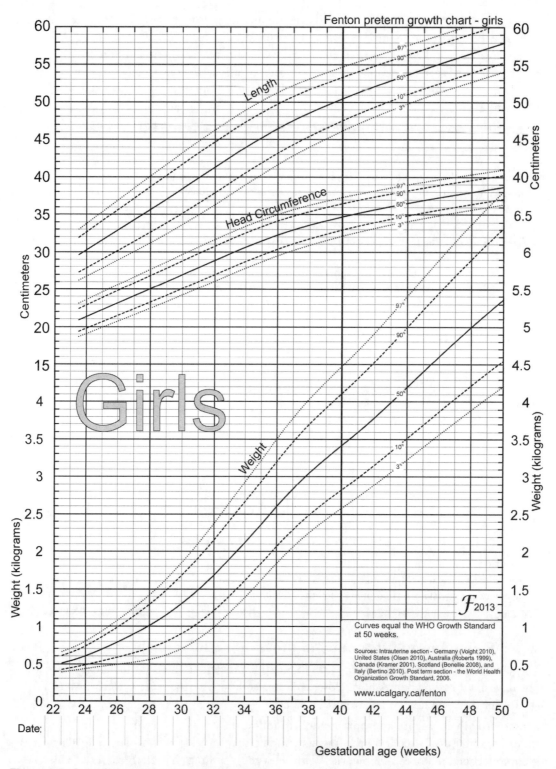

Figure 6.2. Fenton Preterm Growth Charts for Girls and Boys

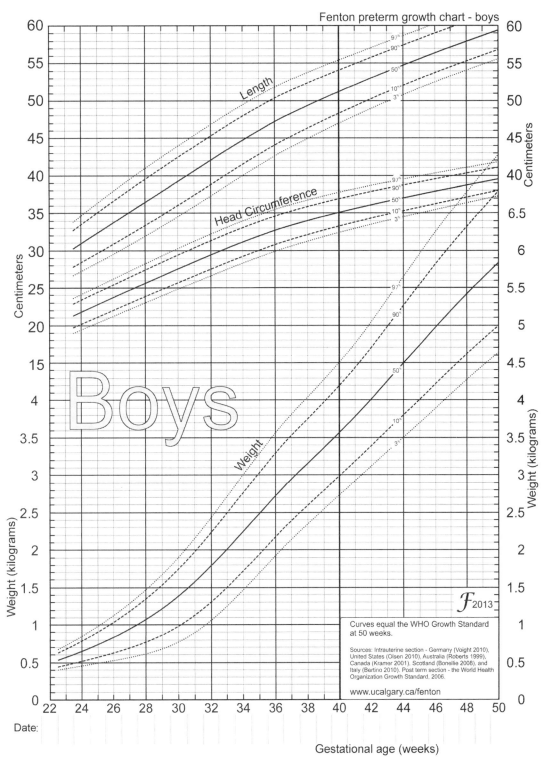

Figure 6.2. Fenton Preterm Growth Charts for Girls and Boys (*continued*)

For babies who are 35 weeks' gestational age and older, there are established, validated curves based on more than 100,000 infants that demonstrate newborn weight loss in the first week and month, depending on the baby's feeding type and delivery method, which can be useful in determining which babies need a formal feeding evaluation and which ones may need supplementation. The NEWT Newborn Weight tool is one such resource, available at www. Newbornweight.org, which can be used to create custom graphs for newborn weight tracking.

8. Which babies need vitamin supplementation?

A. Multivitamins

Vitamins are substances that occur in many foods in small amounts and are necessary for typical metabolic functions. Formulas designed for preterm babies and breast milk supplements, which are both described earlier in this unit, provide vitamins in the amounts necessary for adequate growth of preterm babies.

Preterm newborns of 34 weeks' gestational age or less need to receive a pediatric multivitamin with iron supplementation when discharged home with a feeding plan of

- Preterm discharge formula at volumes less than 24 ounces per day
- Standard or specialty 20 kcal/oz formula
- Unfortified breast milk

Administering vitamin supplements (when needed)

Vitamins and some drugs have high osmolarity. To make them less hyperosmolar, vitamins are administered in the following way:

- A dose of 1 mL/d of an infant multivitamin preparation is administered; for newborns weighing less than 2 kg (<2 lb 6½ oz), start with 0.5 mL/d.
- Vitamins are administered after the baby is tolerating full feedings well.
- The entire volume of vitamins is mixed into one feeding or divided and mixed into several feedings.

Note: Until preterm babies are able to manage full volumes of enteral feedings, try to give medications intravenously or intramuscularly. If these routes of administration are not possible or appropriate, dilute the medications for oral or tube feeding administration in the full volume of milk for a feeding.

B. Vitamin D

All babies should receive at least 400 IU of vitamin D per day. Breastfed babies and babies who are consuming less than 27 oz of standard infant formula per day should be given an oral supplement per AAP guidelines.

 Dilute medications or multivitamins given orally or via tube feedings to decrease their osmolarity. This is especially important for preterm babies.

9. Which babies need iron supplementation?

The AAP recommends that preterm newborns should receive iron supplementation (≥2 mg/kg of elemental iron per day) from 2 weeks until 12 months of age (AAP Committee on Nutrition. *Pediatric Nutrition.* 8th ed. Kleinman RE, Greer FR, eds. American Academy of Pediatrics;

2019: 571). Iron supplements can be started as early as 2 weeks of age, when the baby is tolerating feedings.

- *Non-breastfeeding babies:* Iron supplementation may be given in the form of formula that contains iron or as an additional medication. Formulas described previously that are designed for preterm babies contain iron sufficient to provide 2 mg/kg of elemental iron per day for babies who are receiving full feedings.
- *Breastfeeding babies:* Preterm babies who are receiving plain breast milk, breast milk with fortifier, or less than 24 oz/d of preterm discharge formula should be given 2 mg/kg of liquid ferrous sulfate daily at approximately 2 to 4 weeks of age and continuing through the first 12 months of age. The dose of iron in a preparation of vitamins with iron (10 mg in 1 mL) will provide sufficient iron for preterm breastfed babies until they weigh more than 5 kg (>11 lb).

NOTE: With the practice of delaying cord clamping, it may be that iron supplementation for preterm newborns can be delayed. (It is well established that growing preterm infants are at increased risk for iron deficiency anemia, but timing and dosing of iron supplementation is affected by iron stores and the content of feedings.)

When iron is administered as an additional medication, make certain a baby is tolerating feedings well before beginning supplementation.

Self-test B

Now answer these questions to test yourself on the information in the last section. Refer to the graphs or charts in the unit, as necessary, to answer these questions.

B1. True False Vitamins given orally or through a feeding tube should be diluted with the volume of a full feeding or split over several feedings.

B2. A baby weighing 2,250 g (4 lb 15½ oz) will not ingest more than 30 mL (1 oz) of formula every 4 hours on the third day after birth. What should be done for this baby?

_____

B3. A baby born at 27 weeks' gestational age, with a birth weight of 1,050 g (2 lb 5 oz), weighs this much on the following days:
1,350 g (2 lb 15½ oz) at 30 days
1,450 g (3 lb 3 oz) at 34 days
1,540 g (3 lb 6 oz) at 38 days
1,600 g (3 lb 8½ oz) at 40 days
Is this baby following the expected growth pattern? ____ **Yes** ____ **No**

B4. Vitamins for preterm babies

Yes	No	
____	____	Are unnecessary if a baby is receiving breast milk
____	____	Should be mixed into a baby's feedings
____	____	Should be given separately from a feeding
____	____	May be started when a baby is tolerating feedings well

Check your answers with the list that follows the Recommended Routines. Correct any incorrect answers and review the appropriate section in the unit.

Part 2: Tube Feeding

Objectives

In Part 2 of this unit you will learn

A. To recognize the associated risks of tube feedings

B. When tube feedings should be used

C. When tube feedings should not be used

D. How to feed a baby safely by using a feeding tube

1. What is tube feeding?

Tube feeding is a method of feeding babies who are too sick or too preterm to be fed by mouth. A feeding tube is inserted into the baby's nose or mouth, down the esophagus, and into the baby's stomach. Breast milk or formula is given through this tube.

2. When are tube feedings necessary?

A. Preterm babies (<32–34 weeks' gestational age)
   To be able to be fed successfully via nipple, the baby must be able to coordinate

   - Sucking
   - Swallowing
   - Breathing

   Also, the baby must have developed a gag reflex.

   Preterm babies may be able to do all of these things separately, but babies younger than 32 to 34 weeks' gestational age usually *cannot coordinate* these activities. If sucking, swallowing, and breathing are uncoordinated, or if the gag reflex is not yet present, a baby may aspirate milk while trying to feed.

   Babies at this gestational age will benefit from skin-to-skin time to help develop breastfeeding readiness by smelling, licking, and tasting expressed milk directly from the breast.

B. Certain sick babies (>34 weeks' gestational age)
   Certain conditions in babies older than 34 weeks' gestational age will prevent them from being fed safely via nipple.

   - *Severe neurological problems* may be associated with an absent gag reflex. Any baby with an absent gag reflex should *not* be fed via nipple.
   - *Severe medical problems,* such as sepsis, may make a baby so lethargic that the baby is unable to be fed via nipple. Septic babies also may develop an ileus and may need to receive nothing by mouth and be given intravenous fluids until they are stable and bowel sounds are heard.

C. At-risk babies requiring continuing care
   Babies who were sick and have recovered from their acute illness but are not yet well may need tube feedings. These may include babies who have a gag reflex and are able to coordinate sucking, swallowing, and breathing but tire easily from the exertion of nipple feeding. Tube feedings may be needed to supplement nipple feedings initially for a baby to be able to receive adequate nutrition.

D. Babies with respiratory distress
   Any baby, regardless of gestational age, who has a respiratory rate of more than approximately 60 breaths per minute with evidence of increased work of breathing or who requires oxygen for acute lung disease should *not* receive enteral feedings. These babies should receive nothing by mouth and should be given only intravenous fluids until their work of breathing has returned to normal. Breastfed babies who are designated to receive nothing by mouth or who are receiving tube feedings only can receive oral care by using colostrum or breast milk, as long as they are hemodynamically stable. Oral care with colostrum or breast milk for stable babies prior to the initiation of feedings benefits the developing immune system. If a baby requires long-term intensive care and is still in

mild respiratory distress at several days of age, *cautious* tube feedings may be appropriate. If respiratory distress is severe or prolonged, parenteral nutrition should be provided in a neonatal intensive care unit.

3. How do you decide whether to use a nasogastric or an orogastric tube?

The decision to use a nasogastric or orogastric tube is often based on personal preference. However, the following factors should be considered:

- Nasogastric tubes can usually be taped in place more securely.
- Because of the relatively large oral cavity, babies tend to push orogastric tubes out of their mouths with their tongues. Therefore, orogastric tubes may be more likely to become dislodged during a feeding, thus increasing the chance of aspiration.
- A baby can work on oral feeding with either tube in place, but it is easier for the baby to get a good seal for sucking if a nasogastric tube is in place for supplementation purposes.
- Babies weighing less than 2,000 g (<4 lb 6½ oz) who depend on nasal patency for breathing move significantly less air when one nostril is partially blocked with a nasogastric tube. Orogastric tubes may, therefore, be preferable for small babies who have respiratory distress or apneic spells.

4. How are tube feedings administered?

A feeding tube is inserted through the baby's nose or mouth, down the throat and esophagus, and into the stomach. The upper end of the tube is taped to the baby's lip or cheek to hold the tube in place, and the lower end of the tube lies in the baby's stomach.

A syringe barrel, with plunger removed, is connected to the tube. At each feeding, a calculated volume of milk is placed in the syringe barrel, and gravity causes the milk to drip into the baby's stomach.

The syringe should be changed with each feeding, but the same feeding tube may be used for several feedings. Tube placement should be checked before *every* feeding.

 Do not leave a baby unattended while a tube feeding is being given.

Whenever a radiograph is obtained of a baby with a feeding tube in place, check to be sure the tube tip is 1.5 to 2.0 cm below the lower esophageal sphincter. This location will ensure that the milk flows into the baby's stomach.

Details for all of these steps are given in the Nasogastric Tube Feedings skill unit.

Self-test C

Now answer these questions to test yourself on the information in the last section.

C1. Which of the following babies should have tube feedings instead of oral feedings?

Yes	No	
____	____	A baby born at 31 weeks' gestational age who is large for gestational age without respiratory distress
____	____	An active baby born at 40 weeks' gestational age who requires treatment for hypoglycemia
____	____	A baby born at 35 weeks' gestational age who is appropriate for gestational age with tachypnea, grunting, and retractions and requiring 60% oxygen

C2. List the 3 activities the baby must be able to coordinate to manage nipple feedings successfully.

_____

_____

_____

C3. What reflex must be well developed for the baby to manage nipple feedings safely?

_____

Check your answers with the list that follows the Recommended Routines. Correct any incorrect answers and review the appropriate section in the unit.

5. What is the protocol for tube feedings?

- Use the information in part 1 of this unit to determine the volume of each feeding.
- Before *every* feeding
  - Assess the baby for signs and symptoms of feeding intolerance.
  - Make sure the tube is in the stomach by using a combination of assessment methods, such as measurement at the nares, aspiration and assessment of aspirate contents, and auscultation of injected air (details can be found in the Nasogastric Tube Feedings skill unit).
  - For best practice, it is recommended to not routinely check residuals. A focused physical examination should always be completed. See the focused physical assessment feeding algorithm in Figure 6.3.

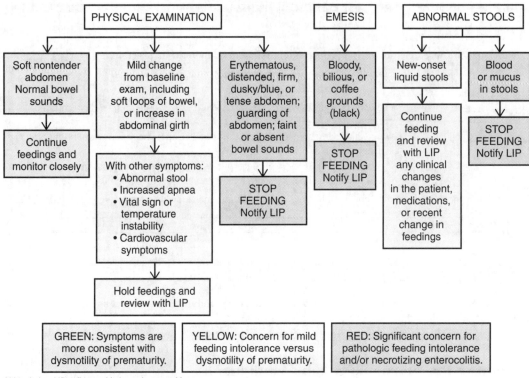

Figure 6.3. Focused Physical Assessment Feeding Algorithm

— If residual checks are still practiced in your institution, follow these steps below:
- If the clinical examination findings are typical and there are no additional signs of feeding intolerance, residuals may not be considered clinically significant in some instances.
  — Volume is less than 2 mL, regardless of feeding volume.
  — Volume is less than 25% for feeding volumes more than 10 mL every 3 hours.
- Refeed the residual milk and stomach contents through the feeding tube. This fluid contains electrolytes and other necessary body chemicals. It is important to replace these stomach contents.

Note: When *first* inserting a gastric tube, there may be a large volume of fluid in the stomach, particularly if a baby is only a few hours old. This residual amniotic fluid may be discarded if it is believed to be interfering with respiratory effort.

- If the residual is more than 25% of feeding volumes greater than 10 mL every 3 hours, consider subtracting the amount from the total to be fed through the tube. If residuals are persistent and increasing in volume, consult your regional perinatal center.

Note: Some institutions will only subtract the residual amount from the next feeding if the residual is more than 50% of the feeding volume.

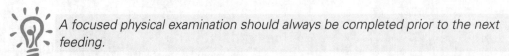

A focused physical examination should always be completed prior to the next feeding.

- Pour the amount of milk for a tube feeding into the syringe barrel and allow gravity to cause it to drip into the baby's stomach.

- Recalculate the volume of milk a baby needs as the baby grows and gains weight. When tube feedings are used, a baby has no control over how much milk is taken with each feeding.

6. When are tube feedings stopped?

A. When they are no longer needed

Continue to observe the baby for indications that the baby is ready to begin oral feeding:

- Strong sucking reflex
- Coordinated sucking and swallowing
- Alertness before feeding and sleep after feeding

All of the following should be documented before tube feedings are stopped and nipple feedings are started:

- The baby must have attained 32 to 34 weeks' gestational age
- The baby must have developed a gag reflex and can coordinate sucking, swallowing, and breathing
- The baby must have no respiratory problems
- The baby must have vital signs, color, and activity within reference range

B. When they are not tolerated

Feeding intolerance may indicate serious intestinal pathology, such as necrotizing entero-colitis or obstruction, or reflect sepsis or poor gastrointestinal motility.

Evidence of successful feeding includes

- Abdominal examination findings within reference range
- Active bowel sounds
- Stooling

Signs of feeding intolerance include

- Emesis
- Bilious aspirates
- Abdominal distension or increase in abdominal girth
- Visible loops of bowel
- Abdominal discoloration
- Grossly bloody, watery, or visually abnormal stools
- Clinical instability or acute deterioration
- Abnormal kidney, ureter, or bladder
- Residuals more than 50% of the full feeding volume or persistent or increasing residuals, if residual checks are still practiced in your institution

When there are signs of feeding intolerance, tube feedings should be held until the baby is evaluated by a physician or nurse practitioner. The decision may be made to interrupt feedings until the cause of feeding intolerance is determined. In the presence of feeding intolerance, consult your regional perinatal center and query additional workup. The baby should be supported with intravenous fluids while not feeding. Orders to give the baby nothing by mouth should be reviewed daily.

In a baby who previously had normal physical examination findings, concerning focused physical examination findings may indicate a serious intestinal problem, such as necrotizing enterocolitis. These babies must be carefully evaluated for signs of feeding intolerance to determine if feedings should continue or if radiographic evaluation is needed.

7. Are any other techniques used to feed preterm babies?

Spoon-feeding, finger feeding, use of an at-breast lactation aid device, and cup feeding are used by some regional perinatal centers as an alternative to an artificial bottle nipple in feeding the preterm baby older than 34 weeks' gestational age who is cleared for oral feeding or receiving breast milk or whose mother's goal is to eventually breastfeed when the baby is able. With any feeding method, the goal is to have the baby associate feeding with rooting, opening the mouth widely, and suckling for a few minutes prior to the release of milk.

Some babies are able to go back and forth between feeding methods with ease from the beginning, but it is not possible to predict which babies will have trouble. No matter the feeding method used, it is best to involve behaviors that will help babies eventually succeed at the breast. Nipple shields can be a useful tool to assist babies with transitioning to the breast from alternate methods of feeding, but these should be used in conjunction with a lactation consultation. Techniques such as spoon-feeding, finger feeding, and cup feeding are considered safe if done properly. For more information, see the current AAP policy statement (*Pediatrics.* 2012;129[3]:e827–e841), and the Academy of Breastfeeding Medicine clinical protocol on supplementation (*Breastfeed Med.* 2009;4[3]:175–182). Updated AAP guidelines are anticipated in 2021.

FEEDING

Recommended Routines

All the routines listed below are based on the principles of perinatal care presented in the unit you have just finished. They are recommended as part of routine perinatal care.

Read each routine carefully and decide whether it is standard operating procedure in your hospital. Check the appropriate blank next to each routine.

Procedure Standard in My Hospital	Needs Discussion by Our Staff	Recommended Routine
_____	_____	1a. Establish a feeding policy for your hospital that includes evidence-based breastfeeding and breast milk handling education, procedures, and support. Sample model hospital policies are available from the AAP (https://www.aap.org/en-us/advocacy-and-policy/aap-health-initiatives/Breastfeeding/Documents/Hospital_Breastfeeding_Policy.pdf) and Academy of Breastfeeding Medicine (*Breastfeed Med.* 2010;5[4]:173–177).
		1b. Establish norms for choice of growth curves, such as Fenton curves for preterm infants and www.newbornweight.org curves for the first week and month for infants older than $35^{0/7}$ weeks' gestation.
_____	_____	2. Establish a policy of withholding feedings and administering intravenous fluids to all babies who • Have a history of maternal hydramnios, until a diagnosis is established • Have excessive mucus, until a diagnosis is established • Have depressed, rapid, or labored respirations • Are vomiting, have distended abdomens, or have not produced stool by 48 hours after birth • Required prolonged resuscitation • Are acutely unstable for any other reason • Have bilious emesis

(continued)

239

_____   _____   3. Establish a policy of withholding nipple feedings, other than pre-suckling and feeding behaviors during skin-to-skin contact with the mother as tolerated, and using tube feedings for babies younger than 32 to 34 weeks' gestational age.

_____   _____   4. Establish a policy for preterm babies of using breast milk (from a baby's own mother), donor breast milk, or isosmolar formulas designed specifically for preterm babies (if breast milk is not available) (https://www.liebertpub.com/doi/full/10.1089/bfm.2017.29047.aje and https://www.hmbana.org/news/blog.html/article/2018/12/19/2019-guide-on-handling-human-milk-has-new-thawing-recommendations-over-1000-cited-references-and-more).

_____   _____   5. Establish a routine for determining the amount and frequency of feedings for babies, according to their gestational age and weight, or the expected weight for babies who are small for gestational age, with an emphasis on cue-based feeding for oral feedings and a minimum number of 8 to 12 feedings per 24 hours, rather than set schedules that do not take into account babies' sleep-wake cycles.

_____   _____   6. Establish a policy of weighing every baby daily and plotting the weight on a growth curve.

_____   _____   7. Establish a policy of providing vitamin and iron supplementation to preterm babies through the use of a formula designed specifically for preterm babies or with supplements added to formula or breast milk.

Self-test Answers

These are the answers to the Self-test questions. Please check them with the answers you gave and review the information in the unit wherever necessary.

Self-test A

A1. The baby may aspirate the milk.

A2. C. Insert an orogastric or nasogastric tube and evaluate for obstruction before feeding.

A3. False *Reason:* Formulas, medications, or vitamins with high osmolarity are more likely to damage the gastrointestinal tract of a newborn, particularly a preterm baby, than isosmolar substances (that have the same osmolarity as breast milk). Formulas designed specifically for preterm babies contain extra calories, vitamins, and minerals in an isosmolar concentration.

A4. Every 2 to 3 hours, 8 to 12 times in a 24-hour period

A5. A. Every 3 to 4 hours
     B. Small for gestational age
     C. 150 mL × 2.3 kg = 345 mL divided into 8 feedings = 43 mL. A small-for-gestational-age baby might also need 24 kcal/oz formula or breast milk to meet caloric and protein needs.

A6. A. Intravenous fluids only

Self-test B

B1. True

B2. Peripheral intravenous line started to supplement the baby's fluid intake; check blood glucose screening tests.

B3. Yes

B4. Yes   No
     ___   _X_   Are unnecessary if a baby is receiving breast milk
     _X_   ___   Should be mixed into a baby's feedings
     ___   _X_   Should be given separately from a feeding
     _X_   ___   May be started when a baby is tolerating feedings well

Self-test C

C1. Yes   No
     _X_   ___   A baby born at 31 weeks' gestational age who is large for gestational age without respiratory distress (tube feedings should be used, unless the baby is breastfeeding, in which case many clinicians would allow the baby to feed at the breast if the baby has demonstrated stable vital signs, color, and activity)

     ___   _X_   An active baby born at 40 weeks' gestational age who requires treatment for hypoglycemia (tube feedings are not necessarily indicated; as long as the blood glucose level has been brought within reference range and the baby is alert, the baby may feed by bottle or breast, in addition to the intravenous glucose therapy used to treat the baby's hypoglycemia)

     ___   _X_   A baby born at 35 weeks' gestational age who is appropriate for gestational age with tachypnea, grunting, and retractions and requiring 60% oxygen (tube feedings should not be given; this baby should be given nothing by mouth and should receive only intravenous fluids for the first several days after birth)

C2. Sucking
     Swallowing
     Breathing

C3. Gag reflex

Unit 6 Posttest

After completion of each unit there is a free online posttest available at www.cmevillage.com to test your understanding. Navigate to the PCEP pages on www.cmevillage.com and register to take the free posttests.

Once registered on the website and after completing all the unit posttests, pay the book exam fee ($15) and pass the test at 80% or greater to earn continuing education credits. Only start the PCEP book exam if you have time to complete it. If you take the book exam and are not connected to a printer, either print your certificate to a .pdf file and save it to print later or come back to www.cmevillage.com at any time and print a copy of your educational transcript.

Credits are only available by book, not by individual unit within the books. Available credits for completion of each book exam are as follows: Book 1: 14.5 credits; Book 2: 16 credits; Book 3: 17 credits; Book 4: 9 credits.

For more details, navigate to the PCEP webpages at www.cmevillage.com.

SKILL UNIT

Nasogastric Tube Feedings

This skill unit will teach you how to insert a nasogastric tube and how to feed a baby by using a nasogastric tube. The techniques for inserting an orogastric tube and using it to feed a baby are almost identical to those for a nasogastric tube. The differences between nasogastric and orogastric tubes are indicated in the appropriate steps.

Study this skill unit and attend a skill session to practice and demonstrate this skill. Then arrange with your coordinator(s) to insert a feeding tube the next time a baby in your hospital needs one.

To master the skill, you will need to demonstrate each of the following steps correctly:

1. Collect and prepare the equipment.

2. Measure the tube.

3. Insert the tube.

4. Check the placement of the tube.

5. Tape the tube in place.

6. Position the baby for a tube feeding.

7. Feed the baby.

Nasogastric Tube Feedings

ACTIONS	REMARKS

Deciding Whether Tube Feeding Is Appropriate

1. Should enteral feeding be used for this baby?

   • Does the baby have acute respiratory distress or other acute illness, particularly during the first few days after birth?

   Yes: Enteral feedings, given with any method, may *not* be appropriate.

   No: Does the baby have any of these conditions?

   — Gestational age younger than 34 weeks

   — Lacks a gag reflex or cannot coordinate sucking, swallowing, and breathing

   — Too weak to feed well via nipple

   — Is recovering from acute respiratory disease and is several days of age or older but is still requiring supplemental oxygen or has an increased respiratory rate

   If yes for any of these conditions: Consider tube feedings or maintain intravenous nutrition.

Preparing to Insert a Nasogastric Tube

2. Collect the following items:

   • 5F or 6.5F Feeding tube

   • 2 Clean syringes

   — 1 Small syringe (5 mL)

   — 1 Large syringe (sized appropriately for the volume of feeding to be given)

   • Stethoscope

   • Tape or a permanent marker

   • Tape to secure the tube to the baby's lip

   • Masking tape or other appropriate method of hanging the feeding syringe

REMARKS:

Select the smallest size tube that will deliver the feeding volume in the desired time.

To check tube placement

To hold the milk for feeding

To mark the length of tube to be inserted when measurement markers are not found on the tube

To hold the barrel of the syringe with milk to the top of the incubator or to the caregiver's or parent's clothing, if the baby will be held during the feeding

ACTIONS   **REMARKS**

Preparing to Insert a Nasogastric Tube (continued)

- Lubricant or sterile water

To lubricate the tube before insertion

- Clear adhesive dressing film (several commercial brands are available)

To protect the baby's lip and cheek from the adhesive tape

- Glove
- Milk to be fed to the baby

Inserting a Nasogastric Tube

3. Measure length of feeding tube needed for the baby.
   - Turn the baby's head to one side (the naris to be used is facing up).
   - Hold the tube as you measure.
   - Begin to measure with the tip of the tube at the opening of the naris into which the tube will be inserted.
   - Keeping the tip in place, extend the tube to the earlobe.
   - Extend the tube from the earlobe to a point midway between the tip of the sternum and the umbilicus.

   Note: When inserting an orogastric tube, measure from the baby's mouth, rather than the nose.

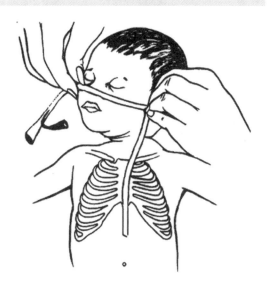

4. If the tube has markers on it, note the one that is closest to the baby's nose. Record it on the baby's chart. As the baby grows, be sure to remeasure often and note the new insertion length.

   If the tube is unmarked, wrap the small piece of adhesive tape around it to mark the point where the tube touches the end of the baby's nose, or mark it with the permanent marker.

ACTIONS   **REMARKS**

Inserting a Nasogastric Tube (continued)

Note: For very-low-birth-weight babies, minimal insertion lengths have been identified.

Only a few hospitals care for babies this size. For those that do, these minimal insertion lengths should be used *only as a guide*. Each baby should be measured and tube placement checked whenever a feeding tube is inserted.

Daily Weight (not birth weight)	<750 g (<1 lb 10 oz)	750–999 g (1 lb 10 oz to 2 lb 3 oz)	1,000–1,249 g (2 lb 3 oz to 2 lb 12 oz)	1,250–1,499 g (2 lb 12 oz to 3 lb 5 oz)
Insertion Length	13 cm	15 cm	16 cm	17 cm

5. Cut a piece of clear adhesive dressing (3 × ½ inches). Place this across the baby's upper lip and the cheek on the side of the naris to be used.

This is used to protect the baby's skin from adhesive tape. The adhesive tape is placed on top of clear adhesive dressing.

6. Prepare adhesive tape that will hold the nasogastric tube to the baby's lip.

  • Cut 2 pieces of ½-inch adhesive tape 4 inches (10 cm) long.

  • Split each piece for half its length.

  • Stick the unsplit section of the tape and one tab across the baby's upper lip (on top of the clear adhesive dressing).

  • Leave half of the split tape loose to wrap around the tube later.

7. Position the baby supine.

If the baby is active, you may need assistance. The baby can be swaddled, when appropriate.

8. Insert the lubricated nasogastric tube into the baby's nose. Continue pushing the tube gently and quickly into the naris and down the throat.

Some babies gag when the tube touches the back of their throat. The gag reflex may be decreased with extension of the nasal pharynx when beginning insertion. Gagging is normal, and you can continue inserting the tube after quickly assessing the baby.

Slightly flexing the baby's head can be helpful after the catheter passes through the pharynx. If the tube comes out of the baby's mouth instead of going down the baby's throat, or if the baby continues to gag, remove the tube and start again.

If the baby turns blue, remove the tube immediately. An uncommon complication of this procedure has occurred—the tube has entered the trachea, rather than the esophagus.

ACTIONS   REMARKS

Inserting a Nasogastric Tube (continued)

9. Stop when the measured marker is at the   Note this measurement before every feeding.
   baby's naris.

Checking the Placement of a Feeding Tube

 The reference standard for assessing appropriate tube placement is radiography. The distal end of the feeding tube should be located just below the 12th thoracic vertebra. If the practitioner is skilled in this procedure, then it is appropriate to use the following methods to check placement, instead of obtaining a radiograph.

10. Assess the condition of the baby,   The status of the newborn is a significant
    especially the respiratory status.   component of confirming placement of
                                                 the tube.

11. Aspirate and assess the stomach fluid.   Note the fluid volume, and refeed it to the
                                                 baby's stomach via the tube.

                                                 The gastric contents can appear clear, off-
                                                 white, grassy green, tan, or brown tinged.
                                                 The intestinal content should be bile stained,
                                                 light to dark golden yellow, or brownish
                                                 green.

                                                 Placing the baby on the left side may
                                                 facilitate obtaining aspirate.

                                                 Injecting air may also move the tube away
                                                 from the baby's stomach wall.

12. Draw 1 to 2 mL of air into the small,
    5-mL syringe.

13. Attach the syringe to the open end of
    the tube.

14. Put a stethoscope over the baby's stomach
    (the upper left quadrant of the abdomen).

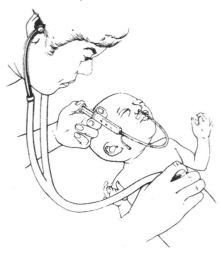

ACTIONS   REMARKS

Checking the Placement of a Feeding Tube (continued)

15. While listening with the stethoscope over the baby's stomach, quickly push in 1 to 2 mL of air with the syringe. Listen for the sound of the air entering the baby's stomach.

    Rumbling heard in the stomach when air is pushed through the tube (often described as a "whoosh") suggests it is in the stomach and not the lungs. However, air may sometimes be heard in the stomach, even when the tube tip is not correctly placed.

16. Withdraw the air from the stomach.

17. Wrap the remainder of the loose end of adhesive tape in a spiral around the tube to hold it in place.

    Note: An orogastric tube may be taped to a baby's cheek, by using the same method described for taping a nasogastric tube to a baby's lip.

    When correct placement has been determined, the tube can be secured.

    If there is any doubt the tube has not been placed correctly, remove it and start over, or request a radiograph before using the tube for feeding.

18. Further stabilize the nasogastric or orogastric tube by curving the tube onto the cheek and taping it to the clear adhesive dressing.

First Feeding Through the Tube

19. Position the baby for feeding; incline the incubator so the baby's head is raised.

    Consider positioning the baby on the right side, because this position aids the emptying of the stomach.

20. Remove the plunger from the large syringe.

21. Attach the barrel of the syringe to the tube.

22. Attach the masking tape to the barrel of the syringe so half of the tape hangs free (or use another preferred method). This half will be used to attach the barrel to the top of the incubator or to the caregiver's clothing.

    If the baby will be held throughout the feeding, the syringe barrel may be taped to the clothing of the caregiver or parent so that the bottom of the barrel hangs a few inches above the baby.

ACTIONS   REMARKS

First Feeding Through the Tube (continued)

23. Pour a measured amount of milk into the barrel of the syringe.

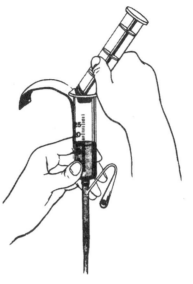

24. Start the flow of milk by allowing gravity to cause the milk to drip.

    • Insert the plunger loosely in the syringe.

    • Push the plunger a little to start the milk.

    • Tilt the plunger to the side to release the vacuum in the barrel.

    • Remove the plunger.

    Do not push the plunger in very far. You must be able to remove the plunger without withdrawing milk from the tube.

25. Tape the barrel to the top of the incubator or caregiver's clothing with the masking tape.

    It is recommended that the baby suck on a pacifier during the feeding. This may be soothing to the baby, may facilitate later nipple feeding, and has been shown to aid gastric motility.

    If the baby is stable and the parents are available, skin-to-skin contact can be done during the feeding.

26. Feed the baby for 15 to 30 minutes.

    Never leave a baby unattended during a tube feeding. If the tube slips out of position, a baby can easily aspirate a large amount of milk. If the milk runs in too fast, a baby may have rapid gastric distension, making it more likely the baby will regurgitate some of the feeding or develop diarrhea.

    Use a 5F or 6.5F feeding tube rather than an 8F tube. An 8F tube allows the milk to run in too quickly.

ACTIONS	REMARKS

First Feeding Through the Tube (continued)

27. When all milk has run into the tube:

- Remove the barrel of the syringe from the tube.

Depending on the volume of milk a baby should receive, you may need to fill the barrel of the 12- or 20-mL syringe more than once during a feeding.

- Leave the tube open.

This allows a "vent" for the baby's stomach and minimizes the chance a baby will aspirate milk or stomach juices. The vent makes it less likely a baby will burp or vomit between feedings.

- Keep the baby in the head-up position for 30 minutes.

Some people prefer to remove the tube after the feeding and insert a new tube before each feeding. Be sure there is no milk left in the syringe or visible in the feeding tube. Then pinch the tube tightly and withdraw it quickly.

Later Feedings With the Tube

28. Position the baby for feeding.

- Incline the incubator so the baby's head is raised.

- Consider positioning the baby on the right side.

29. Check for the correct placement of the tube by using any combination of the following assessment methods: noting the previous measure marker at the naris; listening over the stomach while pushing a small amount of air into the tube; or assessing the baby's abdominal girth.

Always check the position of the tube and the general gastrointestinal status of the baby before *every* feeding. Even a correctly placed tube can slip out of the stomach between feedings.

If there is any doubt the tube is not correctly placed, remove it and start over or request a radiograph before using the tube for feeding.

Measuring the Milk Left in the Stomach From Previous Feeding

30. Attach a 3-, 5-, or 10-mL syringe to the tube and gently pull back the plunger until you feel increased pressure. Withdraw liquid from the stomach until no more fluid can be aspirated.

You are withdrawing residual food and digestive juices left in the stomach from the previous feeding.

31. Observe how much liquid from the previous feeding is in the syringe.

32. Record the amount of liquid from the previous feeding on the patient record.

ACTIONS   **REMARKS**

Measuring the Milk Left in the Stomach From Previous Feeding (continued)

33. This liquid is generally too thick to allow gravity to cause it to drip back into the stomach. Therefore, gently push the liquid back into the tube with the syringe. Push slowly, so the liquid goes in at a rate of 1 to 2 mL per minute.

If you push the liquid back quickly, the baby may vomit.

Generally, you do not want to throw away liquid from the baby's stomach. It contains electrolytes the baby needs to maintain stable body chemistry levels. However, excessive thick mucus or meconium in the stomach may be discarded before the first feeding.

34. Compute the amount of milk needed to complete the feeding.

   Large or repeated aspirates may indicate a baby has an ileus or is otherwise sick.

Consider subtracting the residual amount from the total feeding volume if it is more than 25% of feeding volumes greater than 10 mL every 3 hours.

What Can Go Wrong?

1. The tube may be inserted into the airway instead of the stomach, or the tube may not have been inserted far enough and may thus still be in the esophagus.

The most dangerous consequence of tube feedings is that milk may go into a baby's lungs.

When in doubt, never put fluids into the nasogastric or orogastric tube.

This can happen because the tube is

- Positioned in the esophagus rather than the stomach. The milk may fill the esophagus and overflow into the trachea and lungs.

- Inserted into the trachea rather than down the esophagus, and milk is instilled directly into the lungs.

You must check the placement of a tube before every feeding. Follow your institution's protocol for assessing tube placement.

2. You may overfeed or underfeed the baby.

Calculate volumes carefully. Feed slowly by allowing gravity to cause the milk to drip. When tube feedings are used, the baby has no control over how much milk is taken with each feeding.

3. The tube may perforate the stomach or esophagus.

This is a *rare* complication that may happen during insertion of the tube. Do not force the tube during insertion.

ACTIONS	REMARKS

What Can Go Wrong? (continued)

4. You leave a baby unattended.	The feeding tube may slip or be pulled loose by the baby. If this happens, milk may flow into the baby's lungs. or The milk may stop flowing, causing a delay in the baby receiving the feeding.
5. You fail to check the tube position when a radiograph is obtained.	Whenever a radiograph is obtained of a baby with a feeding tube in place, the position of the tube tip should be noted. Be sure the end and side holes are in the stomach. The distal end should be approximately located at the 12th thoracic vertebra.

Unit 7: Hyperbilirubinemia

Objectives

In this unit you will learn

A. The causes of hyperbilirubinemia and the factors that affect its severity

B. To recognize babies at risk for hyperbilirubinemia

C. To determine the appropriate treatment(s) for hyperbilirubinemia

D. To operate phototherapy lights for maximum effectiveness

E. To assess a baby's risk for severe hyperbilirubinemia

 Recommendations in this unit incorporate American Academy of Pediatrics guidelines given in Pediatrics. *2004;114(1):297–316. Updated guidelines are anticipated in 2021.*

Unit 7 Pretest

Before reading the unit, please answer the following questions. Select the *one best* answer to each question (unless otherwise instructed). Record your answers on the test and check them with the answers at the end of the book.

1. In an otherwise healthy baby, which of the following bilirubin levels would be of most immediate concern to you?
   A. Bilirubin level of 12 mg/dL at 30 hours of age in a full-term baby
   B. Bilirubin level of 8 mg/dL at 2 weeks of age in a breastfeeding baby
   C. Bilirubin level of 9 mg/dL at 10 hours of age in a full-term baby
   D. Bilirubin level of 17 mg/dL in a 3-day-old breastfeeding baby

2. For which of the following babies would you expect the binding capacity of serum protein for bilirubin to be *least* affected?
   A. A baby receiving ceftriaxone
   B. A baby who had a 5-minute Apgar score of 3
   C. A baby with an infection
   D. A baby with hypertension

3. When a baby is jaundiced, which of the following actions is the first you should take?
   A. Begin phototherapy.
   B. Obtain blood samples for laboratory tests.
   C. Restrict feedings.
   D. Perform exchange transfusion.

4. Visible jaundice appearing within 24 hours of birth is usually
   A. Physiological
   B. Caused by human (breast) milk
   C. Caused by bilirubin levels outside of reference range

5. Newborns are more likely than adults to have hyperbilirubinemia because
   A. They have decreased removal of bilirubin by the liver.
   B. Their diet consists of only breast milk or formula.
   C. They have fewer red blood cells.
   D. They have decreased reabsorption of bilirubin in the intestines.

6. The bilirubin of babies with very low Apgar scores may be dangerous at _____ bilirubin level than for a baby with high Apgar scores.
   A. a lower
   B. the same
   C. a higher

7. All of the following complications are possible results of phototherapy, except
   A. Increased number of stools
   B. Anemia
   C. Obstructed nasal breathing
   D. Hyperthermia

(continued)

Unit 7 Pretest (*continued*)

8. All of the following laboratory tests are routine in the investigation of hyperbilirubinemia, except
   A. Platelet count
   B. Coombs (antiglobulin) test
   C. Hematocrit value
   D. Blood smear

9. When treating a baby with phototherapy lights, you would

Yes	No	
____	____	Cover the baby's eyes only for the first 8 hours of phototherapy.
____	____	Discontinue phototherapy immediately if a rash appears.
____	____	Completely undress the baby down to the diaper.
____	____	Restrict the baby's fluid intake.
____	____	Restrict the baby's feedings.

10. **True** **False** All jaundiced babies should receive phototherapy.

11. **True** **False** Jaundice associated with breastfeeding is seen only during the first 3 days after birth.

12. **True** **False** Sepsis increases the risk from hyperbilirubinemia.

1. What is bilirubin?

Bilirubin is formed from hemoglobin as a by-product of the breakdown of red blood cells. It is a waste product that must be eliminated from the body. In high concentrations, bilirubin is toxic to the brain and most tissues of the body.

 Excess bilirubin can cause brain damage.

Bilirubin toxicity is preventable in nearly all cases.

If toxicity occurs, *acute bilirubin encephalopathy* is used to describe the clinical findings during the first weeks after birth; *kernicterus* is used for chronic and permanent clinical findings of bilirubin toxicity, including vision or hearing loss and cerebral palsy.

Bilirubin can be present in the blood in 2 forms:

- Direct-reacting or conjugated form
- Indirect-reacting or unconjugated form

2. How is bilirubin removed from the body?

Elimination of bilirubin occurs in several steps.

A. Bound to serum albumin
Unconjugated bilirubin in the blood is bound to serum albumin and is then transported to the liver.

B. Processed by the liver
In the liver, bilirubin becomes conjugated, so it can be excreted.

C. Excreted in the stool
Conjugated bilirubin is carried in the bile into the intestine, where it is further processed and then excreted in the stool. In newborns, as in fetuses, conjugated bilirubin in the gut can be deconjugated and reabsorbed into the serum as unconjugated bilirubin via a process called *enterohepatic circulation.*

3. How is bilirubin measured and detected?

Laboratories report bilirubin levels as conjugated (also called *direct-reacting*) bilirubin, unconjugated (also called *indirect-reacting*) bilirubin, and total bilirubin (the sum of conjugated and unconjugated levels). Most bilirubin increases in newborns result from increased unconjugated bilirubin levels. In babies, therefore, unconjugated and total bilirubin values are nearly equal to each other. Unless stated otherwise, bilirubin levels given in this unit are total serum bilirubin (TSB) values.

Bilirubin is expressed in milligrams per 100 mL of blood (eg, 5 mg/100 mL). This value may also be noted as 5 mg/dL.

Transcutaneous bilirubin (TcB) may also be measured with any one of several commercially available noninvasive devices. TcB measurement devices can be used as screening tools. They provide valid estimates when the TSB level is less than 15 mg/dL, although some experts use 12 mg/dL as the cutoff for accurate correlation between TcB and TSB values.

Many experts recommend screening all newborns for hyperbilirubinemia with transcutaneous estimation or laboratory measurement at 24 or 36 hours of age prior to discharge from the hospital. While careful clinical examination can help detect most cases of jaundice in babies,

TcB or TSB screening may also be used. The American Academy of Pediatrics (AAP) recommends that all babies be screened with a predischarge bilirubin measurement via either TcB or TSB, and—at a minimum—undergo a careful examination and risk assessment. Whichever method is used, appropriate follow-up after discharge is critical to further assessing the baby's risk for jaundice.

4. What is hyperbilirubinemia?

Hyperbilirubinemia is an increased level of bilirubin in the blood, which causes jaundice. Jaundice is characterized by a yellowish appearance of the skin and, as it progresses, a yellowish coloring of the whites of the eyes.

For reasons that are not entirely clear, babies with increasing bilirubin levels generally show a progression of jaundice from head to toe. If a baby is yellow all over, the bilirubin level is probably higher than if jaundice is visible only in the face. The yellow skin coloring may be seen more easily by pressing your finger on the baby's skin, as if testing capillary refill time. Observe the color of the skin in the blanched area before capillary refill occurs. While visual assessment of jaundice is an important part of the physical examination for all babies, visual assessment alone is not considered a reliable method for determining the bilirubin level.

Jaundice occurs in most newborns and is benign in most cases. Bilirubin may have some protective properties, as it is a powerful antioxidant. Because bilirubin is potentially toxic at higher-than-physiological levels, however, it should be monitored. Assess newborns for jaundice whenever you check their vital signs; however, visual estimation of the *degree* of jaundice can be unreliable—especially in newborns with darkly pigmented skin. If jaundice is present, the only way to know the bilirubin level is to obtain a TcB or TSB measurement.

Phototherapy bleaches the skin, making transcutaneous estimates unreliable when phototherapy is being used. Phototherapy also makes it more difficult to recognize jaundice with visual inspection. TSB (laboratory) measurements should be used for infants who are or have been receiving phototherapy within the previous 24 to 36 hours.

5. What causes hyperbilirubinemia?

Bilirubin is higher in the blood of newborns, as compared with older children and adults, because there is

- *Faster breakdown* of a larger number of red blood cells (overproduction of bilirubin)
- *Less efficient removal* of bilirubin by the liver
- *Increased reabsorption* from the intestines of bilirubin that has been excreted by the liver

Although there are many causes of hyperbilirubinemia (see the Appendix in this unit), the most common are

A. Physiological
   Because of the 3 factors noted previously, approximately 65% of all newborns and 80% of all preterm newborns develop sufficient increases of bilirubin to result in jaundice during the first few days after birth.

B. Hemolytic disease (eg, Rh or ABO incompatibility; glucose-6-phosphate dehydrogenase [G6PD] deficiency; hereditary spherocytosis)
   Hemolysis, the rapid destruction of red blood cells, may result from a variety of conditions. With blood group incompatibility, an antibody from the mother causes hemolysis of the baby's red blood cells. With G6PD enzyme deficiency, or other inherited red blood cell abnormalities, hemolysis results from inherent fragility of the red blood cell.

C. Various neonatal conditions

Any condition that tends to worsen any of the 3 factors noted previously will increase the severity of hyperbilirubinemia. For example,

- Polycythemia, a cephalohematoma, or widespread bruising will intensify overproduction of bilirubin.
- Preterm birth is associated with decreased conjugation of bilirubin by the liver.
- Deconjugation and reabsorption of bilirubin will increase with poor feeding, intestinal obstruction, or ileus.

6. When is bilirubin dangerous to the brain?

Bilirubin is dangerous when it leaves the blood and enters the brain. In the normal state, nearly all bilirubin is bound to serum protein (primarily albumin). The capacity of serum protein to attract and hold bilirubin is called *binding capacity*. When there is an excess amount of bilirubin or an insufficient amount of serum protein, there is not enough binding space, and free bilirubin will result. Free bilirubin enters the brain easily. Under certain circumstances involving severe stress, such as hypoxia or acidosis, the blood-brain barrier is disturbed, and even bilirubin bound to protein may enter the brain and cause damage.

Therefore, bilirubin is most likely to cause brain damage when

- There is too much bilirubin for the serum protein level.
- Serum protein (albumin) levels are low.
- The binding capacity of serum protein is decreased.
- The baby has been severely stressed.

7. What factors influence hyperbilirubinemia?

Some factors increase the likelihood that hyperbilirubinemia will develop. Other factors increase the risk of damage that can occur because of hyperbilirubinemia. Still other factors are likely to influence the risk *of* and *from* hyperbilirubinemia.

A. Increased risk that hyperbilirubinemia will develop
   Hemolysis

   Rapid breakdown of red blood cells may be caused by

- Blood group incompatibility between mother and baby (ABO or Rh).
- G6PD deficiency (inherited enzyme deficiency), which is more common in populations originating from Mediterranean regions, the Middle East, the Arabian peninsula, Southeast Asia, and Africa—but migration and intermarriage have resulted in G6PD becoming more widespread. G6PD deficiency occurs in 11% to 13% of Black males and should be considered if severe hyperbilirubinemia develops, especially because, in general, Black babies have much lower TSB levels than white or Asian babies.
- A variety of neonatal illnesses, such as sepsis.

B. Increased risk of damage from hyperbilirubinemia
   1. Perinatal compromise (eg, hypoxia, acidosis, asphyxia)
   2. Serum albumin level less than 3 g/dL
   3. A sick baby, with any of the following conditions:
      - Significant lethargy
      - Temperature instability
      - Acidosis
      - Poor feeding and/or excessive weight loss

4. Certain drugs

Some medications decrease the serum albumin binding capacity by competing for binding sites. Examples of medications with high binding ratios include

- Salicylates
- Sulfonamides
- Some cephalosporin antibiotics, such as ceftriaxone

C. Increased risk of hyperbilirubinemia *and* associated risks

1. Prematurity

Preterm babies have immature livers, with a decreased ability to process bilirubin. Preterm babies are also more likely to be stressed and are therefore at risk for an impaired blood-brain barrier. They may also be poor feeders owing to being sleepy or having decreased muscle tone and/or lack of coordination. Furthermore, preterm babies often have low serum protein levels and, thus, have fewer bilirubin binding sites, with a resultant increased likelihood of free bilirubin.

2. Sepsis (blood infection)

Hemolysis, hepatocellular damage, poor intake, ileus, or acidosis may occur as a result of sepsis. As noted previously, these factors may increase bilirubin production (hemolysis), decrease bilirubin removal (liver cell damage), increase reabsorption of bilirubin (ileus), or increase risk of hyperbilirubinemia (acidosis).

Preterm birth, perinatal compromise, and infection are 3 important factors that increase the risks associated with hyperbilirubinemia.

Self-test A

Now answer these questions to test yourself on the information in the last section.

A1. What problem can result from hyperbilirubinemia?
_____

A2. What are 3 reasons why newborns have higher bilirubin levels than adults?
_____
_____
_____

A3. What does the binding capacity of serum protein mean?
    A. It is the cohesive property of blood that aids in clotting.
    B. It is the capacity of protein to bind bilirubin to hemoglobin.
    C. It is the capacity of serum protein to attract and hold bilirubin.

A4. **True**   **False**   Under certain conditions, bilirubin bound to protein can enter the brain.

A5. **True**   **False**   Careful visual inspection of a baby's jaundice provides reliable estimation of the serum bilirubin level.

A6. **True**   **False**   Transcutaneous bilirubin measurements are as reliable as serum bilirubin measurements at every bilirubin level.

A7. When is bilirubin dangerous to the brain?
_____

A8. Name at least 2 conditions that can make a given level of hyperbilirubinemia more dangerous.
_____
_____

Check your answers with the list that follows the Recommended Routines. Correct any incorrect answers and review the appropriate section in the unit.

8. What should be done when a baby becomes jaundiced?

If a baby becomes jaundiced during the first 24 hours after birth or is significantly jaundiced at any time, the bilirubin level should be measured. The baby should be examined, and laboratory and other data should be obtained to determine the cause of hyperbilirubinemia. A common mistake is to assume too quickly that jaundice is simply the result of physiological hyperbilirubinemia. There are many causes of an increased bilirubin level. Jaundice should be considered a possible sign of other conditions that may be affecting the baby.

In general, jaundice should not be considered physiological if
- *There is a family history of a first-degree relative having severe jaundice.*
- *It appears in the first 24 hours after birth.*
- *Bilirubin levels increase faster than 0.2 to 0.5 mg/dL per hour.*
- *There is evidence of hemolysis.*
- *Physical examination findings are atypical.*
- *The direct serum bilirubin level exceeds 20% of the total bilirubin level.*
- *Jaundice persists for more than 3 weeks.*

There are 3 kinds of information that should be collected to determine the cause of and appropriate treatment for hyperbilirubinemia.

A. History
- Review prenatal, labor, and delivery histories.
- Review notes for the baby's feeding and output patterns and changes in activity.
- Interview the family for history of first-degree relatives with a history of significant hemolytic disease or jaundice requiring phototherapy.
- Determine baby's ethnicity because enzyme abnormalities, such as G6PD deficiency, and other causes of hyperbilirubinemia are more common in certain ethnicities.

B. Physical examination
- Look for signs of acute or congenital infection (see Unit 8, Infections, in this book).
- Look for areas of accumulated extravasated blood (bruising, cephalohematoma).
- Check the size of the baby's liver and spleen (enlargement suggests the presence of hemolysis).

C. Laboratory tests
- Serum bilirubin (total and conjugated [direct-reacting] bilirubin) levels.
- Mother's and baby's blood group and type.
- Coombs (antiglobulin) test.
- Hematocrit and/or hemoglobin values.
Consider:
- Reticulocyte count.
- Blood smear.
- Other tests as indicated.

A more detailed description of how to determine the causes of jaundice and appropriate treatment is provided in the Appendix in this unit.

9. Does breastfeeding cause jaundice?

There is an association between poor breastfeeding and hyperbilirubinemia in newborns. Two syndromes are discussed. Most experts believe there is considerable overlap between the 2 syndromes.

A. Early-onset jaundice associated with poor feeding
Breastfed babies typically have higher levels of bilirubin than bottle-fed babies in the first several days after birth. The cause of this is not well understood, but it is considered physiological, and if breastfeeding is going well, the higher mean bilirubin levels in breastfed babies should not reach clinical significance. The risk of poor feeding as a contributing factor can be minimized through good breastfeeding support, including

- Family education and realistic expectations
- Feeding within the first hour of birth
- Keeping mother and baby together and responding to all feeding cues rather than a set schedule
- Teaching hand expression to maximize the milk production signaling to the mother's body and the amount of milk transfer
- Lactation consultation to ensure that attachment to the breast is comfortable for the mother, with no nipple compression or rubbing (indicative of attachment effectiveness), and to evaluate for evidence of milk transfer, such as swallowing and the breasts feeling softer or lighter after breastfeeding

If a breastfed baby develops clinically significant jaundice during the first week after birth, after assessing objective criteria to determine whether the baby is receiving adequate intake, such as weight pattern (www.newbornweight.org), output, clinical examination for mucous membranes and skin turgor, observation of feeding for maternal comfort and milk transfer, settling after feedings

- Evaluate the baby as described previously, to rule out other causes of hyperbilirubinemia.
- Encourage and support frequent breastfeeding (at least 8–12 times per 24 hours), and if there is evidence of the baby receiving insufficient intake, assist the mother with increasing her milk production signaling and milk transfer by hand expressing or pumping with each feeding and/or providing the baby with formula supplementation, as needed.
- In an otherwise thriving newborn, only if the bilirubin level is approaching 20 mg/dL or more in an effort to avoid an exchange transfusion would you need to consider temporarily interrupting breastfeeding, substituting formula (perhaps a completely hydrolyzed formula), and initiating phototherapy for 48 to 72 hours to allow the bilirubin level to decline. Every mother should be instructed to pump or express her milk every time the baby receives any formula, to maintain her milk supply. This expressed breast milk may be frozen for later use. As soon as the bilirubin level has begun to stabilize, breastfeeding should be resumed. This is not an indication for completely discontinuing breastfeeding.
  Supplementation with water or glucose water has been shown to be of no value in healthy term or near-term newborns.

B. Physiological late-onset jaundice

As many as 20% to 30% of breastfed babies will continue to have mildly increased levels of bilirubin after birth. The bilirubin level increases progressively and usually reaches a maximum by the fourth or fifth day of age (later in preterm babies) but can persist at a lower level for up to a few weeks. This is probably related to the increased rate of bilirubin reabsorption from the intestines in some breastfed babies or the inhibition of hepatic conjugation by compounds in some human (breast) milk.

If a breastfed baby continues to appear jaundiced or develops clinically significant jaundice during the *second* or *third* week after birth

- If not already done, consider instituting the measures outlined in Section 9A, "Early-onset jaundice associated with poor feeding."
- Fractionate the bilirubin to ensure it is unconjugated hyperbilirubinemia, as would be expected, and not direct or conjugated bilirubin.
- Assess whether the baby is receiving adequate oral intake by looking at the baby's weight gain (www.newbornweight.org) and output.
- Assess the color of the baby's stools. Pale or gray/white or "clay-colored" stools would be concerning for biliary atresia, which would require immediate attention and surgical intervention.
- Assess the baby for any underlying, alternative causes of jaundice, such as family history and infectious diseases, including subclinical urinary tract infections.
- If hyperbilirubinemia persists for more than 3 weeks, the levels may still be within the expected reference range for late-onset physiological jaundice, but consider consultation with regional perinatal center experts, as this is a diagnosis of exclusion.

10. How is hyperbilirubinemia treated?

It is important for babies with pathologic hyperbilirubinemia to receive adequate nutrition and be well hydrated. If there are no contraindications to oral feedings, enteral feedings should continue, to promote the excretion of bilirubin in the stool. If the baby is feeding orally by breast or bottle, effective feeding should be evaluated by

- Observation of feeding.
- Review of daily weight pattern (www.newbornweight.org).
- Assessing urine and stool output.
- Increasing the frequency of feedings and having the mother perform breast compression during feedings and hand expression after feedings, all of which will serve to maximize milk production signaling to her body and ensure that the baby is receiving adequate intake. Unless there is a medical indication (eg, dehydration, hypoglycemia, excessive weight loss) that is not being addressed through adequate breastfeeding management, it is not recommended that formula be added or breastfeeding be interrupted (*Breastfeed Med.* 2010;5[2]:87–93).

A. Phototherapy

Certain types of fluorescent, tungsten halogen, and fiber-optic lights are effective in lowering bilirubin levels in the blood by changing the shape of the bilirubin molecule so that it can be excreted more readily. Phototherapy is useful for term and preterm newborns with physiological jaundice and is commonly used to lower TSB levels.

Phototherapy equipment and lights vary widely, but all can be effective in lowering bilirubin levels. Effectiveness relates to the dose of phototherapy received by the baby. Commercially available devices, or radiometers, are available to measure irradiance emitted by the lights, thereby ensuring that adequate intensity is delivered to the baby.

Because hyperbilirubinemia can be exacerbated by poorly established breastfeeding or infrequent or ineffective breastfeeding, it is important that measures be taken to limit the negative effect phototherapy treatment can have on a baby feeding. Strategies that allow the baby to be held and fed while receiving phototherapy and in the room with the mother, when appropriate, should be implemented to decrease the chances of exacerbating feeding concerns during treatment (*Pediatrics.* 2013;131[6]:e1982–e1985). The baby's feeding and weight patterns, as well as output, should be followed closely, and supplementation with expressed breast milk or formula should be considered only if and when a medical indication of poor intake exists.

B. Intravenous immunoglobulin

Intravenous immunoglobulin has been shown to be effective in preventing the need for an exchange transfusion in babies who have a positive Coombs (antiglobulin) test result for hyperbilirubinemia. For example, intravenous immunoglobulin may prevent the need for an exchange transfusion in a baby with alloimmune hemolytic disease who is receiving intensive phototherapy with increasing bilirubin levels. The recommended dose is 1 g/kg administered over 2 hours. The rate of infusion does not need to be slowly increased when first administering it to a baby. Monitor the baby for adverse reactions (eg, fever, hypotension). Repeat dosing can be considered.

C. Exchange transfusion

Another way to treat hyperbilirubinemia is to exchange the baby's blood with that of an adult donor who has a reference bilirubin level. Although exchange transfusions are more effective than phototherapy in lowering bilirubin levels rapidly, they also have considerably greater risks and are not performed unless intensive phototherapy and other measures fail to lower the bilirubin level.

Self-test B

Now answer these questions to test yourself on the information in the last section.

B1. **True** **False** Phototherapy needs to be started whenever jaundice is detected in a baby.

B2. **True** **False** Breastfed babies are likely to have higher mean bilirubin levels than those of formula-fed babies.

B3. To establish the cause of hyperbilirubinemia, which of the following types of information should always be reviewed?

Yes	No	
____	____	Laboratory test results
____	____	Chest radiograph
____	____	Oxygen saturation level
____	____	History
____	____	Physical examination findings

B4. When is hyperbilirubinemia not physiological? Name at least 2 situations.

_____

_____

B5. **True** **False** A healthy-appearing baby girl is noted to be jaundiced on the first day after birth. She is active and eating well. This is physiological jaundice.

B6. **True** **False** Exchange transfusion is more effective than phototherapy in rapidly lowering bilirubin levels.

B7. **True** **False** Increased incidence of hyperbilirubinemia in breastfed babies may be caused by increased bilirubin reabsorption from the intestines.

B8. Which laboratory tests are performed initially for evaluation of hyperbilirubinemia?

Yes	No	
____	____	Blood smear
____	____	Hematocrit and/or hemoglobin value
____	____	Coombs (antiglobulin) test
____	____	Mother's and baby's blood group

Check your answers with the list that follows the Recommended Routines. Correct any incorrect answers and review the appropriate section in the unit.

---

11. When are babies treated for hyperbilirubinemia with phototherapy?

A. Healthy babies born at 35 or more weeks of gestation (Figure 7.1)

Bilirubin levels should be interpreted according to a baby's age in hours. For the guidelines in Figure 7.1, use *intensive* phototherapy when a baby's TSB exceeds the line indicated for the baby's risk category and age.

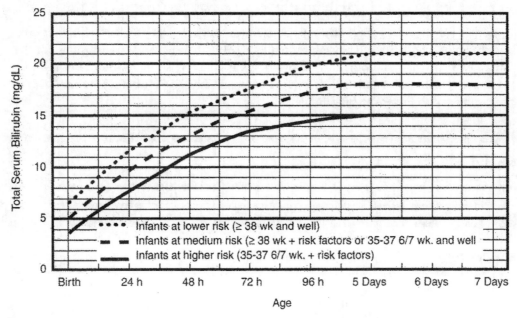

Figure 7.1. Guidelines for Phototherapy for Babies Born at 35 or More Weeks of Gestation
Reproduced with permission from American Academy of Pediatrics Subcommittee on Hyperbilirubinemia. Management of hyperbilirubinemia in the newborn infant 35 or more weeks of gestation. *Pediatrics.* 2004;114(1):304.

Bilirubin levels can be lowered by using phototherapy lights that provide an irradiance of 4 µW/cm²/nm (microwatts per square centimeter per nanometer) or higher.

Intensive phototherapy refers to an irradiance of at least 30 µW/cm²/nm, measured on the baby's skin, directly below the center of the phototherapy lights, and delivered to as much of the baby's skin as possible.

- Use TSB values. Do not subtract conjugated (direct-reacting) bilirubin.
- *Major risk factors*
  — Isoimmune hemolytic disease (ABO, Rh, or certain minor antigens such as anti-c, E, Duffy, and Kell)
  — G6PD deficiency
  — Perinatal compromise
  — Significant lethargy
  — Family history of a first-degree relative who received phototherapy as baby
  — Temperature instability
  — Sepsis
  — Acidosis
  — Albumin level (if measured) less than 3.0 g/dL
- Use the curves based on the baby's risk factors to determine the level at which intensive phototherapy should be started.
- Consider intervening at lower TSB levels for babies who are closer to 35 weeks' gestational age and at higher TSB levels for those closer to 37⁶/⁷ weeks' gestational age.
- If the TSB continues to increase or does not decrease in a newborn who is receiving intensive phototherapy, consider the presence of hemolysis.
- You may consider home phototherapy at TSB levels of 2 to 3 mg/dL below those shown, but home phototherapy should not be used for any baby with risk factors who has not yet shown clinically significant stabilization.

Examples: You would follow the middle, dashed line in Figure 7.1 to determine
— Phototherapy *is not indicated* for a well baby born at 36 weeks'
gestational age with a TSB of 4 mg/dL at 24 hours.
— *Intensive* phototherapy *is indicated* for a well baby born at
36 weeks' gestational age with a TSB of 11 mg/dL at 24 hours.

B. Preterm babies

Management of preterm babies differs from the guidelines noted previously for healthy term, early term, and late preterm newborns. Management decisions are based on the cause of jaundice, the degree of the baby's illness, the risk factors, and the rate of increase of bilirubin levels. The general guidelines recommended for starting phototherapy in preterm newborns are listed in Table 7.1.

C. All babies

When phototherapy is used appropriately, exchange transfusion is *rarely* required for the treatment of hyperbilirubinemia. If, however, intensive phototherapy, maximizing intake, and administering intravenous immunoglobulin (if appropriate) are unsuccessful at preventing the bilirubin level from increasing significantly, an exchange transfusion should be performed, no matter the baby's size or gestational age. Establish a policy of using phototherapy after any exchange transfusion for hyperbilirubinemia.

In some cases, rebound hyperbilirubinemia may occur after an exchange is completed. The baby's bilirubin level should be checked every 4 to 6 hours after an exchange.

Table 7.1. Suggested Use of Phototherapy and Exchange Transfusion in Infants Born at Less Than 35 Weeks of Gestation		
Gestational Age (wk)	Initiate Phototherapy for Total Serum Bilirubin Level (mg dL^{-1})	Initiate Exchange Transfusion for Total Serum Bilirubin Level (mg dL^{-1})
Less than 28$^{0/7}$	5–6	11–14
28$^{0/7}$ to 29$^{6/7}$	6–8	12–14
30$^{0/7}$ to 31$^{6/7}$	8–10	13–16
32$^{0/7}$ to 33$^{6/7}$	10–12	15–18
34$^{0/7}$ to 34$^{6/7}$	12–14	17–19

Adapted with permission from Maisels MJ, Watchko JF, Bhutani VK, Stevenson DK. An approach to the management of hyperbilirubinemia in the preterm infant less than 35 weeks of gestation. *J Perinatol.* 2012;32:660–664.

12. What phototherapy methods should be used?

- *Cover the baby's eyes completely:* The strong lights may cause eye damage if the baby's eyes are not covered.
- *Keep the baby as undressed as possible:* Because the lights affect bilirubin that has collected in the baby's skin, as much of a baby's skin as possible must be exposed to the light for maximum effectiveness.
- *Preserve temperature control:* Phototherapy lights may overheat a baby, especially if cared for in an incubator. Therefore, it is important to check a baby's temperature periodically during phototherapy.

- *Increase the baby's fluid intake, check the body weight and output, and conduct a clinical examination for hydration status frequently:* Phototherapy lights can more than double a baby's stool and evaporative water losses.
- *Provide radiant output (radiant flux or irradiance) at a minimum of 4 μW/cm²/nm:* There is a direct relationship between irradiance and effectiveness of phototherapy in reducing bilirubin levels. Radiant flux should be measured with a radiometer sensor held at the level of the baby's skin, directly below the center of the phototherapy lights. Irradiance measured below the center of the light source will be much higher than that measured at the light periphery. A minimum of 30 μW/cm²/nm, measured at the center of the light source, should be used for babies who require *intensive* phototherapy.
- *Replace bulbs as recommended by the manufacturer or when measurements show inadequate irradiance:* After being used for a number of hours, phototherapy bulbs may lose effectiveness. Perform periodic checks to be sure phototherapy lights provide adequate irradiance.
- *Position phototherapy lights an appropriate distance from the baby:* Phototherapy effectiveness decreases as the distance between the light source and skin increases. However, problems with temperature control (overheating) and lack of clear visibility of the baby may be caused by phototherapy lights placed too close to a baby. Placing fluorescent lights approximately 45 cm (18 in) from the baby has been recommended. Halogen spotlights need to be positioned according to manufacturer recommendations, because burns can result if lamps are placed too close to a baby.
- *Keep the shield that covers the bulbs in place:* This helps to screen the light and reduces the baby's exposure to ultraviolet rays. In addition, a bulb will sometimes burst. The shield prevents glass fragments from falling onto the baby.
- *Use multiple lights to provide additional phototherapy, if needed:* In cases of very high or rapidly increasing bilirubin levels, double or triple lights directed from different angles onto a baby's skin, to expose as much of the skin as possible to phototherapy, are more effective than a single set of lights. Depending on the type of light source used, large term babies may need 2 lights when starting to provide effective therapy over their entire surface area. A fiber-optic phototherapy "blanket" placed under a baby with a conventional phototherapy light(s) over the baby also increases the surface area of the baby exposed to phototherapy and the total radiant flux of the phototherapy.
- *When appropriate, keep mother and baby together and allow for feeding on cue:* Encourage increased frequency of breastfeeding and consider having the mother hand express or pump with each feeding to maximize intake and the signaling of milk production to the mother's body.
- *Explore whether phototherapy may be continued during feeding and skin-to-skin contact.*
- *Continue phototherapy until the bilirubin level falls into the desired range.* Phototherapy may be intermittently stopped for very brief periods (eg, feedings, diaper changes), but otherwise, the therapy should continue uninterrupted.

In summary, consider the following points when providing phototherapy, which is usually administered continuously while the bilirubin level remains above the desired range:

- Keep the baby naked.
- Measure the irradiance (radiant flux) of the phototherapy light(s).
- Provide irradiance of *at least* 4 μW/cm²/nm.
- Provide irradiance of 30 μW/cm²/nm or more if *intensive* phototherapy is needed.

- Position the lights to avoid overheating and to allow clear visibility of the baby.
- Keep the manufacturer's bulb shield in place.
- Use double or triple lights for babies who have high or rapidly increasing bilirubin levels.
- Maximize breastfeeding opportunities and effectiveness; consider having the mother do hand expression or pump her milk with each feeding, to increase signaling and milk production.

In most cases, *brief* interruption of phototherapy during feeding or a portion of parental visiting time will not interfere with phototherapy treatment. It is essential, however, that any interruption be as brief as possible. Treatment can only be effective when the baby is under phototherapy lights for extended periods.

13. What are the complications of phototherapy?

Possible phototherapy complications include

- Eye damage, if the baby's eyes are not covered. (Eye patches should be used.)
- Obstructed nasal breathing, if eye patches slip and cover the baby's nose. (Deaths have occurred from this.)

Use snug-fitting eye covers that will not slip over the baby's nose, check the baby frequently, and educate family members about the importance of keeping the baby's nose free and clear. Consider conducting cardiorespiratory monitoring in babies who cannot be observed closely.

- Skin rash. (Reasons are unknown; continue therapy.)
- Increased water loss through evaporation. (Increase the baby's fluid intake.)
- Hyperthermia. (Monitor the baby's temperature frequently and follow all product guidelines.)
- Other complications, such as bronze baby syndrome due to cholestasis (increased conjugated or direct hyperbilirubinemia, stoppage of bile flow) and severe skin blistering due to congenital photosensitivity, are possible but rare.

14. When is an exchange transfusion needed?

If TSB reaches levels at which brain damage has been reported, despite maximizing the baby's intake and delivering *intensive* phototherapy (including the addition of extra lights to cover more surface area of the baby and the administration of intravenous immunoglobulin, as appropriate), an exchange transfusion should be considered. Significant morbidity, in the form of apnea, bradycardia, cyanosis, vasospasm, necrotizing enterocolitis, thrombosis, and complications of blood transfusions, can occur in association with exchange transfusion. Deaths have occurred. Because exchange transfusions are rarely performed today, risks are difficult to quantify but are likely higher than when exchange transfusions were more common and more providers were skilled in performing them.

Figure 7.2 will help you identify whether a term or near-term baby in your care has a bilirubin level that is approaching the need for an exchange transfusion, and whether regional perinatal center consultation should be considered. The AAP recommends that an exchange transfusion be performed only by trained personnel in a neonatal intensive care unit with full monitoring and resuscitation capabilities (*Pediatrics*. 2004;114[1]:297–316; updated guidelines are anticipated in 2021).

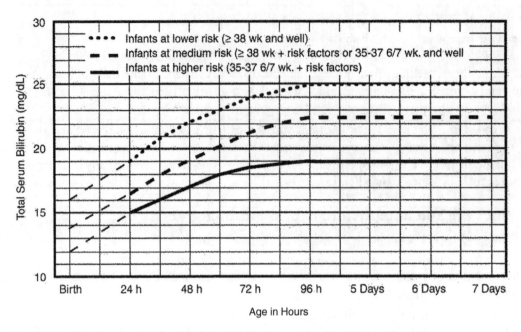

Figure 7.2. Guidelines for Exchange Transfusion in Babies Born at 35 or More Weeks of Gestation
Reproduced with permission from American Academy of Pediatrics Subcommittee on Hyperbilirubinemia. Management of hyperbilirubinemia in the newborn infant 35 or more weeks of gestation. *Pediatrics.* 2004;114(1):305.

- Use TSB values. Do not subtract conjugated (direct-reacting) bilirubin.
- If exchange transfusion is being considered but is not yet decided, obtain a serum albumin level, calculate the bilirubin to albumin ratio, and compare it with the values in Table 7.2. If the bilirubin to albumin ratio exceeds the values in the table, proceed to exchange transfusion. If not, follow other indications in determining the need for exchange. (Do not let a lower bilirubin to albumin ratio delay an exchange that is indicated by other criteria.)
- Risk factors
  - Isoimmune hemolytic disease
  - G6PD deficiency
  - Perinatal compromise
  - Sepsis
  - Temperature instability
  - Significant lethargy
  - Low albumin levels
  - Acidosis
- *Immediate* exchange transfusion is recommended if the baby shows signs of acute bilirubin encephalopathy (ie, hypertonia, arching, retrocollis, opisthotonos, fever, high-pitched cry) or if TSB is more than 5 mg/dL above the lines in Figure 7.2.
- Dashed lines for the first 24 hours in Figure 7.2 indicate uncertainty due to a wide range of clinical circumstances and responses to phototherapy.

Table 7.2. Bilirubin to Albumin Ratio at Which Exchange Transfusion Should Be Considered	
Gestational Age	**TSB (mg/dL)/Albumin (g/dL)**
$>38^{0/7}$ wk	8.0
$35^{0/7}$ to $36^{6/7}$ wk and well baby *or* $>38^{0/7}$ wk if higher risk or isoimmune hemolytic disease or G6PD deficiency	7.2
$35^{0/7}$ to $36^{6/7}$ wk if higher risk or isoimmune hemolytic disease or G6PD deficiency	6.8

Abbreviations: G6PD, glucose-6-phosphate dehydrogenase; TSB, total serum bilirubin.

15. When can phototherapy be stopped?

Skin color is not a reliable index of the degree of hyperbilirubinemia, particularly if a baby is receiving phototherapy. Just because a baby no longer appears jaundiced does not necessarily mean the bilirubin level in the blood has decreased sufficiently to stop treatment.

After starting phototherapy, serum bilirubin levels should be measured at least every 4 to 6 hours in babies who have rapidly increasing bilirubin levels and in preterm babies and sick babies. For otherwise healthy, term newborns who do not have rapidly increasing bilirubin levels, serum bilirubin levels may be checked less frequently. Continue to check serum bilirubin levels until they begin to decline.

It is important to use only TSB rather than TcB measurements when babies are receiving phototherapy. This is because of skin bleaching and the reliability of TcB measurements only for levels below 15 mg/dL, as noted earlier.

The discontinuation of phototherapy is a clinical decision, based on

- Risk factors (eg, history of perinatal compromise, acidosis, illness)
- Adequacy of oral intake and pattern of output
- Serum bilirubin level
- Age of the baby (gestational age at birth and postnatal age)
- Assessment of the baby's risk of severe hyperbilirubinemia

In most cases, if serum bilirubin levels are clearly decreasing and are less than 2 to 3 points below the light level (the bilirubin level at which the phototherapy lights are turned on or off), determined on the basis of plotting on the appropriate phototherapy curve, phototherapy may be discontinued. However, a rebound increase of serum bilirubin may occur. Therefore, bilirubin levels should be checked for at least 12 to 24 hours after phototherapy has been stopped. If a significant rebound increase in bilirubin levels occurs, phototherapy may need to be restarted.

Some health professionals have begun using a calculator to predict the subsequent increase of bilirubin levels prior to stopping phototherapy (BiliTool, available at http://www.bilitool.org/; Chang, *Pediatrics,* March 2017).

16. When is it safe to discharge a baby with hyperbilirubinemia?

Babies who are preterm, have evidence of hemolysis, or have received phototherapy require individual consideration for appropriate timing of discharge and follow-up.

Figure 7.3 is for well newborns born at 36 or more weeks of gestation who have a birth weight of at least 2,000 g (4 lb 6½ oz) or babies born at 35 or more weeks of gestation who have a birth weight of at least 2,500 g (5 lb 8 oz). The babies used to construct the graph had no identifiable risk factors. Figure 7.3 can be used to estimate the likelihood that a baby with a given bilirubin value will reach a level of severe hyperbilirubinemia with a subsequent value. In the figure, *severe* is defined as a bilirubin level higher than that achieved by 95% of well babies at the specified age.

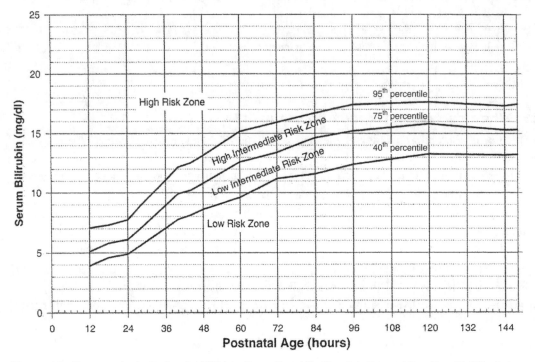

Figure 7.3. Nomogram for the Designation of Risk for Severe Hyperbilirubinemia in Term and Near-Term Well Newborns
Reproduced with permission from Bhutani VK, Johnson L, Sivieri EM. Predictive ability of a predischarge hour-specific serum bilirubin for subsequent significant hyperbilirubinemia in healthy term and near-term newborns. *Pediatrics*. 1999;103(1):9.

To use Figure 7.3, note the baby's exact age in hours when the bilirubin sample was obtained and mark it on the graph. The zone in which the value can be found is used to predict the likelihood of a subsequent bilirubin value reaching a severe level (Table 7.3). This assessment is particularly important for babies who are discharged from the hospital before 72 hours of age.

Table 7.3. Likelihood of Severe Hyperbilirubinemia Based on Bilirubin Plot on Bhutani Curve	
Risk Zone	**Chance of Having Severe Hyperbilirubinemia at Subsequent Sampling (>95th percentile)**
High	54%
High intermediate	21%
Low intermediate	3%
Low	0.6%

Examples

- A 3,000-g (6 lb 10 oz) baby born at 36 weeks' gestational age had a TSB level of 13 mg/dL at 36 hours of age. The value is in the high-risk zone in Figure 7.3, which indicates the baby has a significant risk of having another TSB value in the severe range. This risk for severe hyperbilirubinemia increases as the number of risk factors increases.
- A 2,500-g (5 lb 8 oz) baby born at 37 weeks' gestational age had a TSB level of 8 mg/dL at 36 hours of age. The value can be found in the low-intermediate risk zone, which indicates the baby has a relatively low likelihood of having a subsequent TSB value in the severe range. This risk for severe hyperbilirubinemia increases as the number of risk factors increases.

All newborns discharged up to 48 hours after birth should be evaluated by a health professional within 48 hours of discharge. Use the identified risk zone, as well as a baby's risk factors plus clinical judgments, to determine when and how often the baby's bilirubin level should be checked after discharge. The baby's weight, feeding, and urine and stool outputs should also be assessed.

In general, it is recommended that levels in the high zone be checked again within 6 to 8 hours, levels in the high-intermediate zone be rechecked within 8 to 12 hours, and levels in the low-intermediate zone be rechecked within 12 to 24 hours—especially in newborns who have risk factors.

At discharge, all parents should have received written and verbal explanations of jaundice and the need for further monitoring, as well as a plan for additional monitoring.

Self-test C

Now answer these questions to test yourself on the information in the last section.

C1. Use the graphs in the previous sections to help you answer these questions. For each of the following examples, decide if you should

A. Consider phototherapy.

B. Begin phototherapy.

C. Begin intensive phototherapy.

D. Consider performing an exchange transfusion.

E. Determine that no other action is needed at this time

a. _____ A vigorous baby born at 38 weeks' gestational age has no risk factors but is jaundiced at 30 hours of age, with a bilirubin level of 10 mg/dL.

b. _____ A 1,900-g (4 lb 3 oz) baby born at 33 weeks' gestational age has respiratory distress and a bilirubin level of 10 mg/dL at 36 hours of age.

c. _____ A 3,000-g (6 lb 10 oz), term baby has hemolytic disease from ABO incompatibility and a bilirubin level of 20 mg/dL at 36 hours of age, while undergoing intensive phototherapy since 8 hours of age.

d. _____ A formula-fed baby born at 40 weeks' gestational age has no complications and has a serum bilirubin level of 15 mg/dL at 36 hours of age.

e. _____ A baby born at 36 weeks' gestational age has a serum bilirubin level of 8 mg/dL at 30 hours of age.

f. _____ A baby born at 39 weeks' gestational age had a 1-minute Apgar score of 2 and required prolonged resuscitation, became jaundiced by 12 hours of age, and has a serum bilirubin level of 10 mg/dL.

C2. Name 3 common problems that can develop as a result of phototherapy.

_____

_____

_____

C3. **True** **False** The best way to know when to stop phototherapy is when the baby is no longer jaundiced.

C4. **True** **False** Phototherapy light irradiance should be at least 30 µW/cm^2/nm for intensive phototherapy.

C5. Name the 4 pieces of information that must be considered when deciding when to discontinue phototherapy.

_____

_____

_____

_____

Check your answers with the list that follows the Recommended Routines. Correct any incorrect answers and review the appropriate section in the unit.

HYPERBILIRUBINEMIA

Recommended Routines

All the routines listed below are based on the principles of perinatal care presented in the unit you have just finished. They are recommended as part of routine perinatal care.

Read each routine carefully and decide whether it is standard operating procedure in your hospital. Check the appropriate blank next to each routine.

Procedure Standard in My Hospital	Needs Discussion by Our Staff	Recommended Routine
_____	_____	1. Establish a policy for screening all babies for risk of jaundice on the basis of history, clinical assessment, physical examination, and bilirubin screening.
_____	_____	2. Make sure that every baby receives evidence-based care to establish optimal feeding, that feeding is evaluated and observed for effectiveness prior to discharge, and that appropriate follow-up and management strategies are in place.
_____	_____	3. Establish a policy of defining each case of jaundice as physiological or non-physiological.
_____	_____	4. Establish a policy of investigating the cause of hyperbilirubinemia whenever phototherapy is started.
_____	_____	5. Establish a policy that allows nurses to obtain a transcutaneous bilirubin level or order a total serum bilirubin measurement any time jaundice is noted in a term or preterm newborn or obtain follow-up levels at defined intervals.
_____	_____	6. For all babies receiving phototherapy, establish a policy of • Covering the baby's eyes • Checking the baby's vital signs frequently (consider electronic monitoring) • Monitoring the baby's intake and output and assessing hydration • Limiting interruptions in feeding • Ensuring that the baby's nose is not covered by the eye protection used for phototherapy • Keeping the baby in closer proximity to the mother, if possible

(*continued*)

_____ _____ 7. Establish a policy of obtaining a transcutaneous bilirubin or total serum bilirubin level within 48 hours of birth for term and near-term babies and using Figure 7.3 to predict the course of bilirubin and the likelihood of a subsequent value being in the high-risk zone.

_____ _____ 8. Establish a protocol that all newborns discharged up to 48 hours after birth are evaluated by a health professional within 48 hours after discharge.

Self-test Answers

These are the answers to the Self-test questions. Please check them with the answers you gave and review the information in the unit wherever necessary.

Self-test A

A1. Brain damage

A2. Increased production of bilirubin due to breakdown of more red blood cells, at a faster rate
Less efficient removal of bilirubin by the liver
Increased reabsorption of bilirubin from the intestines

A3. C. It is the capacity of serum protein to attract and hold bilirubin.

A4. True

A5. False   *Reason:* A baby's serum bilirubin level cannot be reliably estimated by the visual assessment of jaundice.

A6. False   *Reason:* Transcutaneous bilirubin and total serum bilirubin levels correlate closely when the bilirubin level is 15 mg/dL or lower. Some experts use 12 mg/dL as the cutoff for accurate correlation. In addition, transcutaneous bilirubin levels should not be used for babies placed under phototherapy lights because the lights can bleach the skin, making transcutaneous bilirubin measurements unreliable.

A7. When it leaves the blood and enters the brain

A8. Any 2 of the following conditions:
- Prematurity
- Sepsis
- Perinatal compromise
- Acidosis
- Illness (lethargy, temperature instability)
- Low serum albumin levels (<3.0 g/dL)
- Certain medications

Self-test B

B1. False   *Reason:* Many babies will not require any treatment. The baby's physical examination, age, weight, risk factors, bilirubin level, and other tests, as indicated, need to be evaluated to determine appropriate treatment.

B2. True

B3.

Yes	No	
X	___	Laboratory test results
___	X	Chest radiograph
___	X	Oxygen saturation level
X	___	History
X	___	Physical examination findings

B4. Any 2 of the following situations:
- It appears in the first 24 hours after birth.
- Bilirubin levels increase faster than 0.5 mg/dL per hour.
- There is evidence of hemolysis.
- Physical examination findings are atypical.
- Direct bilirubin level exceeds 20% of total bilirubin level.
- Jaundice persists for more than 3 weeks.

B5. False   *Reason:* Jaundice is not considered physiological if it appears within 24 hours after birth, even if the baby appears well.

B6. True

B7. True

B8. Yes   No

   X   ___   Blood smear

   X   ___   Hematocrit and/or hemoglobin value

   X   ___   Coombs (antiglobulin) test

   X   ___   Mother's and baby's blood group

Self-test C

C1. a. E. Determine that no other action is needed at this time.

     b. B. Begin phototherapy.

     c. D. Consider performing an exchange transfusion.

     d. C. Begin intensive phototherapy.

     e. A. Consider phototherapy.

     f. C. Begin intensive phototherapy.

C2. Any 3 of the following problems:

- Eye damage (if the baby's eyes are not covered)
- Skin rash
- Nasal obstruction (from an eye patch that has slipped down)
- Increase in stools
- Increase in evaporative water loss
- Hyperthermia

C3. False   *Reason:* Skin color is not a reliable indicator of the degree of hyperbilirubinemia, especially for babies receiving phototherapy. The baby may no longer appear jaundiced but may still have a high serum bilirubin level. Total serum bilirubin (not transcutaneous bilirubin) measurement should be obtained to determine the baby's bilirubin level.

C4. True

C5. Risk factors in the baby's history

Serum bilirubin level

Age of the baby (gestational age at birth and postnatal age)

Assessment of the baby's risk for severe hyperbilirubinemia

Unit 7 Posttest

After completion of each unit there is a free online posttest available at www.cmevillage.com to test your understanding. Navigate to the PCEP pages on www.cmevillage.com and register to take the free posttests.

Once registered on the website and after completing all the unit posttests, pay the book exam fee ($15) and pass the test at 80% or greater to earn continuing education credits. Only start the PCEP book exam if you have time to complete it. If you take the book exam and are not connected to a printer, either print your certificate to a .pdf file and save it to print later or come back to www.cmevillage.com at any time and print a copy of your educational transcript.

Credits are only available by book, not by individual unit within the books. Available credits for completion of each book exam are as follows: Book 1: 14.5 credits; Book 2: 16 credits; Book 3: 17 credits; Book 4: 9 credits.

For more details, navigate to the PCEP webpages at www.cmevillage.com.

Appendix: Identification and Treatment of Jaundice During the First Week After Birth[a]

Physical Examination Findings	Laboratory Findings	Cause	Treatment (in addition to management provided in this unit)
1. Jaundice; healthy-appearing baby, may be preterm	• Negative Coombs (antiglobulin) test result • Hematocrit value, reticulocytes, and smear within reference ranges	Immature liver; decreased conjugation of bilirubin	Ensure the baby is receiving adequate intake.
2. Jaundice; healthy-appearing baby with perhaps some paleness or evidence of tachypnea or mild congestive heart failure	• Direct Coombs (antiglobulin) test: positive result in Rh incompatibility, may be positive result in ABO incompatibility • In Rh and ABO incompatibility: decreased hematocrit value, increased reticulocyte count, and polychromasia seen on smear	Hemolysis secondary to Rh, ABO, or a minor blood group incompatibility	Monitor the baby for anemia in the hospital and after discharge, as antibodies may continue to cause hemolysis for weeks or months.
3. Jaundice; hepatosplenomegaly; lethargy; hypothermia; poor feeding	• Increased direct and unconjugated (indirect-reacting) bilirubin • Perhaps some evidence of hemolysis with decreased hematocrit value, increased reticulocyte count • Negative Coombs (antiglobulin) test result	Sepsis	Obtain cultures; administer antibiotics.
4. Jaundice; ruddy color; frequently SGA or baby of a multi-fetal pregnancy	• Negative Coombs (antiglobulin) test result • Increased hematocrit value • Reticulocytes, smear within reference ranges	Polycythemia with increased bilirubin load from excess red blood cells	Consider treatment of high hematocrit values. (See Unit 9, Identifying and Caring for Sick and At-Risk Babies, in this book.)
5. Jaundice; abnormalities at examination • Hepatosplenomegaly • Possible congenital heart disease, microcephaly, cataracts, hydrocephaly	• Increased direct bilirubin level • Positive viral culture results or antibody increase or positive serology result for syphilis • Negative Coombs (antiglobulin) test result	Congenital viral infection	Provide medical treatment of herpes, toxoplasmosis, or syphilis. (See Unit 8, Infections, in this book.)

(continued)

Appendix: Identification and Treatment of Jaundice During the First Week After Birth[a] (*continued*)

Physical Examination Findings	Laboratory Findings	Cause	Treatment (in addition to management provided in this unit)
6. Jaundice; healthy appearance with the exception of abdominal distension, history of vomiting and delayed or absent stooling	• Increased unconjugated (indirect-reacting) bilirubin level • Negative Coombs (antiglobulin) test result • Smear, reticulocytes within reference range	Bowel obstruction	Provide supportive treatment • IV hydration; give the baby nothing by mouth • NG suction • Abdominal radiography • Surgical consultation
7. Jaundice; healthy-appearing baby with multiple bruises from difficult labor and delivery	• Negative Coombs (antiglobulin) test result • Smear, reticulocytes within reference range	Hemorrhaging under the skin leads to increased breakdown of red blood cells	Follow the clinical course.
8. Jaundice; healthy-appearing baby; possible hepatosplenomegaly; may become acutely ill with hypoglycemia, vomiting, diarrhea, seizures, and clinical signs similar to sepsis	• Increased unconjugated (indirect-reacting) and conjugated (direct-reacting) bilirubin level • Positive urine test result for reducing substances if fed human (breast) milk or formula • Obtain blood sample for measurement of enzyme level	Galactosemia	Remove galactose from the baby's diet; change the baby's diet to formula that contains no galactose or lactose.
9. Jaundice; healthy-appearing baby of Mediterranean, Middle East, Southeast Asian, or African American heritage	• Decreased hematocrit value, increased reticulocyte count, and polychromasia seen on smear • Sudden increase in bilirubin can occur	G6PD deficiency	Test for G6PD. G6PD-deficient babies require intervention at lower TSB levels.

Abbreviations: ABO, major blood group isohemagglutinins; G6PD, glucose-6-phosphate dehydrogenase; IV, intravenous; NG, nasogastric; SGA, small for gestational age; TSB, total serum bilirubin.

[a] For detecting causes of jaundice only during the first few days after birth. If jaundice persists or is late appearing, evaluate further for more rare conditions.

Additional helpful charts and tables are available from the American Academy of Pediatrics at http://shop.aap.org: Phototherapy guidelines for preterm infants (≤ 34⁶ᐟ⁷ weeks of gestation) are shown in Figure 7A.1.

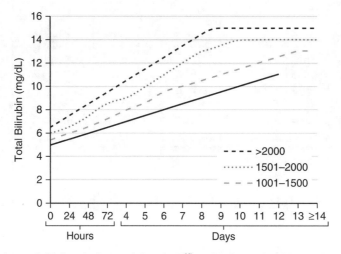

Figure 7A.1. Phototherapy Guidelines for Preterm Infants (≤ 34⁶ᐟ⁷ weeks of gestation). If babies have isoimmune hemolytic disease, acidosis, sepsis, glucose-6-phosphate dehydrogenase, temperature instability, or albumin level < 3 g/dL, consider a lower threshold or curve. When infants become 35⁰ᐟ⁷ weeks' postmenstrual age, consider using AAP Phototherapy Curves for infants 35 weeks and older.
Curves for < 1,000 g derived from Morris BH, Oh W, Tyson JE, et al. Aggressive vs. conservative phototherapy for infants with extremely low birth weight. *N Engl J Med.* 2008;359:1885–1896. Other birth weight group curves modified from Wallenstein MB, Bhutani VK. Jaundice and kernicterus in the moderately preterm infant. *Clin Perinatol.* 2013;40:679–688, Maisels MJ, Watchko JF, Bhutani VK, Stevenson DK. An approach to the management of hyperbilirubinemia in the preterm infant less than 35 weeks of gestation. *J Perinatol.* 2012;32:660–664, and Management of hyperbilirubinemia in the newborn infant 35 or more weeks of gestation. *Pediatrics.* 2004;114:297–316.

Exchange and Intravenous Immunoglobulin (IVIG) Guidelines for Preterm Infants (≤ 34⁶ᐟ⁷ weeks' gestation)

Consider if bilirubin levels or rate of rise are high. If isoimmune hemolytic disease, consider 1 g/kg IVIG over 2 hours. Also may consider adding other therapies such as phenobarbital (5 mg/kg) for 3 days; ursodiol (10 mg/kg/day) (*J Pediatr Gastroenterol Nutr.* 2016;62:97–100), or probiotics (*Saccharomyces boulardii* 250 mg/day) (*J Clin Diagn Res.* 2016;10:SC12–SC15; *J Matern Fetal Neonatal Med.* 2013;26:215–221).

Unit 8: Infections

Objectives

In this unit you will learn

A. Why newborns can easily become infected

B. Which babies are at risk for infection

C. The types of neonatal infections

D. The clinical signs and laboratory findings suggestive of infection

E. What to do when infection is suspected

F. The importance of the appropriate use of antibiotics

G. How to control the spread of infections in the nursery

Note: Certain recommendations, guidelines, and charts in this unit are adapted from material published by the American College of Obstetricians and Gynecologists and the American Academy of Pediatrics in the following sources:

For more detailed discussion of specific perinatal infections and their management, consult

- American Academy of Pediatrics, American College of Obstetricians and Gynecologists. *Guidelines for Perinatal Care.* 8th ed. American Academy of Pediatrics; 2017
- American Academy of Pediatrics. *Red Book: 2021 Report of the Committee on Infectious Diseases.* Kimberlin DW, Barnett ED, Lynfield R, Sawyer MH, eds. 32nd ed. American Academy of Pediatrics; 2021

For a detailed description of infection control procedures to prevent transmission of blood-borne and nosocomial pathogens, see the recommendations of the Centers for Disease Control and Prevention.

- Siegel JD, Rhinehart E, Jackson M, Chiarello L; Healthcare Infection Control Practices Advisory Committee. *2007 Guideline for Isolation Precautions: Preventing Transmission of Infectious Agents in Healthcare Settings.* http://www.cdc.gov/hicpac/pdf/isolation/Isolation2007.pdf. Accessed October 15, 2019.

Unit 8 Pretest

Before reading the unit, please answer the following questions. Select the *one best* answer to each question (unless otherwise instructed). Record your answers on the test and check them with the answers at the end of the book.

1. Which of the following signs most commonly indicates a newborn has a systemic infection?
   A. A low body temperature
   B. An increased body temperature
   C. Persistent cough
   D. Skin rash

2. Which of the following statements is true?
   A. Medication is available to cure babies with congenital rubella.
   B. An infected baby will always have a white blood cell count outside of reference range.
   C. An infected baby may develop metabolic acidosis.
   D. Gentamicin should be administered via rapid intravenous push to obtain therapeutic blood levels.

3. Of the following procedures, what is the first thing that should be done for a baby suspected of having a systemic infection?
   A. Begin antibiotic therapy.
   B. Wash the baby with diluted hexachlorophene (pHisoHex).
   C. Obtain blood cultures.
   D. Administer intravenous γ-globulin.

4. Which of the following procedures is most effective in controlling the spread of infection in the nursery?
   A. Have everyone wear hospital scrub clothing.
   B. Require handwashing between handling babies.
   C. Put all babies in incubators.
   D. Have everyone wear masks.

5. What is one reason babies become infected more often than adults?
   A. The level of complement in the blood is excessively high.
   B. They are exposed to more virulent organisms.
   C. They have fewer white blood cells.
   D. Their immune system is immature.

6. **True** **False** Babies with mild localized staphylococcal infections require only mild soap and water washes of the affected area and application of an antibiotic ointment.

7. **True** **False** An umbilical arterial catheter increases a baby's risk for infection.

8. **True** **False** Neonatal group B β-hemolytic streptococcal sepsis is rarely a life-threatening infection.

9. **True** **False** Even if a baby shows no sign of infection, congenital syphilis should be treated with intravenous antibiotics for 10 to 14 days.

(*continued*)

Unit 8 Pretest (*continued*)

10. **True   False**   Hepatitis B virus vaccine is recommended only for babies with mothers who test positive for hepatitis B surface antigen.

11. **True   False**   Antiretroviral treatment of HIV-positive women during pregnancy and labor can dramatically reduce the number of babies who become infected with HIV.

12. **True   False**   Gonococcal conjunctivitis is a localized infection that requires systemic antibiotic treatment.

13. For each of the following conditions, determine if it places the baby at risk for developing an infection:

    Yes   No

    ____   ____   Rupture of membranes 24 hours prior to delivery

    ____   ____   Active labor for 24 hours

    ____   ____   Father's skin colonized with staphylococcal epidermidis

14. A pregnant woman's membranes ruptured 36 hours before delivery. Twenty-four hours after birth, the baby has a reduced temperature and low activity level.

    Yes   No

    ____   ____   The baby was at risk for infection at the time of birth.

    ____   ____   Reduced temperature is a clinical sign of infection in babies.

    ____   ____   This baby probably has a localized infection.

    ____   ____   The first actions to take are to begin supportive care and obtain cultures from this baby.

    ____   ____   You should obtain blood cultures and promptly begin antibiotics.

    ____   ____   Ampicillin alone is an appropriate treatment for this baby.

A newborn with systemic infection (sepsis) has a very high probability of dying or being permanently damaged if the infection is not suspected and treated quickly.

1. Why do babies become infected?

A. Defense mechanisms are immature
Babies are less capable of handling infections than older children and adults because babies' immune systems are immature and slower to respond to immune threats.

B. Antibodies against specific microorganisms have not developed
Normally, while in utero, a fetus is not exposed to any microorganisms and thus does not have the opportunity to develop resistance to specific infectious agents.

C. Immunoglobulin G (IgG) antibody levels may be low (if the baby is preterm)
Some of the maternal antibodies (IgG type) are normally transferred across the placenta to the fetus during the third trimester. If a baby is significantly preterm, there will be a decreased amount of maternally acquired antibodies.

D. All babies have low amounts of immunoglobulin M (IgM) antibody
One type of maternal antibody (IgM) is too large to be transferred across the placenta. Therefore, all newborns, term and preterm, are deficient in IgM antibodies.

2. How are types of infections grouped?

A. Acute life-threatening infection of the blood (sepsis, septicemia)
There is a high mortality rate for babies with acute, life-threatening infections of the blood. Also, infections of the blood in newborns can become an infection of the spinal fluid (meningitis). The most common causative organisms are bacterial.

- Gram-positive bacteria (eg, group B β-hemolytic streptococcus [GBS])
- Gram-negative bacteria (eg, *Escherichia coli*, *Klebsiella*)
- Gram-variable bacteria (eg, *Listeria*)

Viral infections (eg, herpes simplex virus [HSV], cytomegalovirus [CMV]) can also cause severe blood infections in the newborn but are less common.

B. Localized infections
Infections in this category are confined to a specific area or part of the baby. These infections are usually not life-threatening but may become so if not treated properly. The most common conditions are

- Staphylococcal pustulosis
- Abscess
- Omphalitis (infection of the umbilical stump)
- Conjunctivitis
- Wound infections

C. Congenital infections

These infections are associated with an infection of the pregnant woman during pregnancy. The fetus acquires the infection in utero. If infected early in pregnancy, the fetus may develop cataracts, congenital heart disease, or other abnormalities. If infected late in pregnancy or at the time of delivery, a baby may be born with symptoms of an acute systemic infection or become sick within the neonatal period or even be asymptomatic. Common intrauterine infections are often referred to as TORCHS infections.

- *Toxoplasmosis*
- *Other* (eg, varicella, Coxsackie virus B, HIV)
- *Rubella*
- *Cytomegalovirus*
- *Herpes simplex*
- *Syphilis*

In addition to these infections, it is also known that many babies born to women who tested positive for hepatitis B surface antigen (HBsAg) will become infected with hepatitis B virus (HBV), unless treatment is started soon after birth.

Although TORCHS infections may be diagnosed on the basis of the effect they have already had on the baby prior to birth, identification of the infecting agent is important because appropriate therapy may alter the outcome.

D. Hospital-acquired infections

Hospital-acquired infections (also called *nosocomial infections*) often result in systemic, life-threatening illness in newborns. Babies who require continued hospitalization are at risk for nosocomial infections. There are several reasons for this.

- Likelihood of needing a greater number of invasive procedures.
- Longer period to be exposed to a greater number of health workers, who may have also cared for other babies and for patients in other hospital areas.
- Inadequate use of infection control measures, such as standard precautions and proper handwashing.
- Overuse or misuse of some antibiotics, which then allows resistant strains of bacteria to develop. *Nationwide, infections with drug-resistant organisms are a serious and increasing problem.*

Self-test A

Now answer these questions to test yourself on the information in the last section.

A1. Inadequate handwashing by hospital staff may result in a newborn developing this type of infection: _____.

A2. Why do babies become infected? (Choose as many as appropriate.)
- **A.** Their immune systems are immature.
- **B.** They cannot receive antibiotics routinely used in adults.
- **C.** They have not built up antibodies against specific organisms.
- **D.** If preterm, their maternally acquired antibody levels will be low.

A3. For each of the following infections, determine the general type or category:
- **A.** Acute, systemic (blood) infection
- **B.** Localized infection
- **C.** Congenital intrauterine infection
- _____ *Escherichia coli* infection
- _____ Staphylococcal pustulosis
- _____ Conjunctivitis
- _____ Group B β-hemolytic streptococcus infection
- _____ Cytomegalovirus

A4. True False Sepsis (blood infection) is rarely life-threatening in babies.

A5. True False Overuse of antibiotics is one reason drug-resistant forms of bacteria develop.

A6. True False Prolonged hospitalization increases a baby's risk for infection.

Check your answers with the list that follows the Recommended Routines. Correct any incorrect answers and review the appropriate section in the unit.

3. Which babies are at risk for infection?

To be at risk for infection means having been exposed to certain conditions or circumstances that predispose a baby to developing an infection.

A. Life-threatening systemic infections
   The following conditions place a baby at risk for developing a systemic infection:
- Rupture of amniotic membranes longer than 18 hours
  Note: Although less common, it is also possible for a fetus to become infected through intact membranes (ascending infection).
- Labor longer than 20 hours
- Maternal fever (temperature 38.0°C [100.4°F] or higher) during labor
- Maternal illness (eg, varicella, gastroenteritis, urinary tract infection)
- Preterm delivery
- Woman with genital herpes simplex lesions at the time amniotic membranes rupture
- Vagina or rectum colonized with GBS, history of a previous baby with GBS infection, or maternal GBS urinary tract infection at any time during this pregnancy
- Invasive procedure or any foreign body, such as an umbilical catheter
- Prolonged hospitalization (more than several days)

B. Localized infections

Babies are at risk for developing localized infections if subjected to any of the following conditions:

- High staphylococcal colonization rates in other newborns in the nursery
- Any puncture site, such as from an intravenous (IV) or fetal monitoring scalp electrode, or even "heel sticks"
- Staphylococcal, gonococcal, or chlamydial infections predisposing the baby to conjunctivitis (eye infection)

C. Congenital intrauterine infections

The following conditions during pregnancy or at delivery place a baby at risk for becoming infected in utero:

- Pregnant woman contracts rubella (German measles).
- Pregnant woman has syphilis (or undergoes seroconversion to positive findings).
- Pregnant woman is exposed to cat litter (cats are frequently carriers of *Toxoplasma gondii*).
- Pregnant woman has active genital herpes (intrauterine infection is extremely rare; infection is usually acquired after rupture of the membranes, during labor, or at birth).
- Pregnant woman contracts CMV.
- Pregnant woman contracts varicella.
- Pregnant woman tests positive for HBsAg.
- Pregnant woman tests positive for HIV antibody.

4. How do you know a baby is infected?

It is difficult to diagnose infections in babies because the signs and symptoms usually seen with infections in older children and adults are frequently absent or the opposite of what you would expect in infants. The single best clue is if the baby is known to have risk factors for infection.

Clinical signs must also be taken into account when infection is considered or suspected. The most frequent clinical signs seen in an infected baby are changes in vital signs, color, feeding pattern, or general activity.

Certain laboratory studies can also help determine whether a baby is infected. In addition, cultures should be obtained at the first suspicion of sepsis. Although results will not be available for up to several days, positive culture results will provide strong evidence the baby is infected and guide you in adjusting therapy to provide the most appropriate antibiotics.

A. Life-threatening systemic infections (sepsis)
1. Risk factors
Newborns are at risk for developing systemic infection if subjected to any of the conditions listed in Section 3A.
2. Clinical signs
The signs and symptoms of systemic infection may be subtle and easily missed. Any change in vital signs is concerning for the possibility of sepsis.
- Respiratory difficulty (grunting, nasal flaring, retracting, tachypnea, or an apnea spell)
Respiratory symptoms are the most common signs and may mimic respiratory distress syndrome or transient tachypnea of the newborn.

- Marked increase or decrease in heart rate
- Unexplained hypotension
- Reduced body temperature (or, less commonly, an increased body temperature)
- Pale, gray, or mottled color; poor capillary refill
- Poor feeding
- Change in activity (either reduced activity levels [lethargy or decreased tone] or irritability)
- Abdominal distension, vomiting
- Jaundice
- Seizure activity

3. Laboratory findings

An infected baby may or may not have laboratory findings outside reference range. Even if laboratory findings are within reference range, sepsis should be suspected if the baby appears sick at examination. The laboratory studies most strongly associated with sepsis include

- White blood cell (WBC) count with the number of total neutrophils outside (above or below) the shaded area in Figure 8.1
- Ratio of immature to total polymorphonuclear (PMN) WBCs of more than 0.2 (20%) (a poor predictive value for sepsis but a normal ratio may be reassuring in ruling out sepsis)
- The number of immature neutrophils (bands) expressed in absolute terms (total WBC count times the percentage of bands) exceeding the reference limits as in Figure 8.2
- Low blood pH or serum bicarbonate level (an infected baby may develop a gray color from poor perfusion; low blood pH or serum bicarbonate level may result from this poor perfusion)
- Low platelet count and coagulation values outside reference range
- Unexplained hypoglycemia or hyperglycemia

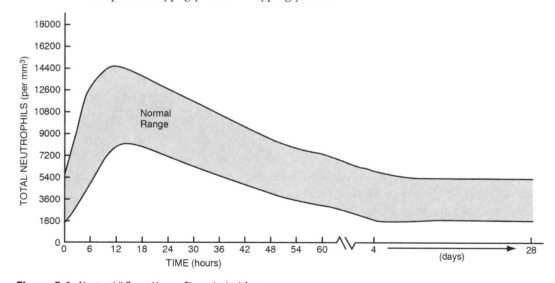

Figure 8.1. Neutrophil Count Versus Chronological Age

Adapted with permission from Manroe BL, Weinberg AG, Rosenfeld CR, Browne R. The neonatal blood count in health and disease. I. Reference values for neutrophilic cells. *J Pediatr.* 1979;95(1):89–98.

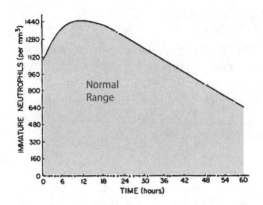

Figure 8.2. Immature Neutrophil Count in the First
60 Hours After Birth
Adapted with permission from Manroe BL, Weinberg AG, Rosenfeld
CR, Browne R. The neonatal blood count in health and disease.
I. Reference values for neutrophilic cells. *J Pediatr.* 1979;95(1):89–98.

Many of these findings are also seen in sick but noninfected neonates. Additionally, neonates born to women with preeclampsia can have clinically significant leukopenia (low WBC count) or neutropenia (low PMNs) without being infected. Because timing is so important in the identification and initiation of drug therapy for systemic infections, *you cannot wait for culture results to differentiate between infectious and noninfectious conditions.* You must rely on your knowledge of risk factors and observation of clinical signs to suspect neonatal systemic infection.

Example of WBC count outside reference range: An 18-hour-old baby develops respiratory distress and is suspected of having pneumonia. His laboratory results are as follows:

White blood cell count	5,000
Neutrophils	1,650 (33%)
Bands	750 (15%)
Juveniles (metamyelocytes, myelocytes, promyelocytes)	200 (4%)
Lymphocytes	2,400 (48%)
Total immature cells (bands + juveniles)	950 (19%)
Total polymorphonuclear cells (neutrophils + bands + juveniles)	2,600 (52%)

This baby's total neutrophil count (sum of PMNs, bands, and juveniles) is less than 7,200, which is below the reference range for a baby 18 hours old, as shown in Figure 8.1. The ratio of total immature cells (sum of bands and juveniles) to total PMN cells for this baby is 19% to 52% or 0.37 (37%), which is greater than 0.2 (20%). Both of these findings, in conjunction with the respiratory distress, suggest that the baby has a high likelihood of being infected.

Note: A baby who has had severe perinatal compromise or has recently been stressed (eg, after circumcision) may have laboratory findings suggestive of sepsis without being infected.

B. Localized infections

Localized infections in the neonate are easier to diagnose than systemic infections.

1. Risk factors

Newborns are at risk for localized infection if subjected to any of the conditions listed in Section 3B.

2. Observational factors

Clinical signs and symptoms of localized infections are easily recognizable.
- Swelling at the infected site
- Warmth of the infected area
- Erythema (redness) of the infected site
- Pustules
- Conjunctivitis (red, swollen, watery, or pus-filled eye[s])

Localized infections must be promptly detected and treated. If not properly managed, a localized infection may quickly develop into a systemic, life-threatening infection.

C. Congenital intrauterine infections

Babies with congenital intrauterine infections may seem extremely ill, but more often they have subtle findings or are asymptomatic.

1. Risk factors

Newborns are at risk for congenital intrauterine infections if their mothers had any of the conditions listed in Section 3C. Refer to this list, as well as Book 2: Maternal and Fetal Care, Unit 3, Infectious Diseases in Pregnancy, for additional information on maternal and neonatal management. *Most babies with congenital infections, however, have no maternal history to indicate an infection.*

2. Observational factors

A newborn with congenital infection may have any or all of the signs of a baby with sepsis. Other findings may include
- Spots of bleeding within the skin (petechiae or purpura)
- Blisters on the skin (vesicles)
- Jaundice lasting more than several days (conjugated [direct-reacting] and unconjugated [indirect-reacting] forms of bilirubin may be increased; see Unit 7, Hyperbilirubinemia, in this book)
- Enlarged liver or spleen with other evidence of liver injury, such as increased transaminase levels (liver cellular enzymes)
- Rapidly enlarging head or a particularly small head
- Cataracts or abnormal retinas
- Poor response to sound
- Rash
- Pneumonia
- Anemia
- Thrombocytopenia (low platelet count)
- Lymphadenopathy (enlarged lymph nodes)

3. Laboratory findings

Blood and other samples obtained to test for many congenital intrauterine infections may take several weeks to yield positive results. Most of the tests involve measuring the level of antibody in the baby's and the mother's blood at the time of illness and again during the first few weeks after birth. Consult your state infectious disease laboratory for the proper technique and timing for obtaining these samples.

D. Hospital-acquired infections
1. Risk factors
   The babies at highest risk for nosocomial infection are babies who
   - Are hospitalized for more than several days
   - Require invasive procedures
2. Clinical signs
   Hospital-acquired infections are usually systemic infections. Babies with nosocomial infections therefore exhibit the clinical signs listed in Section 4A2.
3. Laboratory findings
   These findings are listed in Section 4A3 for systemic infections. Hospital-acquired infections, however, are more likely to be caused by drug-resistant organisms. Drug-resistant bacteria grown from a baby's cultures will show resistance to the usual antibiotics. Check culture results and antibiotic sensitivities carefully. Consider consultation with infectious disease experts about appropriate antibiotics.

Self-test B

Now answer these questions to test yourself on the information in the last section.

B1. What does "at risk for infection" mean?
   A. There are certain predisposing conditions that make it likely the baby will become infected.
   B. The baby will give infections to other people.
   C. The baby will definitely become sick because of exposure to other infected babies.

B2. Name at least 3 conditions that put a newborn at risk for sepsis.

_____

_____

_____

B3. Name 2 conditions that would put a baby at risk for localized infections.

_____

_____

B4. What is (are) the best clinical sign(s) that a baby may have a systemic infection?
   A. Change in heart rate
   B. Reduced temperature
   C. Reduced activity
   D. All of the above

B5. What are the common clinical signs of localized infections?

_____

_____

_____

_____

B6. Name at least 2 conditions occurring during pregnancy that put the baby at risk for a congenital infection.

_____

_____

B7. **True   False**   Results of white blood cell count and differential can reliably indicate whether a baby has bacterial sepsis.

Check your answers with the list that follows the Recommended Routines. Correct any incorrect answers and review the appropriate section in the unit.

5. What should be done if a baby is suspected of being infected?

From the time the first clinical sign(s) appear(s) or you become suspicious that a baby may have sepsis, you have a short amount of time to obtain cultures and initiate drug therapy.

As soon as you suspect a baby is septic, immediately begin supportive care, obtain blood cultures, and then begin antibiotic therapy.

Drug therapy must be initiated as quickly as possible after obtaining cultures. Do not wait for culture results before starting drug therapy.

When the culture results are known (typically in 2–3 days), antibiotic therapy can be stopped or adjusted, according to the culture results, antibiotic sensitivities, and the baby's clinical condition.

A. Systemic life-threatening infections

The 5 actions noted in Box 8.1 should be taken immediately.

Box 8.1. Actions to Take Immediately in a Baby Suspected of Having Life-Threatening Infection

1. Provide supportive care *quickly*.
2. Obtain cultures and laboratory tests *quickly*. At least 1 mL of blood (preferably more) should be obtained when acquiring blood cultures. Aerobic blood culture should be prioritized over anaerobic cultures.
3. Administer antibiotics *as soon as possible*.
4. Adjust the antibiotics according to culture results.
5. Monitor the antibiotic levels, if indicated.

More details for these 5 steps are as follows:

1. Supportive care

    As soon as a baby is suspected of having a systemic infection, the following actions should be taken immediately:

    - Connect the baby to a heart rate monitor and pulse oximeter.
    - Establish an IV line for
        — Fluids (unstable babies suspected of having sepsis should be given nothing by mouth until their vital signs are stable)
        — Antibiotics and possible emergency medications
    - Check all vital signs frequently (heart rate, respirations, temperature, blood pressure).
    - Perform frequent blood glucose screening tests to check for hypoglycemia and hyperglycemia.

2. Culture and laboratory tests

    Once supportive care has been started, appropriate laboratory studies should be conducted and cultures obtained. Essential studies for all babies in whom sepsis is suspected include

    - Blood cultures
    - WBC count with differential

- Chest radiography, if the baby has signs of respiratory distress
- Platelet count

Consider C-reactive protein (CRP) or procalcitonin (*Ann Clin Biochem.* 2002; 39[Pt 2]:130–135) levels as early markers of infection. Serum values of CRP exceeding 7.5 mg/L, or procalcitonin values exceeding 2.5 mcg/L, particularly when serial measurements show an increase, are potentially suggestive of systemic infection. CRP levels peak 48 hours after the start of infection. However, CRP levels have also been associated with an increase in antibiotic usage/duration and hospital days. Consider these markers if antibiotics are started and there is uncertainty as to whether to stop or continue antibiotics after 48 to 72 hours. A low CRP level is a better indicator of an infant not having an infection than a high CRP level is at suggesting the infant has an infection (a strong negative predictive value). It may also be helpful to check blood pH and serum bicarbonate levels.

Additional studies for babies sufficiently stable to tolerate the procedure(s) include
- Lumbar puncture (for cerebrospinal fluid glucose levels, protein levels, microscopic examination, and culture; consider HSV polymerase chain reaction [PCR] study if there are concerns for HSV infection)
- Blood glucose tests (obtained at the same time as lumbar puncture for comparison with cerebrospinal fluid glucose levels)

Note: Many experts advise delaying a lumbar puncture until a baby is stable because early therapy will not be changed by the results, and the procedure can be very stressful for a baby.

3. Antibiotic therapy

 If a baby is suspected of having a systemic infection, obtain blood cultures and then immediately begin antibiotics. Do not wait for laboratory and culture reports before starting antibiotics.

Antibiotics should be selected to be effective against gram-positive and gram-negative organisms. A general suggestion for choice of antibiotics (Table 8.1) is

ampicillin (gram-positive organisms, including GBS, *Listeria*)	and	**gentamicin** (gram-negative organisms)

Table 8.1. Antibiotic Therapy: Recommended Dosing			
Postmenstrual Age (wk)	Postnatal Days	Dose	Interval[a]
Ampicillin	0–7	100 mg/kg/dose	q12h
	≥8	100 mg/kg/dose	q6–8h
Gentamicin[b]			
≤29[c]	0–7	4 mg/kg/dose	q48h
	8–28	4 mg/kg/dose	q36h
	≥29	4 mg/kg/dose	q24h
30–34	0–7	4 mg/kg/dose	q36h
	≥8	4 mg/kg/dose	q24h
≥35	ALL	4 mg/kg/dose	q24h

Ampicillin dosing is based only on postnatal days and not on postmenstrual age.

[a] Follow a different schedule involving longer intervals for extremely preterm babies and other babies with clinically significant perinatal compromise.

[b] **Gentamicin monitoring:** Measure peak level with positive culture results and troughs when treating >48 hours. Obtain peak concentrations 30 minutes after end of infusion and trough concentrations just prior to the third dose. If the patient has serious infection or significant changes in renal status, consider measuring serum concentration 24 hours after dose administration prior to infusing subsequent doses. This is especially important for infants with renal compromise.

Goal peak: 5–12 mcg/mL   Goal trough: 0.5–2 mcg/mL

[c] Use corrected postmenstrual age when choosing dosing. Use <29-week dose if significant asphyxia, patent ductus arteriosus, or treatment with indomethacin.

Gentamicin administered intravenously should be infused over 30 minutes. Avoid bolus infusion of gentamicin to minimize the drug's ototoxic and nephrotoxic complications. If IV access is not obtainable, gentamicin may be administered via intramuscular injection. Ampicillin may be administered via slow IV push or intramuscular injection.

The infection control service in each hospital should monitor prevalent organisms and, if resistant organisms appear, the choice of first-line antibiotics should be adjusted. For example, cephalosporins are used in some hospitals. Vancomycin is often administered to babies who develop infections later during their hospitalization.

If the baby is infected with a known organism (ie, the infecting organism has been identified and confirmed), antibiotics specific for that organism should be started while other antibiotics are discontinued. Also, when culture results demonstrate that a specific organism is resistant to a specific antibiotic, antibiotic therapy should be changed accordingly.

Note: In addition to ruling out infection by a drug-resistant organism, the use of acyclovir for treatment of possible HSV infection should be considered for babies who become more ill while receiving antibiotic therapy or who develop signs of sepsis, including an increased temperature, at several days of age. Consult regional perinatal center staff.

Use only antibiotics that culture and sensitivity results indicate are effective against the particular infecting organism.

If culture results demonstrate the infecting organism is resistant to a particular antibiotic, either do not use that drug or discontinue its use if already initiated.

If infection is proven or strongly suspected from clinical and laboratory findings, IV antibiotic therapy is usually administered for 7 to 14 days, depending on the type of organism and the severity of illness. Consult an infectious disease expert for the duration of antibiotic therapy, if needed.

If blood cultures show no growth for 36 to 48 hours after attainment and the baby appears well, you might elect to stop antibiotic therapy at that time.

B. Localized infections

The *general principles* of treating localized infections in adults also apply to babies.

- Incision and drainage of abscesses (the material from an abscess should be cultured and a Gram stain prepared)
- Débridement of wound infections
- Culture, Gram stain, and topical treatment of conjunctivitis, except that gonococcal and chlamydial local infections or conjunctivitis will require systemic therapy

Because an abscess may sometimes form at the site where a scalp electrode was placed for fetal monitoring during labor, some experts advise a scrub with antimicrobial soap to the electrode site for all babies who received internal fetal heart rate monitoring. This is not a treatment measure but is used to help prevent development of a scalp abscess.

 Localized infections are much more likely to develop into systemic life-threatening infections in babies than in adults and must therefore be treated promptly and thoroughly.

1. Chlamydial (conjunctivitis, pneumonia)

Topical prophylaxis with silver nitrate, erythromycin, or tetracycline routinely used to prevent gonococcal ophthalmia will *not* reliably prevent chlamydial conjunctivitis. Chlamydial conjunctivitis is treated with systemic erythromycin, administered orally. Babies born to women with untreated or incompletely treated chlamydia infection should be monitored for development of disease. Prophylactic antibiotics are not recommended; neither is cesarean delivery.

If chlamydial conjunctivitis develops, treat it with

- Erythromycin 12.5 mg/kg per dose (50 mg/kg/d) administered orally, every 6 hours for 14 days

Erythromycin therapy is only about 80% effective, however, so follow-up of infected infants is required, and a second course of treatment may be necessary. Erythromycin may be poorly tolerated in some babies, in which case oral azithromycin may be used after the neonatal period.

Treatment with azithromycin should be

- Azithromycin 20 mg/kg daily, administered orally for 3 days

Any infant that tests positive for chlamydial conjunctivitis should also be tested for gonorrhea. Additionally, any infant treated with either erythromycin or azithromycin should be followed up for signs and symptoms of hypertrophic pyloric stenosis.

Chlamydial pneumonia can develop from infection acquired at the time of delivery. Onset of symptoms is usually between 2 and 19 weeks after birth. Treatment is oral erythromycin or sulfonamides.

2. Gonococcal (conjunctivitis, scalp abscess)

Topical antibiotic treatment is not adequate when localized gonococcal infection is present. Systemic antibiotic therapy should be used. Because of the high frequency of penicillin-resistant *Neisseria gonorrhoeae*, ceftriaxone is the preferred antibiotic treatment, although resistance is becoming more common. Treat the baby with

- Ceftriaxone 50 mg/kg (not to exceed 125 mg), one dose, administered intramuscularly or intravenously

  Ceftriaxone should be administered cautiously to babies younger than 1 month—especially preterm babies—owing to the displacement of bilirubin from albumin and the risk of kernicterus. Cefotaxime, 100 mg/kg, administered intravenously or intramuscularly, is recommended for babies with hyperbilirubinemia who are being treated for gonococcal infections.

- Cefotaxime 100 mg/kg, one dose, administered intramuscularly or intravenously

Because topical treatment is inadequate by itself and unnecessary when systemic antibiotic therapy is used, there is no need to use ophthalmic antibiotic ointment for babies with gonococcal conjunctivitis. Instead, those babies should have their eyes irrigated frequently with sterile saline, until the discharge is eliminated.

 If local infection becomes disseminated (eg, sepsis, joint infection), a much longer course of therapy is recommended. Consult an infectious disease expert.

3. Staphylococcal pustulosis

- *Mild:* Thoroughly wash the affected area with mild soap. Follow this cleansing with application of a topical antibiotic ointment, such as mupirocin or bacitracin.

  Note: Epidemic *Staphylococcus aureus* outbreaks in newborn nurseries require special measures. Soaps containing chlorhexidine or alcohol-based rubs are indicated for hand hygiene during outbreaks. However, other measures may also be appropriate. Consult an infectious disease expert.

- *Moderate or severe:* Provide therapy for mild localized infection, *plus* obtain blood cultures and administer oral, intramuscular, or IV antistaphylococcal antibiotics (eg, nafcillin, cefazolin, vancomycin). Be certain to check culture sensitivities because drug-resistant organisms are becoming more common (Kaplan SL. Suspected *Staphylococcus aureus* and streptococcal skin and soft tissue infections in neonates: evaluation and management. UpToDate; 2020).

Self-test C

Now answer these questions to test yourself on the information in the last section.

C1. **True** **False** It is necessary to know the bacterial culture results before beginning antibiotic therapy for a baby suspected of being septic.

C2. What are the 4 supportive procedures that must be initiated if a baby is suspected of having a systemic infection?

_____

_____

_____

_____

C3. What are the 4 essential tests or studies that should be performed for all babies suspected of having a life-threatening infection?

_____

_____

_____

_____

C4. What other tests may be helpful in evaluating a baby with a severe, life-threatening infection?

_____

_____

_____

C5. In selecting antibiotics to administer when an infection is suspected, what 2 general types of organisms need to be considered?_____ and _____

C6. Which of the following statements best describes the treatment of localized infections?
   A. Follow the same procedure as for adults.
   B. Make sure the infection does not spread, by washing the baby with harsh soaps.
   C. The same procedures used on adults apply, but special care must be taken to keep the infection from developing into a systemic, life-threatening infection.

C7. What is a first-line drug to use against gram-negative organisms? _____

C8. **True** **False** Chlamydial conjunctivitis can be treated effectively with an ophthalmic preparation of erythromycin.

C9. **True** **False** If gonococcal conjunctivitis develops, treatment with systemic ceftriaxone or cefotaxime is recommended.

C10. **True** **False** Mild staphylococcal pustulosis infections require treatment with systemic antibiotics.

Check your answers with the list that follows the Recommended Routines. Correct any incorrect answers and review the appropriate section in the unit.

C. Congenital infections

Babies with congenital rubella and certain other infections require special isolation precautions. Women with varicella-zoster virus (chickenpox) infection near the time of delivery, as well as their babies, might require special precautions, depending on the timing of the infection. Many congenital intrauterine infections and some acquired during the birth process (perinatal acquisition) require particular isolation precautions and cannot be treated with specific drug therapy. For these and other infectious diseases not discussed in the following text, consult the resources listed at the beginning of this unit or regional perinatal center staff.

1. Cytomegalovirus
   - *Transmission and risk:* Congenital infection can cause varying degrees of illness in the baby, with primary (first-time) maternal infection, especially early in pregnancy, carrying the highest risk of damage to the fetus. Most babies are not symptomatic at birth, but some will go on to demonstrate hearing loss or learning disability in childhood.
     Infection also can occur as a result of passage through an infected birth canal, ingestion of CMV-positive breast milk, or transfusion of CMV-positive blood. Most babies infected during or shortly after birth do not develop signs of infection. Preterm babies are at greater risk for illness than term babies.
   - *Clinical findings:* Babies with symptomatic CMV infection may present with fetal growth restriction, jaundice (especially conjugated [direct-reacting] hyperbilirubinemia), thrombocytopenia, purpura ("blueberry muffin" rash), hepatosplenomegaly, microcephaly, cerebral calcifications, chorioretinitis, or cataracts.
   - *Diagnosis and treatment:* Viral culture of urine or saliva is used to confirm CMV infection. Neonatal treatment is appropriate for many situations. Consult regional perinatal center staff.
   - *Precautions:* Standard precautions for blood and body fluids are indicated. Meticulous handwashing is particularly important for pregnant women who are caring for patients with known CMV infection. Keep in mind, however, that about 1% of all live-born babies are infected in utero and excrete CMV at birth, but only a small fraction of those babies are recognized as having CMV disease.
   - *Follow-up:* Regardless of their initial clinical presentation, babies with congenital CMV infection, as well as babies with infection acquired soon after birth, should undergo long-term follow-up, with assessment of hearing, vision, psychomotor development, and learning abilities.

2. Hepatitis B virus
   - *Transmission and risk:* Infected persons carry HBV in all body fluids. The virus is transmitted primarily by intimate (usually sexual) contact and less often by transfusion of contaminated blood (rare in the United States) or sharing of needles by drug users. More than one-third of adults who test positive for HBsAg have no easily identified risk factor.

     Routine testing at the first prenatal visit is recommended for *all* women. Vaccination during pregnancy should be offered to HBsAg-negative women. Women who were not screened during pregnancy should be tested when admitted for delivery.

     Transplacental transmission from the pregnant woman to her fetus occurs but is uncommon. Neonatal infection seems to result mainly through direct contact with the mother's blood at the time of delivery. The rate of transmission to the newborn is not affected by whether the woman is a chronic carrier or has an acute infection at the time of delivery or by the route of delivery (cesarean or vaginal delivery). If a baby was not infected at delivery, postnatal transmission through close personal contact between mother and child is likely during early childhood.

     If untreated, more than half the babies born to women with hepatitis B infection will become infected, and up to 25% of those babies will develop fatal liver disease (chronic active hepatitis, cirrhosis, or hepatocellular carcinoma) and die prematurely.
   - *Precautions:* For babies of HBsAg-positive women, the baby should be cleansed promptly of maternal blood after delivery. Standard precautions should be used by health professionals.
   - *Treatment* (Tables 8.2 and 8.3): Transmission of HBV infection can be prevented for approximately 95% of babies born to HBsAg-positive women by the administration of HBV vaccine and hepatitis B immunoglobulin, with the first dose administered within 12 hours of birth.

     The HBV vaccine alone is also highly effective in preventing infection and is recommended for *all* newborns, regardless of whether the mother is HBsAg positive or negative. In either case, a series of 3 doses is required.

 All newborns should receive hepatitis B vaccine (American Academy of Pediatrics, American College of Obstetricians and Gynecologists. Guidelines for Perinatal Care. 8th ed. American Academy of Pediatrics; 2017:490).

Babies born to HBsAg-positive women should also receive hepatitis B immunoglobulin.

Table 8.2. Hepatitis B Immunoprophylaxis According to Newborn Birth Weight[a]		
Maternal Status	**Newborn < 2,000 g (4 lb 6½ oz)**	**Newborn ≥ 2,000 g (4 lb 6½ oz)**
HBsAg positive	Hepatitis B vaccine + HBIG (within 12 h of birth)	Hepatitis B vaccine + HBIG (within 12 h of birth)
	Continue vaccine series beginning at 1–2 mo of age according to recommended schedule for babies born to HBsAg-positive mothers (see Table 8.3).	Continue vaccine series beginning at 1–2 mo of age according to recommended schedule for babies born to HBsAg-positive mothers (see Table 8.3).
	Immunize with 4 vaccine doses; do not count birth dose as part of vaccine series.	
	Check anti-HBs and HBsAg after completion of vaccine series.[b] • HBsAg-negative newborns with anti-HBs levels ≥ 10 mIU/mL are protected and need no further medical management. • HBsAg-negative newborns with anti-HBs levels < 10 mIU/mL should be reimmunized with 3 doses at 2-mo intervals and retested.	Check anti-HBs and HBsAg after completion of vaccine series.[b] • HBsAg-negative newborns with anti-HBs levels of 10 mIU/mL are protected and need no further medical management. • HBsAg-negative newborns with anti-HBs levels < 10 mIU/mL should be reimmunized with 3 doses at 2-mo intervals and retested.
	Newborns who are HBsAg positive should receive appropriate follow-up, including medical evaluation for chronic liver disease.	Newborns who are HBsAg positive should receive appropriate follow-up, including medical evaluation for chronic liver disease.
HBsAg status unknown	Test mother for HBsAg immediately after admission for delivery.	Test mother for HBsAg immediately after admission for delivery.
	Hepatitis B vaccine (by 12 h of birth)	Hepatitis B vaccine (within 12 h of birth)
	Administer HBIG if mother tests HBsAg positive or if mother's HBsAg result is not available within 12 h of birth.	Administer HBIG (within 7 days) if mother tests HBsAg positive; if mother's HBsAg status remains unknown, some experts would administer HBIG (within 7 days).
	Continue vaccine series beginning at 1–2 mo of age according to recommended schedule based on mother's HBsAg result (see Table 8.3).	Continue vaccine series beginning at 1–2 mo of age according to recommended schedule based on mother's HBsAg result (see Table 8.3).
	Immunize with 4 vaccine doses; do not count birth dose as part of vaccine series.	

(continued)

	Table 8.2. Hepatitis B Immunoprophylaxis According to Newborn Birth Weight[a] (*continued*)	
Maternal Status	**Newborn < 2,000 g (4 lb 6½ oz)**	**Newborn ≥ 2,000 g (4 lb 6½ oz)**
HBsAg negative	Delay first dose of hepatitis B vaccine until 1 mo of age or hospital discharge, whichever is first.	Hepatitis B vaccine at birth[c]
	Continue vaccine series beginning at 1–2 mo of age (see Table 8.3).	Continue vaccine series beginning at 1–2 mo of age (see Table 8.3).
	Follow-up anti-HBs and HBsAg testing is not needed.	Follow-up anti-HBs and HBsAg testing is not needed.

Abbreviations: anti-HBs, antibody to hepatitis B surface antigen; HBIG, hepatitis B immune globulin; HBsAg, hepatitis B surface antigen.

[a] Extremes of gestational age and birth weight are no longer a consideration for timing of hepatitis B vaccine doses.

[b] Test at 9 to 18 months of age, generally at the next well-child visit after completion of the primary series. Use a testing method that allows determination of a protective concentration of anti-HBs (10 mIU/mL).

[c] The first dose may be delayed until after hospital discharge for a newborn who weighs at least 2,000 g (≥4 lb 6½ oz) and whose mother is HBsAg negative, but only if a physician's order to withhold the birth dose and a copy of the mother's original HBsAg-negative laboratory report are documented in the newborn's medical record.

Adapted with permission from American Academy of Pediatrics. Hepatitis B. In: Kimberlin DW, Brady MT, Jackson MA, Long SS, eds. *Red Book: 2018 Report of the Committee on Infectious Diseases*. 31st ed. American Academy of Pediatrics; 2018:420.

Table 8.3. Hepatitis B Vaccine According to Maternal Hepatitis B Surface Antigen Status[a,b]

Maternal HBsAg Status	Single-Antigen Vaccine		Single-Antigen + Combination	
	Dose	**Age**	**Dose**	**Age**
Positive	1[c]	Birth (<12 h)	1[c]	Birth (<12 h)
	HBIG[d]	Birth (<12 h)	HBIG	Birth (<12 h)
	2	1–2 mo	2	2 mo
	3[e]	6 mo	3	4 mo
			4[e]	6 mo (Pediarix) or 12–15 mo (Comvax)
Unknown[f]	1[c]	Birth (<12 h)	1[c]	Birth (<12 h)
	2	1–2 mo	2	2 mo
	3[e]	6 mo	3	4 mo
			4[e]	6 mo (Pediarix) or 12–15 mo (Comvax)
Negative	1[c,g]	Birth (before discharge)	1[c,g]	Birth (before discharge)
	2	1–2 mo	2	2 mo
	3[e]	6–18 mo	3	4 mo
			4[e]	6 mo (Pediarix) or 12–15 mo (Comvax)

Abbreviations: HBIG, hepatitis B immune globulin; HBsAg, hepatitis B surface antigen.

[a] Centers for Disease Control and Prevention. A comprehensive immunization strategy to eliminate transmission of hepatitis B virus infection in the United States: recommendations of the Advisory Committee on Immunization Practices (ACIP) part 1: immunization of infants, children, and adolescents. *MMWR Recomm Rep.* 2005;54(RR-16):1–31. http://www.cdc.gov/mmwr/preview/mmwrhtml/rr5416a1.htm. Accessed October 14, 2019.

[b] See Table 8.2 for vaccine schedules for preterm newborns weighing <2,000 g (<4 lb 6½ oz).

[c] Recombivax HB or Engerix-B should be used for the birth dose. Comvax and Pediarix (combination vaccines) cannot be administered at birth or before 6 weeks of age.

[d] Hepatitis B immunoglobulin (0.5 mL) administered intramuscularly in a separate site from the vaccine.

[e] The final dose in the vaccine series should not be administered before 24 weeks (164 days) of age.

[f] Mothers should have blood drawn and tested for HBsAg as soon as possible after admission for delivery; if the mother is found to be HBsAg positive, the newborn should receive HBIG as soon as possible but no later than 7 days of age.

[g] On a case-by-case basis and only in rare circumstances, the first dose may be delayed until after hospital discharge for a newborn who weighs at least 2,000 g (≥4 lb 6½ oz) and whose mother is HBsAg negative, but only if a physician's order to withhold the birth dose and a copy of the mother's original HBsAg-negative laboratory report are documented in the newborn's medical record.

Adapted with permission from American Academy of Pediatrics. Hepatitis B. In: Kimberlin DW, Brady MT, Jackson MA, Long SS, eds. *Red Book: 2018 Report of the Committee on Infectious Diseases.* 31st ed. American Academy of Pediatrics; 2018:422.

3. HSV infection (human herpesvirus)

- *Transmission and risk:* Congenital HSV infection is rare. Transmission to the baby most often occurs during passage through the birth canal, with active lesions present. There is a very low risk of infection to babies born vaginally or via cesarean delivery to women with a history of recurrent genital herpes but who have no symptoms at the time of delivery.

 If a woman has clinically active genital herpes simplex infection when labor begins, prompt cesarean delivery is recommended if the membranes rupture at or near term.

There is no evidence that there is a duration of rupture of membranes beyond which the fetus does not benefit from cesarean delivery. Therefore, a cesarean delivery is recommended at any time after rupture of the membranes. If the fetus is significantly preterm, infectious disease and maternal-fetal medicine expertise is recommended.

Neonatal HSV infection is uncommon; however, if it occurs it carries a high risk of permanent neurological damage or death.

- *Clinical findings:* Neonatal HSV infection can present in different ways.
  — *Systemic disease* involves the liver, lungs, skin, and other organs, including the central nervous system. More than one-third of these babies do not have the vesicular lesions characteristic of herpes. HSV infection should be considered if a baby who is several days of age or who was born after prolonged rupture of membranes develops respiratory distress, seizures, temperature instability (especially fever), increased alanine transaminase levels, and other signs of sepsis.
  — *Infection localized to the central nervous system* appears at presentation with seizures, lethargy, irritability, poor feeding, temperature instability, or bulging fontanels.
  — *Disease localized to the skin, eyes, or mouth* may include conjunctivitis, keratitis, or chorioretinitis. Vesicles or ulcers can be seen on the skin or in the mouth.

Symptoms may be present at birth, especially if rupture of the membranes was prolonged, or may occur as late as 4 to 6 weeks after birth. Onset of systemic disease is usually during the first 2 weeks after birth.

- *Diagnosis:* HSV cultures or PCR assays should be obtained from skin lesions (if present), mouth, conjunctivae, and anus. Blood and cerebral spinal fluid samples should be sent for HSV PCR. Positive cultures obtained 12 to 24 hours after delivery are indicative of infection, rather than contamination from maternal exposure. Immunodiagnostic techniques involving vesicle scrapings are available in some institutions. Serologic testing is of little value when an acute infection is suspected.

- *Treatment:* Consult perinatal regional center experts whenever a baby appears ill at birth after a vaginal delivery involving active maternal disease. If treatment with IV acyclovir is recommended, it should be started promptly. In addition to cultures, other tests may be advisable. Recommendations to treat asymptomatic babies may be made on the basis of culture results. Consultation with infectious disease experts and, often, care at a regional perinatal center is generally recommended for these babies.

Neonatal illness is treated with acyclovir 20 mg/kg/dose administered intravenously every 8 hours for 14 to 21 days, depending on whether the disease is limited to the skin, eyes, or mouth or is disseminated. The dosing interval should be increased if renal or hepatic function is impaired, and renal and hepatic function should be monitored, regardless of the function when therapy is initiated.

- *Precautions:* Contact precautions should be used by health professionals. Newborns known to have been exposed to active HSV lesions and their mothers should be isolated from all other babies. Postnatal infection through direct contact with lesions (around an adult's mouth or a mother's breasts) or through indirect contact from the hands of family or health professionals can occur.

  A private room for the mother, with continuous rooming-in, may be used as long as the baby is not ill and the mother uses good handwashing technique. The mother should use a clean barrier whenever she handles her baby to be sure the baby does not come into contact with lesions or potentially infectious material. If the mother or another family member has "cold sores," a disposable surgical mask should be worn whenever the baby is touched or held, until the lesions have crusted and dried. Even with a mask, nuzzling and kissing the baby should be avoided until the lesions have cleared. If there are no breast lesions, the mother may breastfeed safely.

- *Follow-up:* Parents and health professionals need to be alert to the possibility of the onset of HSV illness at several weeks of age in high-risk babies. Consideration should be given to delaying circumcision beyond 1 month of age in male newborns, because herpes infection is more likely to occur at the site of skin trauma.

4. HIV

- *Transmission and testing:* A history of substance abuse, multiple sexual partners, or sexually transmitted infection(s) may indicate an increased risk for HIV. However, with increasing heterosexual transmission, there may be no apparent risk factors. While universal HIV testing is recommended for all pregnant women, infected babies continue to be born to undiagnosed women. Treatment of a pregnant woman who is HIV positive can

  — Delay the onset of active disease for the woman.

  — Dramatically reduce the likelihood that the virus will be passed to the baby.

 Routine testing of all pregnant women for HIV infection is recommended (for more information on HIV testing, see American Academy of Pediatrics, American College of Obstetricians and Gynecologists. Guidelines for Perinatal Care. 8th ed. American Academy of Pediatrics; 2017).

Rapid testing should be offered to any woman in labor if she was not tested during pregnancy or if her result is not known.

If a woman's HIV status during pregnancy or postpartum is unknown, HIV testing of the newborn is important for care of the baby (American Academy of Pediatrics, American College of Obstetricians and Gynecologists. Guidelines for Perinatal Care. 8th ed. American Academy of Pediatrics; 2017:503).

Nearly all babies born to women who are HIV positive—even babies not actually infected with the virus—will test positive at birth because of antibodies acquired in utero from the mother.

Babies born to women who are HIV positive should be tested at 1 month and at 4 to 6 months of age. Nearly 100% of HIV-infected babies can be identified by 4 to 6 months of age. Early antiviral therapy is indicated for all babies who are exposed to HIV.

- *Precautions:* After delivery, all blood and maternal body secretions should be removed from the baby's skin. There is no need to isolate the mother or the baby, although standard precautions should be used. If desired, the baby may room-in with the mother. Breastfeeding should be discouraged, however, because the virus can be transmitted through breast milk.

- *Treatment:* Combination antiretroviral therapy or monotherapy with zidovudine administered during pregnancy and labor has been shown to reduce mother-to-child transmission by two-thirds.

Cesarean delivery, performed before the onset of labor and before rupture of the membranes, may be of particular benefit to babies whose mothers have a high viral RNA load of 1,000 copies/mL or more at the time of delivery.

If antenatal and intrapartum zidovudine treatment were used, continue zidovudine therapy for the baby. Even if a woman did not receive antepartum or intrapartum zidovudine, recommended neonatal therapy, starting within 12 hours of birth, is as follows:

— 35 weeks' gestational age and older: zidovudine 4 mg/kg, twice daily, for the first 4 to 6 weeks of age, starting as soon as possible after birth.

— 30 weeks to 35 weeks' gestational age: zidovudine 2 mg/kg, twice daily, for 14 days; then increase to 3 mg/kg, twice daily, to complete a total of 6 weeks of treatment. Newborns unable to take oral medications should be treated with IV zidovudine 1.5 mg/kg, twice daily, and subsequently switched to the oral regimen as soon as possible.

— Younger than 30 weeks' gestational age: zidovudine 2 mg/kg, twice daily, for 28 days; then increase to 3 mg/kg, twice daily, to complete a total of 6 weeks of treatment. Newborns unable to take oral medications should be treated with IV zidovudine 1.5 mg/kg, twice daily, and subsequently switched to the oral regimen as soon as possible.

In mothers who did not receive antiretroviral treatment before the onset of labor, a 2- or 3-drug neonatal treatment regimen has resulted in a lower rate of maternal-to-child HIV transmission. A preferred regimen is as follows:

— Zidovudine: dosed as previously described.

— Nevirapine: 3-dose regimen. The first dose is administered as soon as possible after birth; the second dose is administered 48 hours after the first dose; and the third dose is administered 96 hours after the second dose. Dosing is based on birth weight.
  - 1,500 (3 lb 5 oz) to 2,000 g (4 lb 6½ oz): 8 mg total for each dose
  - More than 2,000 g: 12 mg total for each dose

Consult the 2021 *Red Book* (https://shop.aap.org/red-book-2021-report-of-the-committee-on-infectious-diseases-32nd-edition-paperback/) or access http://aidsinfo.nih.gov for up-to-date treatment regimens.

Arrange for comprehensive follow-up care for HIV-positive babies, their mothers, and their families.

 Evaluation, monitoring, and management of babies born to women who are HIV positive can be complex. Information changes rapidly. Consult with infectious disease experts. In addition, refer to www.cdc.gov and http://aidsinfo.nih.gov.

5. Syphilis
- *Transmission:* Over the past several years, there has been a nationwide increase in congenital syphilis. Transmission to the fetus can occur at any stage in the woman's illness and at any time during pregnancy. High-risk patients whose serologic screening result was negative earlier in the pregnancy should be rescreened in the third trimester or at delivery.

 No newborn should be discharged from a hospital without determination of the mother's serologic status for syphilis (American Academy of Pediatrics, American College of Obstetricians and Gynecologists. Guidelines for Perinatal Care. 8th ed. American Academy of Pediatrics; 2017:543; and American Academy of Pediatrics. Red Book: 2021 Report of the Committee on Infectious Diseases. Kimberlin DW, Barnett ED, Lynfield R, Sawyer MH, eds. 32nd ed. American Academy of Pediatrics; 2021).

- *Precautions:* **Contact precautions should be used until penicillin therapy has been administered for at least 24 hours.** Parents, visitors, and health professionals should use gloves when handling the baby during this time.
- *Evaluation* (Figure 8.3)
  1. Whom to evaluate?
     Any baby, if syphilis in the woman was
     — Untreated or inadequately treated
     — Treated with a non-penicillin regimen (eg, erythromycin) or an inadequate penicillin dose
     — Treated appropriately with penicillin, but the expected decrease in nontreponemal antibody titer did not occur
     — Treated less than 1 month before delivery
     — Treated, but the treatment or penicillin dose was not documented
     — Treated but with insufficient serologic follow-up to be able to assess the response to treatment and the current infection status

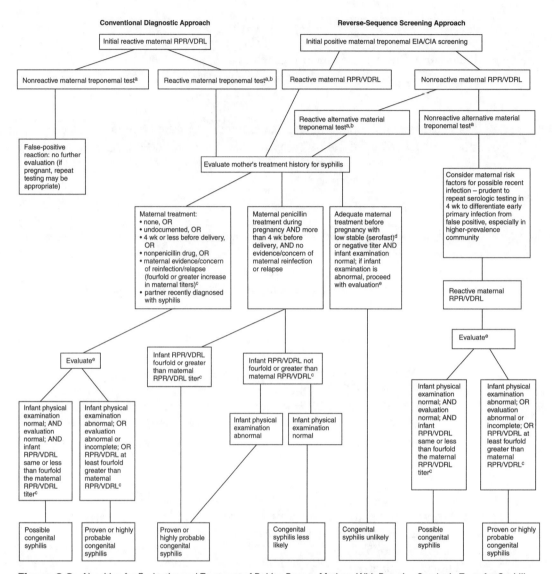

Figure 8.3. Algorithm for Evaluation and Treatment of Babies Born to Mothers With Reactive Serologic Tests for Syphilis
Abbreviations: EIA, enzyme immunoassay; RPR, rapid plasma reagin; VDRL, Venereal Disease Research Laboratory.

[a] *Treponema pallidum* particle agglutination (TP-PA) (which is the preferred treponemal test), fluorescent treponemal antibody absorption (FTA-ABS), or microhemagglutination test for antibodies to *T pallidum* (MHA-TP).

[b] Test for HIV antibody. Infants of HIV-infected mothers do not require different evaluation or treatment for syphilis.

[c] A 4-fold change in titer is the same as a change of 2 dilutions. For example, a titer of 1:64 is 4-fold greater than a titer of 1:16, and a titer of 1:4 is 4-fold lower than a titer of 1:16. When comparing titers, the same type of nontreponemal test should be used (eg, if the initial test was an RPR, the follow-up test should also be an RPR).

[d] Stable VDRL titers 1:2 or less or RPR 1:4 or less beyond 1 year after successful treatment are considered low serofast.

[e] Complete blood cell and platelet count; cerebrospinal fluid examination for cell count, protein, and quantitative VDRL; other tests as clinically indicated (eg, chest radiographs, long-bone radiographs, eye examination, liver function tests, neuroimaging, and auditory brainstem response). Reproduced with permission from American Academy of Pediatrics. Syphilis. In: Kimberlin DW, Brady MT, Jackson MA, Long SS, eds. *Red Book: 2018 Report of the Committee on Infectious Diseases*. 31st ed. American Academy of Pediatrics; 2018.

2. What to include?

- *Physical examination:* Clinical findings suggestive of congenital syphilis include unexplained jaundice, rash, hepatosplenomegaly, pneumonia, anemia, lymphadenopathy, and thrombocytopenia. Most infected babies, however, are asymptomatic.
- *Nontreponemal serologic test* of the baby's blood (cord blood testing is unreliable because of high false-positive and false-negative results)
- *Lumbar puncture* with testing of cerebrospinal fluid for Venereal Disease Research Laboratory (VDRL) cells and protein
- *Radiographs* of the long bones
- *Other tests* as indicated, such as chest radiography, complete blood cell count, liver function tests, ophthalmologic examinations, and auditory brainstem response tests.

 Babies can have congenital syphilis without displaying any clinical signs of infection.

If untreated, syphilis will cause irreversible damage to a baby's brain and other organs, although the damage may not become apparent until many years after birth.

- *Tests:* Two types of serologic tests, nontreponemal (VDRL, rapid plasma reagin, and automated reagin test) and treponemal (microhemagglutination assay—*Treponema pallidum* and fluorescent treponemal antibody absorption), are used to detect an infection, but neither type of test by itself is sufficient to establish a diagnosis.
- *Treatment:* If a baby had risk factors that prompted evaluation for congenital syphilis, treatment should be administered if
  — Infection is documented.
  — Tests results cannot rule out infection.
  — The baby cannot be fully evaluated.
  — Adequate follow-up cannot be ensured.

Follow the treatment guidelines in Table 8.4.

Table 8.4. Recommended Treatment of Neonates (≤4 Weeks of Age) With Proven or Possible Congenital Syphilis		
Clinical Status	**Evaluation**	**Antimicrobial Therapy**
Proven or highly probable disease	CSF analysis for VDRL, cell count, and protein CBC and platelet count Other tests as clinically indicated (eg, long-bone radiography, liver function tests, ophthalmologic examination)	Aqueous crystalline penicillin G, 100,000–150,000 U/kg per day, administered as 50,000 U/kg per dose, IV, every 12 h during the first 7 days of age and every 8 h thereafter for a total of 10 days (preferred) **OR** Penicillin G procaine, 50,000 U/kg per day, IM, in a single dose for 10 days
Physical examination within reference range and serum quantitative nontreponemal titer the same or less than 4-fold the maternal titer (a) (i) Mother was not treated or was inadequately treated or has no documented treatment;	CSF analysis for VDRL, cell count, and protein CBC and platelet count Long-bone radiography	Aqueous crystalline penicillin G, IV, for 10 days, as above **OR**
(ii) mother was treated with erythromycin or other non-penicillin regimen; (iii) mother received treatment 4 wk before delivery; (iv) maternal evidence of reinfection or relapse (4-fold or greater increase in titers)	None	Penicillin G procaine, 50,000 U/kg per day, IM, in a single dose for 10 days **OR**
(b) (i) Adequate maternal therapy given >4 wk before delivery; (ii) mother has no evidence of reinfection or relapse		Penicillin G benzathine, 50,000 U/kg, IM, in a single dose Clinical, serologic follow-up, and penicillin G benzathine, 50,000 U/kg, IM, in a single dose
(c) Adequate therapy before pregnancy and mother's nontreponemal serologic titer remained low and stable during pregnancy and at delivery	None	None

Abbreviations: CBC, complete blood cell count; CSF, cerebrospinal fluid; IM, intramuscular; IV, intravenous; VDRL, Venereal Disease Research Laboratory.

Derived from American Academy of Pediatrics. Syphilis. In: Kimberlin DW, Brady MT, Jackson MA, Long SS, eds. *Red Book: 2018 Report of the Committee on Infectious Diseases*. 31st ed. American Academy of Pediatrics; 2018:782.

- *Follow-up:* Newborns treated for congenital syphilis should undergo follow-up evaluations at 1, 2, 4, 6, and 12 months of age, with nontreponemal tests performed at 2 to 4, 6, and 12 months after treatment ended or until the tests become nonreactive or the titer has decreased 4-fold. Titers should decline by 3 months of age and become nonreactive by 6 months of age. Consider repeat treatment if titers remain stable, including persistently low titers. Newborns who had cerebrospinal fluid findings outside reference range and neurosyphilis require more extensive and longer-term follow-up. Expert consultation is recommended for these babies.

6. Toxoplasmosis

- *Transmission and risk:* Toxoplasmosis infection is rarely recognized in a pregnant woman because the illness is self-limited and mild, with nonspecific symptoms often described as a "cold." Feces of infected cats and meat of infected sheep, pigs, and cattle harbor the organism, with human infection usually resulting from exposure to cat feces or ingestion of raw or undercooked meat. Reinfection is uncommon and occurs only in immunosuppressed persons because the first infection normally confers lifelong immunity. Babies born to women with HIV and toxoplasmosis infection are at significantly increased risk for becoming infected.

  Maternal infection early in pregnancy is more likely to cause severe symptoms than infection late in pregnancy. More than 70% of babies with congenital infection have no symptoms at birth, although visual impairment, learning disability, or intellectual disability may become apparent months or years later.

- *Clinical findings:* Neonatal symptoms of congenital toxoplasmosis may include hepatosplenomegaly, jaundice, thrombocytopenia, anemia, seizures, microcephaly, hydrocephalus, intracranial calcifications, or lymphadenopathy.

- *Diagnosis and treatment:* Consult regional perinatal center neonatal and infectious disease experts. Serologic tests are the primary diagnostic methods. Availability and interpretation of sensitive and specific assays usually require specialized expertise. Treatment requires multiple drugs administered over a prolonged period. Investigational drugs may be appropriate in some circumstances.

- *Precautions:* Standard precautions are recommended.

7. Rubella

- *Transmission and risk:* The likelihood of transplacental transmission of rubella is very high during the first trimester and somewhat lower later in pregnancy. Maternal infection, especially early during the first trimester, carries a high risk of spontaneous abortion, fetal death, or congenital rubella syndrome. Second-trimester infection may be less harmful, but growth restriction, intellectual disability, or deafness is possible. Third-trimester infection is associated with less risk for fetal harm. Some infected babies display little or no clinical evidence of infection at birth but may demonstrate hearing defects, abnormal neuromuscular development, learning deficits, or behavioral disturbances later in childhood.

313

- *Clinical findings:* Congenital rubella syndrome typically includes serious eye disorders (cataracts, glaucoma) as well as auditory, cardiac, and neurological disorders. Fetal growth restriction, microcephaly, hepatosplenomegaly, thrombocytopenia, and purpuric skin lesions (blueberry muffin rash) may also occur.
- *Diagnosis and treatment:* Consult your local regional perinatal center and/or infectious disease specialist. Treatment is supportive.
- *Precautions:* Contact isolation is indicated for children with proven or suspected congenital rubella until they are at least 1 year of age or they have 2 cultures negative for rubella virus at least 1 month apart after the age of 3 months.

8. Tuberculosis (TB)
   - *Transmission and risk:* Congenital TB is rare, but in utero infection can occur when there is maternal bacillemia.
   - *Clinical findings:* Infants are generally asymptomatic if TB is acquired perinatally.
   - *Diagnosis and treatment:* If a newborn is suspected of having congenital TB, a tuberculin skin test (TST), chest radiography, lumbar puncture, and cultures should be performed promptly. TST test results are generally negative in perinatal acquired TB; thus, treatment should be initiated regardless of TST results. Consult infectious disease experts and the regional perinatal center for treatment and follow-up plans.
   - *Precautions:* Precautions for the infant depend on maternal findings.
     — *Mother with positive TST results and normal chest radiographic findings –* Asymptomatic mothers require no separation from the infant. The infant does not need evaluation or therapy.
     — *Mother with clinical signs and/or symptoms and abnormal chest radiographic findings suggestive of TB –* Infants should be evaluated for congenital TB. Mother and infant should be separated until appropriate therapy is provided to the mother. Mothers should also wear a mask and adhere to infection control measures.
     — *Mother with positive TST results, abnormal chest radiographic findings, but no clinical evidence of TB –* Infants are likely at very low risk of TB infection and do not require separation.

9. Varicella-Zoster
   - *Transmission and risk:* Fetal infection with varicella-zoster virus during the first or second trimester can result in fetal death or varicella embryopathy, characterized by limb hypoplasia, scarring of the skin, and eye and/or nervous system damage. Fetal infection from maternal varicella beyond the second trimester is less likely. Maternal varicella infection between 5 days before and 2 days after delivery is associated with a high infant mortality rate. This is because there is little time for the infant to transplacentally acquire maternal antibodies to the disease.
   - *Diagnosis and treatment:* Diagnosis is typically established clinically; however, varicella can be identified by using various diagnostic tests of lesions. Consult infectious disease experts. VARIZIG is the treatment of choice for newborns exposed to varicella who can receive treatment within 10 days of exposure. If VARIZIG is not available, IV immunoglobulin (400 mg/kg) should be administered. Consult your regional perinatal center for up-to-date treatment guidelines.

- *Precautions*: Airborne and contact precautions are recommended for all infants born to mothers with varicella until 21 days of age or up to 28 days of age if VARIZIG or IV immunoglobulin was administered. Infants should be separated from their mothers until the mother's vesicles have dried. If the infant is born with lesions, the mother and infant can be isolated together. Infants with varicella embryopathy without active skin lesions do not need isolation.

10. Coronavirus disease 2019 (COVID-19 or SARS-CoV-2)

- *Transmission and risk*: In late 2019, a novel coronavirus spread across the world, causing a global pandemic. At the time of this writing, there is much that we have yet to learn about COVID-19 and its effect on newborns and infants. It appears that children, neonates included, are less likely than adults to be clinically affected by the virus; however, there have been case reports of both term and preterm infants with respiratory distress after delivery from a mother who tested positive for the virus. The clinical presentation has varied from severe pneumonia to mild respiratory distress; however, most newborns who have tested positive remain asymptomatic. Other reported signs have included fever, cough, lethargy, rhinorrhea, diarrhea, and vomiting. The current understanding is that SARS-CoV-2 is transmitted primarily through respiratory droplets, either during or shortly after delivery. It is unknown whether transplacental passage occurs, and if it does, what effect this has on the infant.

- *Diagnosis and treatment*: At the time of this writing, there is no specific treatment that has been recommended for infants and newborns who have tested positive for COVID-19. Current recommendations from the American Academy of Pediatrics include testing infants for COVID-19 24 hours after birth for SARS-CoV-2 RNA via PCR if their mother tested positive within 14 days of delivery or if the mother is a person under investigation for COVID-19. An additional test at 48 hours of age is recommended if the initial test result is negative. For the most complete up-to-date recommendations on diagnosis and treatment, consult your referral neonatologist, infectious disease experts, or the Centers for Disease Control and Prevention (www.cdc.gov).

- *Precautions*: Current recommendations indicate that all infants born to mothers with confirmed or suspected COVID-19 should also be suspected as being infected until laboratory tests are available. Infants with presumed COVID-19 should not be cohorted with other infants, and health professionals should use appropriate personal protective equipment (PPE) owing to the risk of aerosolization. For the most complete, up-to-date PPE recommendations and precautions, consult your local infectious disease expert or the Centers for Disease Control and Prevention (www.cdc.gov).

D. Hospital-acquired infections

Care for babies with nosocomial infections is the same as for any baby who has a systemic infection. Because hospital-acquired infections are more likely to be caused by drug-resistant organisms, pay close attention to culture results and antibiotic sensitivities and adjust antibiotic therapy accordingly.

6. How do you care for a baby whose mother received antibiotics during labor?

Women may receive antibiotics during labor for the prevention of early-onset GBS disease. See Book 2: Maternal and Fetal Care, Unit 3, Infectious Diseases in Pregnancy, for a description and flow diagram of recommended intrapartum antibiotic therapy.

It has been shown that penicillin or ampicillin administered during labor (intrapartum prophylaxis [IAP]) to women at risk for transmitting GBS disease decreases the number of babies who become infected. Neonatal GBS infection can cause life-threatening, systemic illness. Three potential options for early-onset sepsis risk assessment for infants born at least 35 weeks' gestational age are presented in Figure 8.4. For infants born at less than 35 weeks' gestational age, blood cultures should be performed and empirical antibiotics started in the setting of preterm labor, prelabor rupture of membranes, or any concern for intraamniotic infection (such as chorioamnionitis); if there was an indication for GBS IAP but antibiotics were not administered to the mother; or if the infant has any respiratory or cardiovascular instability.

Although intrapartum antibiotics are administered to help prevent neonatal GBS disease, a small number of babies will still become infected. However, routine administration of antibiotics to all newborns born to women who received intrapartum antibiotics for the prevention of GBS infection is not recommended.

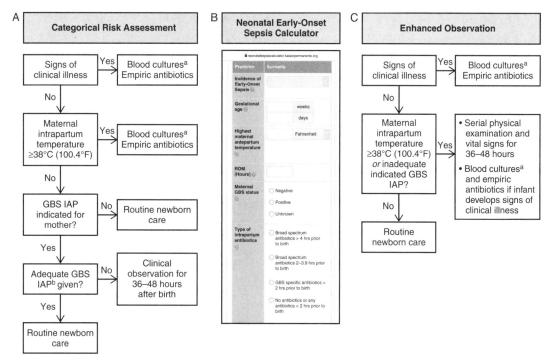

Figure 8.4. Options for Early-Onset Sepsis Risk Assessment Among Infants ≥ 35 Weeks' Gestational Age

A, Categorical risk assessment. B, Neonatal early-onset sepsis calculator. The screenshot of the Neonatal Early-Onset Sepsis Calculator (https://neonatalsepsiscalculator.kaiserpermanente.org/) was used with permission from Kaiser-Permanente Division of Research. C, Enhanced observation.

Abbreviations: GBS, group B β-hemolytic streptococcus; IAP, intrapartum prophylaxis.

[a] Consider lumbar puncture and cerebrospinal fluid culture before initiation of empirical antibiotics for infants who are at the highest risk of infection, especially those with crucial illness. Lumbar puncture should not be performed if the infant's clinical condition would be compromised, and antibiotics should be administered promptly and not deferred because of procedure delays.

[b] Adequate GBS IAP is defined as the administration of penicillin G, ampicillin, or cefazolin ≥ 4 hours before delivery.

Reproduced with permission from Puppolo KM, Lynfield R, Cummings JJ; American Academy of Pediatrics Committee on Fetus and Newborn, Committee on Infectious Diseases. Management of infants at risk for Group B streptococcal disease. *Pediatrics.* 2019;144(2):e20191881.

7. How do you provide for infection control in the nursery?

GOOD HANDWASHING and use of waterless antiseptic agents are the most important techniques for preventing the spread of infection.

A. Health professionals

Because the screening of pregnant women for the presence of HIV or hepatitis infections is recommended but not mandatory, and because physical examination does not allow the identification of adults or newborns infected with these viruses, blood and body fluid precautions should be used for *all* patients. These precautions will also help protect patients and health professionals against the spread of other bacterial and viral pathogens.

Standard precautions should be used at all times. Many hospital protocols specify that gloves should be worn for *every* contact with patients or with patient equipment that may involve

- Blood
- Any body fluid, secretion, or excretion, *except sweat,* regardless of whether it contains visible blood
- Non-intact skin
- Mucous membranes

When handling more than one baby, gloves should be changed between them. In addition, the use of gloves does not replace handwashing or the use of waterless antiseptic agents. Gloves may be defective or may become torn with wear. Therefore, wash your hands with water and an antiseptic solution or rub your hands with a waterless antiseptic agent each time you change your gloves.

Protective gowns and eyewear, masks, or face shields are recommended when exposure to splashed blood or body fluids is likely, such as in the delivery room or during suctioning and other such procedures.

Standard (blood and body fluid) precautions should be used consistently
- *For all patients*
- *By all health professionals*
- *At all times*

In addition to protecting themselves from infection, all health workers need to be vigilant in preventing transmission of infection between babies and from personnel or other patients to babies. Hospital-acquired infections can and should be prevented. This is of increasing importance in light of the growing problem of drug-resistant organisms.

Certain illnesses require transmission-based precautions (airborne, droplet, or contact) in addition to standard precautions used for all patients. Consult with the sources listed at the beginning of this unit or the infection control staff in your hospital.

The importance of GOOD HANDWASHING and use of waterless antiseptic agents cannot be overstated in preventing transmission of infections from
- *Baby to baby*
- *Personnel to baby*
- *Baby to personnel*

B. Babies

For babies with "closed space" infections (eg, sepsis, meningitis, urinary tract infections), good handwashing technique should suffice for prevention of the spread of these infections.

Certain babies are more likely to be shedding organisms and, ideally, should be isolated from other babies. These include babies with

- Diarrhea
- Bacterial or viral pneumonia
- Open infections, such as wound infections
- Staphylococcal disease, such as pustulosis and abscess
- Congenital infections

It may be impractical to isolate such babies in a separate room, particularly if a baby is critically ill. Physical separation within the nursery is acceptable, although separate staffing is recommended. In general, pregnant women should not care for babies who have congenital viral infections.

A small number of infections are transmitted by airborne droplets, and babies with these infections should be isolated from the nursery altogether. These include babies with

- Chickenpox (varicella-zoster virus)
- Congenital TB

See Book 2: Maternal and Fetal Care, Unit 3, Infectious Diseases in Pregnancy, for further discussion of maternal and neonatal management of TB and chickenpox.

 Each hospital should have written protocols for the control of infections in the obstetric area and the nursery. You should be familiar with these procedures.

C. Use of antibiotics

The appropriate use of antibiotics will help curtail the development of drug-resistant organisms. Care should be taken to use first-line antibiotics initially. For example, do not use vancomycin when ampicillin would be equally effective. Switch to other antibiotics only when culture sensitivities indicate the first choice is not effective against the specific infecting agent or a patient develops new signs of infection while receiving first-line antibiotics.

Promptly discontinue use of any antibiotic shown to be ineffective against a particular organism.

Self-test E

Now answer these questions to test yourself on the information in the last section.

E1. What is the single most important thing that can be done to prevent the spread of infection?

_____

E2. Blood and body fluid precautions should be used for
- **A.** All babies
- **B.** Babies with a known viral infection
- **C.** Babies of HIV-positive mothers
- **D.** Babies of all mothers who received no prenatal care

E3. What should be done if a culture report indicates that gram-positive infecting bacteria are not sensitive to an antibiotic a baby is receiving?
- **A.** Stop antibiotics and begin acyclovir.
- **B.** Increase the dose of the antibiotic.
- **C.** Continue use of the antibiotic and begin the use of another antibiotic known to be effective against gram-positive organisms.
- **D.** Stop the antibiotic and begin the use of another antibiotic known to be effective against gram-positive organisms.

E4. **True**   **False**   The use of gloves eliminates the need for handwashing.

E5. Infection control means to:

Yes	No	
____	____	Prevent the transmission of organisms from an infected baby to other babies in the nursery.
____	____	Wash hands before and after caring for each baby.
____	____	Keep all babies with proven infections in isolation.
____	____	Prevent the transmission of organisms between health professionals and patients.
____	____	Prevent the transmission of organisms from an infected baby to health professionals.
____	____	Use broad-spectrum antibiotics for all at-risk patients.

Check your answers with the list that follows the Recommended Routines. Correct any incorrect answers and review the appropriate section in the unit.

INFECTIONS

Recommended Routines

All the routines listed below are based on the principles of perinatal care presented in the unit you have just finished. They are recommended as part of routine perinatal care.

Read each routine carefully and decide whether it is standard operating procedure in your hospital. Check the appropriate blank next to each routine.

Procedure Standard in My Hospital	Needs Discussion by Our Staff	Recommended Routine
_____	_____	1. Establish a system to periodically review the use of infection control measures and ensure that good handwashing or use of a waterless antiseptic agent and standard precautions are used *at all times*.
_____	_____	2. Establish a mechanism to invoke additional transmission-based precautions, as appropriate, for individual patients.
_____	_____	3. Establish a system for ensuring that maternal risk factors for infection are reliably transferred to a baby's chart and that the baby's health professionals are notified.
_____	_____	4. Establish a policy of performing a blood culture before starting antibiotic therapy.
_____	_____	5. Establish a routine of withholding feedings, starting an intravenous line, and attaching an electronic heart rate monitor and pulse oximeter for all babies in whom sepsis is suspected.
_____	_____	6. Establish written protocols for management of babies and pregnant or postpartum women with suspected or proven contagious diseases.
_____	_____	7. Establish a system to provide hepatitis B immunization for *all* babies, according to recommendations for baby's birth weight and maternal hepatitis B surface antigen status.
_____	_____	8. Consider establishing a policy to provide antimicrobial cleansing of the scalp electrode site for all babies who received internal fetal heart rate monitoring.

Self-test Answers

These are the answers to the Self-test questions. Please check them with the answers you gave and review the information in the unit wherever necessary.

Self-test A

A1. Inadequate handwashing by hospital staff may result in a newborn developing a(n) *hospital-acquired or nosocomial* infection.

A2. A, C, and D

A3. ___A___ *Escherichia coli* infection

    ___B___ Staphylococcal pustulosis

    ___B___ Conjunctivitis

    ___A___ Group B β-hemolytic streptococcus infection

    _A, C_ Cytomegalovirus

A4. False   *Reason:* There is a high mortality rate for babies with sepsis. Also, blood infections in babies may develop into meningitis, which may result in severe damage.

A5. True

A6. True

Self-test B

B1. A. There are certain predisposing conditions that make it likely the baby will become infected.

B2. Any 3 of the following conditions:
- Rupture of membranes longer than 18 hours (although uncommon, it is also possible for a fetus to become infected through intact membranes [ascending infection])
- Labor longer than 20 hours
- Maternal fever (temperature of 38.0°C [100.4°F] and higher) during labor
- Maternal illness (eg, varicella, gastroenteritis, urinary tract infection)
- Preterm delivery
- Pregnant woman with genital herpes simplex virus (HSV) lesions at the time the membranes rupture
- Birth canal or rectum colonized with group B β-hemolytic streptococcus (GBS) or history of a previous baby with GBS infection or GBS bacteriuria at any time during this pregnancy
- Invasive procedure or any foreign body, such as an umbilical catheter
- Prolonged hospitalization (more than several days)

B3. Any 2 of the following conditions:
- High staphylococcal colonization rates in other newborns in the nursery
- Puncture site
- Staphylococcal, gonococcal, or chlamydial infections predisposing a baby to conjunctivitis

B4. D. All of the above

B5. Swelling at the infected site

Warmth of the infected area

Erythema of the infected site

Pustules

Red, swollen, watery, or pus-filled eye(s), if conjunctivitis

B6. Any 2 of the following conditions:
- Rubella (German measles), syphilis, varicella, or cytomegalovirus infection in the mother during pregnancy
- Maternal exposure to cat litter during pregnancy

- Mother with active genital HSV infection at the time of delivery
- Mother who tests positive for hepatitis B surface antigen
- Mother who tests positive for HIV

B7. False *Reason:* A baby with sepsis may have laboratory findings within reference ranges. In a baby with risk factors or clinical signs of sepsis, the white blood cell (WBC) count and differential findings, if outside reference range, may provide further evidence of sepsis. However, a baby who experienced perinatal compromise or who was stressed may have a WBC count and differential outside reference ranges, without being infected.

Self-test C

C1. False *Reason:* While blood cultures should be performed before antibiotics are started, antibiotic therapy should not be delayed until culture results are known. As soon as a baby suspected of being septic is stabilized and blood cultures are performed, antibiotics should be started. Many institutions believe this should be done immediately (within 1 hour of birth) or, if the baby becomes sick later, within 1 hour of when sepsis is first suspected. If necessary, the antibiotics used may be readjusted once the culture and sensitivity results are known.

C2. Connect the baby to a cardiac monitor and pulse oximeter.
Establish an intravenous line; consider giving the baby nothing by mouth.
Check vital signs frequently.
Perform blood glucose screening tests frequently.

C3. Blood culture
Chest radiography, if there are signs of respiratory distress
White blood cell count and differential
Platelet count

C4. Blood pH and serum bicarbonate levels
C-reactive protein or procalcitonin levels
Lumbar puncture (for stable babies able to tolerate procedure) with simultaneous blood glucose level checks

C5. *Gram positive* and *gram negative*

C6. C. The same procedures used on adults apply, but special care must be taken to keep the infection from developing into a systemic, life-threatening infection. (Gonococcal, chlamydial, and certain staphylococcal infections, however, also require systemic therapy.)

C7. *Gentamicin*

C8. False *Reason:* Chlamydial conjunctivitis requires treatment with systemic erythromycin or a sulfonamide antibiotic.

C9. True

C10. False *Reason:* Mild staphylococcal pustulosis can be washed with mild soap and treated with a topical antibiotic. Moderate or severe infections require those measures, plus systemic treatment with suitable antibiotics.

Self-test D

D1. True
D2. False *Reason:* Most babies with congenital syphilis show no signs or symptoms of the infection at birth. Only a few infected babies will have characteristic findings.

D3. True
D4. True

D5. False   *Reason:* The risk of neonatal herpes infection is very low when a woman with a history of herpes infections delivers vaginally and no active lesions are present at the time of delivery. The risk of neonatal herpes infection is much higher if active lesions are present whcn vaginal delivery occurs, regardless of the time since membrane rupture.

D6. True

D7. True

D8. True

D9. True

Self-test E

E1. Good handwashing before and after handling each baby

E2. A. All babies

E3. D. Stop the antibiotic and begin use of another antibiotic known to be effective against gram-positive organisms.

E4. False   *Reason:* Gloves may be defective or may become damaged. Hands should be washed each time gloves are changed.

E5.

Yes	No	
X	___	Prevent transmission of organisms from an infected baby to other babies in the nursery.
X	___	Wash hands before and after caring for each baby.
___	X	Keep all babies with proven infections in isolation.
X	___	Prevent the transmission of organisms between health professionals and patients.
X	___	Prevent the transmission of organisms from an infected baby to health professionals.
___	X	Use broad-spectrum antibiotics for all at-risk patients.

Unit 8 Posttest

After completion of each unit there is a free online posttest available at www.cmevillage.com to test your understanding. Navigate to the PCEP pages on www.cmevillage.com and register to take the free posttests.

Once registered on the website and after completing all the unit posttests, pay the book exam fee ($15) and pass the test at 80% or greater to earn continuing education credits. Only start the PCEP book exam if you have time to complete it. If you take the book exam and are not connected to a printer, either print your certificate to a .pdf file and save it to print later or come back to www.cmevillage.com at any time and print a copy of your educational transcript.

Credits are only available by book, not by individual unit within the books. Available credits for completion of each book exam are as follows: Book 1: 14.5 credits; Book 2: 16 credits; Book 3: 17 credits; Book 4: 9 credits.

For more details, navigate to the PCEP webpages at www.cmevillage.com.

Unit 9: Identifying and Caring for Sick and At-Risk Babies

Objectives

In this unit you will

A. Review the concepts taught in Book 1: Maternal and Fetal Evaluation and Immediate Newborn Care, Unit 1, Is the Mother Sick? Is the Fetus Sick?, and Unit 4, Is the Baby Sick? Recognizing and Preventing Problems in the Newborn.

B. Review the situations in which *anticipation* of problems is most important.

C. Review the situations in which *immediate action* is most important.

D. Learn how to *decide what to do first* when a sick baby has more than one problem.

E. Work through a *realistic clinical case example* to apply the information learned in the previous units to the care of newborns in your hospital.

Unit 9 Pretest

Before reading the unit, please answer the following questions. Select the *one best* answer to each question (unless otherwise instructed). Record your answers on the test and check them with the answers at the end of the book.

1A. A 4,000-g (8 lb 13 oz) baby girl is born in your hospital to a woman who was diagnosed with glucose tolerance outside reference range at 24 weeks of gestation. She underwent cesarean delivery at 36 weeks because of stress test results outside reference range. The Apgar scores of the baby were 8 at 1 minute and 9 at 5 minutes. The baby is pink and active, with the following vital signs: pulse, 140 beats per minute; respirations, 40 breaths per minute and unlabored; temperature, 36.5°C (97.7°F); blood pressure, 46/36 mm Hg. What should be done for this baby?

Yes	No	
____	____	Give the baby supplemental oxygen.
____	____	Do a gestational age and size examination.
____	____	Perform a blood glucose screening test.
____	____	Start an intravenous line and administer 8 mL of 10% glucose.
____	____	Repeat vital sign checks frequently.

1B. It is quite likely this baby is

Yes	No	
____	____	Small for gestational age
____	____	Preterm
____	____	Large for gestational age
____	____	Post-term

1C. The baby is at risk for developing

Yes	No	
____	____	Hypoglycemia
____	____	Diarrhea
____	____	Meconium aspiration
____	____	Respiratory distress syndrome
____	____	Neonatal diabetes mellitus

1D. At 2 hours of age, the baby's vital signs are within reference ranges, and she continues to look well. By this time, assuming that no further information is available, which of the following actions should have been taken already or would now be appropriate to take?

Yes	No	
____	____	Start oral feedings (breast or bottle).
____	____	Begin antibiotic therapy.
____	____	Place the baby under phototherapy lights.
____	____	Repeat blood glucose screening tests.
____	____	Give the baby supplemental oxygen.
____	____	Treat this baby like she is a healthy baby.

(continued)

Unit 9 Pretest (*continued*)

2A. An 1,800-g (3 lb 15½ oz), 3-day-old baby with an estimated gestational age of 33 weeks has been in your care in the nursery. She has been feeding well, has had no respiratory problems, and is appropriate size for gestational age. Because of her size and gestational age, she has been continuously connected to a cardiorespiratory monitor. Between feedings, she suddenly becomes apneic, cyanotic, and limp, with a heart rate of 50 beats per minute. She does not resume breathing with vigorous stimulation. For each item, mark the line in the one most appropriate column.

Do Immediately	Do in Next Several Minutes	Not Indicated	
_____	_____	_____	Perform a blood glucose screening test.
_____	_____	_____	Administer epinephrine 0.5 mL (1:10,000).
_____	_____	_____	Connect an oximeter to the baby.
_____	_____	_____	Assist ventilation with bag and mask.
_____	_____	_____	Stimulate the baby with warm water.
_____	_____	_____	Obtain a hematocrit value.
_____	_____	_____	Check the baby's blood pressure.
_____	_____	_____	Perform a blood gas analysis.
_____	_____	_____	Take the baby's temperature.

2B. What are the possible reasons for this baby's difficulties?

Yes	No	
____	____	Common problem of preterm birth
____	____	Sepsis
____	____	Hypoglycemia
____	____	Aspirated formula
____	____	Blood oxygen level too high

This unit is an expansion of the concepts you learned in Book 1: Maternal and Fetal Evaluation and Immediate Newborn Care. It is also a review of many of the ideas you learned in previous units.

To determine if a baby is sick, at risk, or well, do the following 2 things:

- Review the baby's history.
- Examine the baby.

1. How do you know a baby is well?

A. History

Consider all the risk factors you have learned about for each of the perinatal periods.

- Maternal history
- Labor and delivery history
- Neonatal history

B. Physical examination

A well baby

- Is $37^{0/7}$ to $42^{6/7}$ weeks' gestational age at birth
- Is an appropriate weight for gestational age
- Has the following findings within reference ranges
    — Heart rate
    — Respirations
    — Temperature
    — Blood pressure
    — Color
    — Activity
    — Feeding pattern
- Passes meconium within the first 24 hours after birth
- Urinates within the first 24 hours after birth

 A well baby has no risk factor in any of the perinatal periods; is term and appropriate for gestational age; has vital signs, color, activity, feeding, and stool and urine output within reference ranges; and has no abnormal clinical features, such as vomiting, respiratory distress, apnea, blood in the stool, abdominal distension, or seizures.

2. How do you know a baby is at risk?

An at-risk baby is one who has a higher chance of developing problems because of risk factors in the baby's history or the baby's size or gestational age. An at-risk baby's well-being depends on

- Continued careful assessment
- Anticipation of problems that are likely to occur
- Prevention of these problems or immediate treatment of them, should they occur

 An at-risk baby needs continued monitoring for potential problems but does not need immediate treatment for any problem.

A. History
1. Abnormal prenatal or neonatal history
Consider all of the risk factors for each of the perinatal periods.
- Maternal history
- Labor and delivery history
- Neonatal history
2. Previously sick baby
Babies who were sick but now have vital signs, color, activity, and feeding patterns within reference ranges are also at-risk babies.

B. Physical examination
An at-risk baby

- Is preterm or post-term
and/or

- Is large for gestational age (LGA) or small for gestational age
- Has the following findings within reference ranges
  — Heart rate
  — Respirations
  — Temperature
  — Blood pressure
  — Color
  — Activity
  — Feeding pattern
- Passes meconium within the first 24 hours after birth
- Urinates within the first 24 hours after birth

 An at-risk baby has vital signs, color, activity, feeding, and stool and urine output within reference ranges but is preterm or post-term, and/or is large for gestational age or small for gestational age, and/or has prenatal or neonatal risk factors, and/or is a baby recovering from having been sick.

3. How do you know a baby is sick?

A. History
A sick baby may be in any of the following groups:

- A well baby, without any identified risk factors, who suddenly develops vital signs, color, activity, or feeding pattern outside reference range
- An at-risk baby whose condition deteriorates
- A baby sick from birth

B. Physical examination

The items to consider in your initial examination include

Heart examination:

- Tachycardia (>180 beats per minute)
- Bradycardia (<100 beats per minute)
- Persistent murmur

Respirations:

- Tachypnea (sustained respiratory rate > 60 breaths per minute)
- Gasping
- Apnea
- Grunting, abnormal cry, retracting, nasal flaring, or stridor

Temperature:

- High
- Low
- Unstable

Blood pressure:

- Hypotension
- Prolonged capillary refill time
- Weak pulses

Color:

- Cyanotic
- Pale, gray, or mottled
- Red
- Jaundiced

Activity:

- Tremors, irritability, seizures
- Floppy, decreased muscle tone
- Little response to stimulation

Feeding:

- Poor feeding
- Abdominal distention
- Recurrent vomiting

 A sick baby has vital signs, color, activity, or feeding pattern outside reference range and needs immediate action to stabilize the baby, investigate the cause, and treat the abnormality.

Self-test A

Now answer these questions to test yourself on the information in the last section.

A1. List 3 "categories" of babies who require different types of care.

_____
_____
_____

A2. Well babies are term and appropriate for gestational age. List 3 other characteristics of well babies.

_____
_____
_____

A3. At-risk babies have vital signs within reference ranges. List 4 other characteristics at-risk babies may have.

_____
_____
_____
_____

A4. List 6 characteristics sick babies may have.

_____
_____
_____
_____
_____
_____

Check your answers with the list near the end of the unit. Correct any incorrect answers and review the appropriate section in the unit.

4. What should you do for a well baby?

A well baby may become sick. For this reason, you should *routinely assess* the condition of all well babies by checking their temperatures, heart rates, and respiratory rates at least once every 8 hours. Color, activity, and feeding pattern should be carefully assessed. If a well baby does become sick, this will be evident by changes in vital sign(s), color, activity, or feeding pattern.

5. What should you do for an at-risk baby?

The key to management of an at-risk baby is to *anticipate problems* so that they may be avoided or corrected quickly. To do this, you should perform certain tests frequently to *monitor risk factors*. For example, an LGA baby is at risk for hypoglycemia. You would anticipate this and perform blood glucose screening tests.

6. What should you do for a sick baby?

Once you have determined a baby has vital signs, color, tone, activity, or feeding pattern outside reference range and have therefore classified the baby as sick, you must *act quickly* to correct these abnormalities.

You need to do the following 4 things when caring for sick babies:

1. *Call for help.*
2. *Treat the immediate life-threatening problem(s)* by checking the baby's *airway, breathing, and circulation, and then stabilize* the baby *(resuscitation ABCS).*
3. *Determine why* the baby is sick and *treat the cause* when it is found.
4. *Monitor risk factors* so potential problems can be prevented or treated promptly.

For example

- An LGA baby suddenly turns blue and has a seizure. (*Call for help* per your hospital's protocol. For example, this may be a verbal shout to someone outside the room, pushing an emergency alarm button, or activating a voice technology or mobile communication device.)
- You immediately establish a patent airway, assist with ventilation, and give the baby oxygen as necessary, until the baby has good breath sounds and is pink. (*Treat the immediate problem.*)
- You then perform a blood glucose screening test and check the baby's vital signs. You attach an oximeter and cardiorespiratory monitor to the baby. You find the blood glucose screening test result is 0 to 20 mg/dL. (*Determine why the baby is sick.*)
- You quickly obtain a blood sample for blood glucose determination, insert a peripheral intravenous line or umbilical venous catheter, administer 10% glucose (2 mL/kg), and then begin a constant infusion of 10% glucose. (*Treat the cause of the abnormality [See Book 1, Maternal and Fetal Evaluation and Immediate Newborn Care, Unit 8, Hypoglycemia].*)
- Twenty minutes later, you perform another blood glucose screening test and find the level is 80 to 120 mg/dL. You continue to perform blood glucose screening tests every 30 to 60 minutes for several hours, and then at longer intervals. (*Monitor the risk factors.*)

7. How do you decide what to treat first?

Care of sick babies may seem extremely complicated. At times, it may seem difficult to decide what action to take first when a baby with multiple risk factors suddenly becomes apneic or cyanotic or has a seizure. Remember, no matter what the cause of the problems, the first thing you should *always* do is call for help and check the baby's *airway, breathing, and circulation, and then stabilize* the baby.

Remember the Resuscitation ABCS

Airway: Make sure there is no obstruction to airflow into the baby's lungs.

Breathing: Assist the baby's breathing with bag and mask, or endotracheal tube and bag breathing, as necessary.

Circulation: Check the baby's heart rate and blood pressure. If these are outside the reference ranges, take immediate action to correct them.

Then

Stabilize

1. Check
   - All vital signs
   - Hematocrit values
   - Blood glucose screening levels
2. Restore these values to within reference range or as close as possible.

3. Connect a cardiorespiratory monitor to the baby and a pulse oximeter to assess the need for supplemental oxygen.

4. Decide exactly what other problems or risk factors the baby has and begin evaluation and treatment of those.

8. What should you *avoid* doing when caring for at-risk and sick babies?

You have learned many actions you should take to care for at-risk and sick babies. Certain actions, however, may make these babies worse. What follows is a list of *don'ts*.

A. Feeding

Sick babies should *not* be fed by mouth or tube until their vital signs are stable. In general, sick babies should have intravenous fluids started early and continued for several days. A sick baby may aspirate if fed by mouth. Later, after the baby's vital signs have stabilized, tube feedings might be considered, unless there are concerns about possible gastrointestinal injury. Mothers should be assisted in expressing and storing breast milk for a sick baby.

B. Bathing

Sick and at-risk babies should *not* be bathed until their vital signs have been stable for several hours; even then, a bath is not a necessary part of the baby's care. The vernix (the material covering the baby's skin before birth) may help to prevent infection and does not need to be washed off quickly after birth. Baths should be delayed until the baby is completely stable because a bath can be stressful and can easily cause a baby to become hypothermic.

C. Administering oxygen

Sick babies *do not always* require supplemental oxygen. Oxygen given to sick, preterm babies who have typical lungs has been associated with eye damage (retinopathy of prematurity). Always confirm the need for oxygen with oximetry and adjust the inspired oxygen to aim for an 88% to 92% Spo$_2$ range, setting oximeter alarm limits to 85% to 95%. If a baby is clearly cyanotic, however, oxygen should be given while the oximeter is being connected.

D. Removing oxygen

Sick babies who are acutely ill and require oxygen to maintain acceptable saturation levels should *not* be removed from supplemental oxygen for radiographs, weighing, or any other reason, regardless of how brief it may be. Abrupt decreases in inspired oxygen can result in desaturation that will be very difficult to reverse.

E. Gestational age assessment and physical examination

Sick babies should *not* undergo a detailed physical and neurological examination until their vital signs are stable. Sick babies require gentle care; any excessive stimulation may cause them to become sicker. When the baby is stable, a gentle examination may be done.

Whenever possible, multiple interventions (eg, checking the temperature, changing a diaper) should be done at the same time (clustering of care) to avoid disturbing the baby any more often than is essential.

F. Handwashing

Sick and preterm babies are more susceptible to infections than healthy babies. By far, the most common way infections are transmitted among babies and from staff members to babies is lack of careful handwashing or lack of consistent use of a waterless antiseptic agent (alcohol-based hand rub).

Do not forget to wash your hands or use a waterless antiseptic hand rub before and after entering a patient room or care area and before and after examining or caring for a baby.

 Cleansing of the hands and taking standard precautions are needed at all times, for all babies, by all health professionals.

9. How do you determine why a baby is sick?

You need to assess the baby's

- *Risk factors:* You should learn the risk factors (if any) for every baby delivered in your hospital. This includes reviewing each baby's prenatal, labor and delivery, and neonatal history.
- *Vital signs and observations:* Temperature, pulse, respirations, and blood pressure should be checked at least once an hour, for every sick baby. At-risk babies also require frequent checking of vital signs. Color, tone, and activity should be assessed carefully and routinely.
- *Laboratory tests:* The appropriate tests depend on a baby's risk factors or illness. Proper care of an at-risk or sick baby requires appropriate tests be done, even if a baby "looks OK."

Self-test B

Now answer these questions to test yourself on the information in the last section.

B1. What are the resuscitation ABCS that help you decide what to do first when caring for sick babies?

A. _____

B. _____

C. _____

S. _____

B2. What are 6 things you should not do for sick babies?

_____

_____

_____

_____

_____

_____

B3. What are the 3 main sources of information you use to assess why a baby is sick?

_____

_____

_____

Check your answers with the list near the end of the unit. Correct any incorrect answers and review the appropriate section in the unit.

Subsection: Vital Signs and Observations

Review the *observe*, *think*, and *act* categories for each vital sign, as well as color, activity, and feeding.

A. Heart Rate (reference range is approximately 120–160 beats/min)[a]		
Observe	**Think**	**Act**
Tachycardia (>180 beats/min)	• Hypovolemia • Anemia • Acidosis • Sepsis • Hyperthermia • Congestive heart failure • Arrhythmia	• Attach an oximeter and adjust the FIO_2 to achieve $SpO_2 = 88\%–92\%$. • Check hematocrit value, blood pressure, blood gas, temperature. • Consider cultures and antibiotics. • Obtain an electrocardiogram if the heart rate is >220 beats/min.
Bradycardia (<100 beats/min)	• Hypoxia • Hypothermia[b] • Acidosis • Sepsis • Congenital heart block	• Attach an oximeter and adjust the FIO_2 to achieve $SpO_2 = 88\%–92\%$. • Give oxygen if the saturation level is below target range. • Check arterial blood gas and temperature. • Consider cultures and antibiotics. • Obtain an electrocardiogram if bradycardia is persistent when the baby is awake and active.

Murmurs	• Functional
	• Congenital heart disease
		• If a murmur persists, obtain a chest radiograph and echocardiogram, if available.
		• If a baby is cyanotic
		  — Give oxygen and check oximetry and arterial blood gas values.
		  — Consult cardiology or regional perinatal center staff.

[a] Newborn heart rates are variable and should be counted for *1 full minute*. Assess the whole baby when interpreting a high or low heart rate.

[b] Warm a severely chilled baby according to guidelines in Book 1: Maternal and Fetal Evaluation and Immediate Newborn Care, Unit 7, Thermal Environment.

B. Temperature (reference is approximately 37.0°C [98.6°F])		
Observe	**Think**	**Act**
Hyperthermia (> 37.5°C [> 99.5°F])	• Overheated environment • Sepsis (rarely)	• Check environmental temperature. • Consider cultures (bacterial and/or viral) and therapeutics (antibiotics and/or antivirals).
Hypothermia (< 36.5°C [< 97.7°F]) or unstable temperature	• Sepsis • Shock • Acidosis • Excessive heat loss • Necrotizing enterocolitis	• Check environmental temperature. • Check and correct routes of heat loss. • Check blood pressure, blood gas values, white blood cell count with differential. • Warm the baby.[a] • Consider cultures and antibiotics. • Consider abdominal radiography.

[a] Warm a severely chilled baby according to guidelines in Book 1: Maternal and Fetal Evaluation and Immediate Newborn Care, Unit 7, Thermal Environment.

C. Blood Pressure (reference range varies according to gestational and postnatal age)[a]		
Observe	**Think**	**Act**
Below reference range	• Shock from blood loss • Sepsis • Acidosis • Poor oxygenation • Poor cardiac output	• Check arterial blood gas values, hematocrit value, white blood cell count with differential. • Attach an oximeter and adjust the FIO_2 to achieve SpO_2 = 88%–92%. • Administer a volume expander (10 mL/kg) slowly, if indicated (suspected hypovolemia). • If blood loss is suspected, send a blood sample for type and crossmatch. • Consider cultures and antibiotics.

[a] Refer to the graphs in Unit 4, Low Blood Pressure (Hypotension), in this book.

D. Respirations (reference range is approximately 20–60 breaths per minute)[a]		
Observe	**Think**	**Act**
Grunting, flaring, retractions, tachypnea (sustained respiratory rate >60 breaths per minute), or stridor	• Respiratory distress syndrome • Transient tachypnea • Meconium aspiration • Pneumonia • Pneumothorax • Airway obstruction • Sepsis • Shock • Hypoglycemia • Polycythemia • Anemia • Hypothermia • Hyperthermia • Diaphragmatic hernia • Tracheoesophageal fistula • Congenital heart disease	• Attach an oximeter and adjust the FIO_2 to achieve $SpO_2 – 88\%–92\%$. • Check blood pressure, arterial blood gas values, blood glucose screening levels, hematocrit value, chest radiograph, temperature, WBC count with differential. • Roughly estimate the baby's gestational age and size. • Review the maternal and neonatal history. • Consider cultures and antibiotics. • Consider providing assisted ventilation.
Gasping	Severe acidosis	• Attach an oximeter and adjust the FIO_2 to achieve $SpO_2 = 88\%–92\%$. • Obtain blood gas values; especially check the pH level. • Consider providing assisted ventilation.
Apnea	• Worsening respiratory distress • Low blood oxygen level • Hypoglycemia • Sepsis • Other clinically significant illness (eg, necrotizing enterocolitis) • Shock • Acidosis • Low calcium level • Low sodium level • Central nervous system disorder • Cold-stressed baby who is overheated when rewarmed[b] • Preterm	• Attach an oximeter and adjust the FIO_2 to achieve $SpO_2 = 88\%–92\%$. • Consider providing assisted ventilation. • Check the baby's blood pressure, temperature, blood glucose screening levels, hematocrit value, arterial blood gas values, chest radiograph, calcium level, sodium level, WBC count with differential. • Consider lumbar puncture. • Obtain cultures and start antibiotics. • Review the maternal and neonatal history.
Severe respiratory distress at birth	• Choanal atresia • Diaphragmatic hernia • Pierre Robin sequence	• Attempt to pass a nasogastric tube. If a nasogastric tube will not pass, place an oral airway. • Sunken abdomen: Intubate and ventilate with bag, insert nasogastric tube, position baby in 45° head-up angle, obtain chest radiograph. Intubate trachea rather than providing face-mask ventilation. • Place baby prone; consider placing a large-bore (12F) nasopharyngeal tube.

Abbreviation: WBC, white blood cell.

[a] Newborn respiratory rates are variable and should be counted for *1 full minute*. Assess the whole baby when interpreting a high or low respiratory rate.

[b] Warm a severely chilled baby according to guidelines in Book 1: Maternal and Fetal Evaluation and Immediate Newborn Care, Unit 7, Thermal Environment.

338

E. Color		
Observe	**Think**	**Act**
Cyanotic (confirm with oximetry)	• Respiratory distress • Hypoxia • Hypoglycemia • Acidosis • Hypothermia • Sepsis • Heart disease • Pneumothorax (especially with sudden cyanosis)	• Give the baby oxygen and adjust the F_{IO_2} to achieve $SpO_2 = 88\%–92\%$. • Ventilate as indicated. • Check temperature, arterial blood gas values, hematocrit value, blood glucose screening level, chest radiograph, echocardiogram (if available), WBC count with differential. • Consider cultures and antibiotics.
Pale, pallor	• Shock • Anemia • Sepsis	• Attach an oximeter and adjust the F_{IO_2} to achieve $SpO_2 = 88\%–92\%$. • Check blood pressure, hematocrit value, arterial blood gas values, WBC count with differential. • Administer a volume expander or packed red blood cells, as indicated. • Consider cultures and antibiotics.
Red	• Polycythemia • Overheating • Severe hypothermia	• Check hematocrit values. • Check the baby's temperature and the environmental temperature.
Yellow (jaundiced)	• Liver immaturity or injury • Hemolysis • Sepsis	• Check the baby's vital signs, bilirubin level, smear of peripheral blood, Coombs (antiglobulin) tests, reticulocytes, mother's and baby's blood type. • Consider cultures and antibiotics. • Assess the baby's hydration. • Assess the baby's feeding pattern. • Investigate signs of congenital infections. • Assess the baby's medication history.
Mottled, gray	• Acidosis • Hypotension • Hypothermia • Sepsis	• Attach an oximeter and adjust the F_{IO_2} to achieve $SpO_2 = 88\%–92\%$. • Check arterial blood gas values, blood pressure, temperature, WBC count with differential. • Consider cultures and antibiotics. • Consider obtaining a chest radiograph for pneumothorax.

Abbreviation: WBC, white blood cell.

F. Activity		
Observe	**Think**	**Act**
Decreased muscle tone or decreased reflex irritability, lethargy	• Sepsis • Hypoglycemia • Acidosis • Shock • Birth trauma • Central nervous system hemorrhage • Intrapartum maternal medications	• Consider cultures and antibiotics. • Consider lumbar puncture. • Check blood pressure, WBC count with differential, blood gas values, blood glucose screening level, hematocrit value. • Review maternal medications during labor. • Consider cranial ultrasonography.

Increased activity (tremors, irritability, seizures[a])	• Hypoglycemia
	• Low serum calcium level
	• Meningitis
	• Complications of perinatal compromise
	• Drug withdrawal
		• Check blood glucose screening level, serum calcium level.
		• Consider lumbar puncture.
		  — *High WBC count:* Culture spinal fluid and treat baby with antibiotics.
		  — *Bloody:* Suspect traumatic lumbar puncture or possible birth injury.
		• Assess maternal drug history.
		• Consider toxicology screen of baby's urine and meconium.

Abbreviation: WBC, white blood cell.

[a] Treat definite seizures *immediately*. Give phenobarbital 20 mg/kg intravenously. Be prepared to ventilate the baby if respiratory depression occurs. Provide a maintenance dose of 3.5 to 5.0 mg/kg/d. Check serum levels and readjust the dose as necessary to maintain a serum level of 15 to 40 mcg/mL.

G. Feeding		
Observe	**Think**	**Act**
Poor intake	• Sepsis • Complications of perinatal compromise	• Check temperature, hematocrit value, arterial blood gas values, blood pressure, blood glucose screening level. • Consider cultures and antibiotics. • Start IV line.
Recurrent vomiting, abdominal distension, bloody stools	• Sepsis • Gastrointestinal obstruction • Necrotizing enterocolitis	• Check temperature, blood pressure, hematocrit value, arterial or venous blood gas values (check the pH level especially), blood pressure, blood glucose screening level, WBC count with differential. • Consider cultures and antibiotics. • Pass a nasogastric tube (8F) and connect it to low constant suction. • Obtain chest and abdominal radiographs. • Withhold feedings. • Start an IV line.
Excessive mucus or difficulty feeding	Tracheoesophageal fistula	• Insert a nasogastric tube (8F) and connect it to low constant suction. • Obtain a radiograph; look for the nasogastric tube coiled in a blind pouch. • Do *not* administer barium or dye. • Do not feed the baby enterally; start an IV. • Position the baby at a 45° head-up angle.
Recurrent, excessive residual amount found in stomach before tube feeding	• Necrotizing enterocolitis • Sepsis • Ileus	• Do not feed the baby enterally; start an IV line. • Check temperature, hematocrit value, arterial blood gas level, blood glucose screening level, WBC count with differential. • Consider cultures and antibiotics. • Consider abdominal radiography and nasogastric tube drainage.

Abbreviations: IV, intravenous; WBC, white blood cell.

Subsection: Tests and Results

Selected tests and guidelines for responding to results are discussed as follows. For other blood tests and how to interpret and respond to results, such as bilirubin levels, see the other units in this book.

A. Blood Gas Values (See also Unit 1, Oxygen, and Unit 2, Respiratory Distress, in this book.)
Blood gas assessments are used to measure the oxygen, carbon dioxide, and pH levels of the blood. An arterial blood gas analysis is needed to measure blood oxygen levels. However, a venous or capillary blood gas analysis provides a fair estimate of carbon dioxide, pH, and bicarbonate levels.

If a pulse oximeter is used, less frequent arterial blood gas determinations may be needed, depending on the stability of oxygenation level and the need to evaluate pH and carbon dioxide levels.

Acceptable Blood Gas Values

Arterial		Capillary		Venous	
PaO_2	45–65 mm Hg[a]	PO_2	Unreliable	PO_2	Unreliable
pH level	7.30–7.40	pH level	7.25–7.35	pH level	7.25–7.35
$PaCO_2$	40–50 mm Hg	PCO_2	45–55 mm Hg	PCO_2	45–55 mm Hg
HCO_3^-	19–22 mEq/L	HCO_3^-	19–22 mEq/L	HCO_3^-	19–22 mEq/L

[a] There is controversy among experts as to the appropriate range of PaO_2 and oxyhemoglobin saturation levels. Know the acceptable range for your hospital. Also, the target range will be different immediately after birth. (See Book 1: Maternal and Fetal Evaluation and Immediate Newborn Care, Unit 5, Resuscitating the Newborn.)

Blood Gas Test Results and Recommended Responses

Test	Blood Gas Result Outside Reference Range	Action
PaO_2	>80 mm Hg (high)	Lower the oxygen concentration. Follow the oxygenation trend with pulse oximetry.
	<40 mm Hg (low)	Increase the oxygen concentration. Follow the oxygenation trend with pulse oximetry.
$PaCO_2$	>60 mm Hg	Consider noninvasive ventilation or intubation and invasive ventilation if the $PaCO_2$ continues to increase and the pH level is <7.25.
	<35 mm Hg (low)	Look for the reason for hyperventilation. Consider the possibility of metabolic acidosis or low PaO_2.
pH level	<7.25 (low)	If a baby's ventilation is adequate and the bicarbonate level is <15–16 mEq/L, consider administering sodium bicarbonate while determining and treating the cause of acidosis.[a]
		If $PaCO_2$ is >60 mm Hg, consider providing assisted ventilation.
HCO_3^- (Bicarbonate)	<16 mEq/L (low)[a]	If $PaCO_2$ is within reference range or low, consider administering sodium bicarbonate while determining and treating the cause of metabolic acidosis.[a]
		If $PaCO_2$ is >60 mm Hg, do not administer sodium bicarbonate. Treat high $PaCO_2$ with assisted ventilation and recheck blood gas values.

[a] Severe metabolic acidosis (pH level < 7.20 with serum bicarbonate level < 15–16 mEq/L) indicates severe illness. The cause must be determined and treated. Intravenous sodium bicarbonate therapy may be considered but, as a general rule, is not recommended unless

• Serum bicarbonate level is < 15–16 mEq/L.

• $PaCO_2$ level is < 40–45 mm Hg.

• There is adequate spontaneous or assisted ventilation.

• Cause of acidosis is being assessed and treated.

B. Oxyhemoglobin Saturation and PaO_2

The precise relationship of oxygen saturation and PaO_2 is affected by several factors, such as gestational age, age since birth, and whether the baby has received a blood transfusion.

Oxyhemoglobin Saturation	PaO_2
Low: 0%–85%	0–45 mm Hg
Desirable range: 88%–92%[a]	45–65 mm Hg
High: 95%–100%	75–600 mm Hg

[a] Although the optimum target SpO_2 is 88% to 92%, this narrow range is difficult to maintain precisely. Many neonatal units set oximeter alarms at 85% to 95% and try to aim for the middle of this range.

Figure 9.1 shows an approximation of the curve that could be constructed from the results of blood drawn from a slightly preterm baby during the first few days after birth. For some babies, simultaneous measurements of PaO_2 and oxygen saturation levels may generate results quite different than those predicted with the graph.

Oxyhemoglobin saturation as measured with a pulse oximeter is most valuable for detecting *low* blood oxygen levels. It is *not* a sensitive measure for *high* blood oxygen levels and provides no information about pH, carbon dioxide, and serum bicarbonate levels.

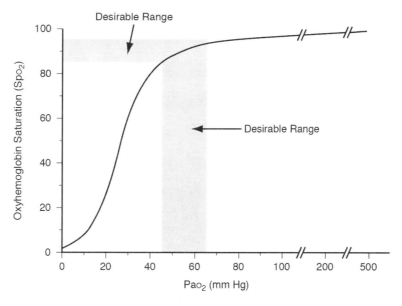

Figure 9.1. Relationship of PaO_2 and SpO_2

C. Blood Glucose Screening Test

Blood Glucose Screening Test (reference range is 45–130 mg/dL)	
Screening Test Results	**Actions**
<25 mg/dL	1. Obtain blood for glucose testing. 2. Start an IV with 10% glucose. Administer 2 mL/kg over 5–10 minutes. 3. Maintain the IV at 5 mL/kg/h. 4. Perform another screening test or blood glucose level check within 15–30 minutes. If the test result remains <25 mg/dL, a higher glucose administration rate (increased volume or concentration) will be needed. 5. Begin frequent feedings as soon as the blood glucose level is within reference range, the baby is stable, and the baby is able to feed. 6. Monitor the baby with frequent blood glucose screening tests.

Between 25 and 45 mg/dL	1. Obtain blood for glucose testing.
	2. Begin early, frequent feedings (immediately or within 4 hours of birth).
	3. Supplement with IV 10% glucose if either of the following conditions occurs:
	  • Feedings are not tolerated.
	  • Blood glucose level remains 25–45 mg/dL.
	4. Monitor with frequent blood glucose screening tests.

Between 45 and 90 mg/dL	Begin early, frequent feedings (within 4 hours of birth).

Abbreviation: IV, intravenous.

D. Electrolytes

Electrolytes are usually checked in any baby who experienced perinatal compromise, had seizures, has a gastrointestinal problem, or requires intravenous fluids for more than 24 hours. There may be other abnormalities of electrolytes as a result of complex disease processes. These abnormalities are not discussed here.

Electrolytes	Reference Ranges[a]
Sodium	133–148 mEq/L
Potassium	4.5–6.6 mEq/L
Chloride	100–115 mEq/L
Bicarbonate	19–22 mEq/L
Calcium (total)	8–11 mg/dL
Calcium (ionized)	4.0–4.7 mg/dL

[a] Reference ranges may vary from laboratory to laboratory. Check the ones used by your laboratory.

Electrolytes	
Result Outside Reference Range[a]	**Action**
Low sodium level	Decide if the baby has received too much IV fluid in the face of poor urinary output. Decide if the baby has not received enough sodium or is losing sodium (eg, through stool or ileostomy).
High sodium level	Suspect the baby may have received too much sodium in the form of IV fluids or sodium bicarbonate. Stop excess sodium from being administered. Suspect the baby (especially a very preterm baby) may be dehydrated and consider increasing the fluid intake.
Low bicarbonate level	See the Blood Gas Test Results and Recommended Responses Table earlier in this section.
Low calcium level	Low calcium levels are not uncommon in preterm babies or in babies who required prolonged resuscitation and received sodium bicarbonate. In general, if the total serum calcium level is < 7 mg/dL or the ionized calcium level is < 3.5 mg/100 mL and there are any symptoms of hypocalcemia (seizures or jitteriness), treatment is recommended. You should administer 200 mg/kg of calcium gluconate (*slowly*, intravenously) as a starting dose, or 500 mg/kg/d intravenously as a maintenance dose. When calcium is administered intravenously, you must *monitor the baby's heart rate*. If the heart rate begins to decrease during the infusion, *stop the infusion*. You also should provide calcium supplementation by central venous line or *make certain the IV is not infiltrated* because calcium may cause severe tissue damage.

Abbreviation: IV, intravenous.

[a] Reference ranges may vary from laboratory to laboratory. Check the ones used by your laboratory.

E. Hematocrit Value (reference range is 45%–65% on the first day after birth in a baby born at term)

The hematocrit or hemoglobin value of a baby's blood tells you if the baby has anemia or polycythemia. Depending on results, you may want to give blood or even take blood away.

When evaluating the baby for polycythemia, *obtain hematocrit samples only from a vein*. A sample obtained from a heel stick may be extremely inaccurate during the first several days after birth.

Hematocrit Value	
Result Outside Reference Range	**Action**
High: > 65%–70%	*Polycythemia:* May lead to sludging of blood in the capillary beds of the lungs and brain. If the baby has symptoms or if the high value has been confirmed by a repeat determination, a reduction or dilutional exchange transfusion can be performed to lower the hematocrit value by removing some of the baby's blood and replacing it with physiological (normal) saline solution. See Book 4: Specialized Newborn Care, Unit 2, Exchange, Reduction, and Direct Transfusions.
Low: < 30%	*Anemia:* Type and crossmatch the baby's blood and consider administering packed red blood cells (10 mL/kg) if the baby is in distress (increased heart rate, respiratory distress) or if the hematocrit value is decreasing rapidly. See Unit 4, Low Blood Pressure (Hypotension), in this book.

F. Platelet Count (reference range is 150,000–450,000/mm^3)

Characteristically in newborns, the platelet count will decrease acutely in response to a variety of illnesses and then may become abnormally high as the baby recovers. The baby's platelet count may also be low because of certain maternal drugs; specific maternal conditions, such as pregnancy-related hypertension; or an antibody that the mother may have made against the baby's platelets.

Platelet Count	
Result Outside Reference Range	**Action**
< 150,000/mm^3	*Thrombocytopenia:* Decreasing platelet counts can be an indicator of illness, such as infection. Administration of platelets is usually not necessary, however, unless the count becomes extremely low or the baby shows signs of bleeding. Platelet counts < 100,000/mm^3 are outside reference range at any gestational age. • Look for signs of infection and consider conducting other tests for infection. • Review maternal history for low platelet count, preeclampsia, bacterial or viral infection or other illness, or drugs associated with low platelet counts. • Recheck the platelet count. Monitor the baby and obtain further studies, depending on the results and the baby's clinical condition.
< 50,000/mm^3	If the platelet count is < 50,000/mm^3 and there are signs of bleeding (eg, petechiae, gastrointestinal blood, oozing needle puncture sites), consider administering platelets. Consult with your regional perinatal center about appropriate diagnostic studies that should be obtained prior to a platelet transfusion.
< 25,000/mm^3	Many experts advise administering platelets if the count is < 25,000/mm^3, even if there is no evidence of bleeding. Consult with regional perinatal center staff about appropriate diagnostic studies that should be obtained prior to a platelet transfusion.

G. Spinal Fluid Tests

Spinal fluid is obtained via a lumbar puncture, usually because infection (eg, meningitis) is suspected. Several tests may be performed on the fluid. White blood cells, red blood cells, and bacteria can be identified with a microscope. Spinal fluid glucose and protein levels can be measured. If you suspect infection, spinal fluid should be cultured.

Spinal Fluid	Reference Ranges (During the First Day After Birth)
White blood cells	0–26 per mm^3
Red blood cells	0–600 per mm^3
Glucose level	38–64 mg/dL
Protein level	40–140 mg/dL

Spinal Fluid Tests	
Result Outside Reference Range	Action
Increased white blood cell count	Consider infection. Culture the fluid and treat the baby with antibiotics.
Increased red blood cell count	Consider birth trauma, central nervous system hemorrhage, or a traumatic lumbar puncture. Central nervous system imaging, such as head ultrasonography or brain magnetic resonance imaging, should be considered.
Bacteria	Consider infection. Culture the fluid and treat the baby with antibiotics.
Low glucose level	Consider low blood glucose level or infection. Culture the fluid and treat the baby with antibiotics. Perform a blood glucose screening test and manage the baby's condition, according to the results.
High protein level	Consider birth trauma, a central nervous system hemorrhage, or infection for which central nervous system imaging may be performed or additional testing for infection may be conducted.

H. Urine Tests

Urine may be examined under a microscope to determine if there are red blood cells, white blood cells, or bacteria in the urine. When infection is suspected, a urine sample obtained via bladder catheter or suprapubic tap should be cultured.

Urine Tests	
Result Outside Reference Range	Action
White blood cells	Consider infection. Obtain cultures. Consider beginning antibiotics.
Red blood cells	Consider severe perinatal compromise. Consider restricting fluids.
Bacteria	Consider infection. Consider obtaining blood and urine cultures and beginning antibiotics.

I. Radiographs
  1. Chest radiographs

  Chest radiographs help determine the cause of respiratory distress and the severity of the problem.
  2. Abdominal radiographs

  Abdominal radiographs help decide the cause of vomiting, "spitting," abdominal distension, or a sunken abdomen. If an umbilical catheter is in place, it will be visible on the radiographs and should be checked for proper positioning.

Chest Radiographs	
Result Outside Reference Range	**Action**
Respiratory distress syndrome	Treat as indicated in Unit 2, Respiratory Distress, in this book. Cannot be distinguished from bacterial pneumonia and sepsis. Consider obtaining cultures and starting antibiotics.
Transient tachypnea of the newborn	Treat respiratory distress as indicated in Unit 2, Respiratory Distress, in this book.
Pneumothorax	A small pneumothorax may not need treatment if blood gas levels are within reference ranges and the baby is in no distress. Otherwise, insert a needle and aspirate air if the baby is in distress and a chest tube is not immediately available; when available, insert a chest tube and connect it to an underwater seal and appropriate suction apparatus.
Pneumonia	Obtain cultures. Treat with antibiotics.
Meconium aspiration	Treat respiratory distress as indicated in Unit 2, Respiratory Distress, in this book. Consider obtaining cultures and starting antibiotics.
Diaphragmatic hernia	Insert a ≥ 8F nasogastric tube and aspirate air from the baby's stomach. Leave the tube in place and connected to suction. Do not use bag-and-mask assisted ventilation. Intubate if the baby is in respiratory distress.
	Consult regional perinatal center staff immediately about surgery and possible transport of the baby to an extracorporeal membrane oxygenation (ECMO) center.
Esophageal atresia or tracheoesophageal fistula	Insert an 8F sump tube (Replogle) into the baby's esophageal pouch. Connect it to suction or aspirate air and fluid frequently. Position the baby in a 45° head-up position. Do not feed the baby, and do not administer barium or dye. Consult a pediatric surgeon immediately.
Abnormal heart configuration	Obtain • Arterial blood gas levels • Blood pressure in the baby's arms and legs (4 extremities) • Echocardiogram • Pre-ductal and post-ductal pulse oximetry values (right hand and one leg)

Abdominal Radiographs	
Result Outside Reference Range	**Action**
Intestinal obstruction	Stop feedings. Insert a nasogastric sump tube (Replogle) and connect it to suction. Consult a pediatric surgeon immediately.
Necrotizing enterocolitis (dilated loops of bowel with air in the intestinal wall)	Give the baby nothing by mouth. Insert a nasogastric tube and connect it to suction. Obtain cultures and begin antibiotics. Monitor the baby's vital signs. Record all intake and output. Consult your regional perinatal center.
LOW-lying umbilical arterial catheter found outside the desired L3-L4 location • Too high (above the third lumbar vertebra) or • Too low (below the fourth lumbar vertebra)	Adjust or replace the catheter so the tip lies between the third and fourth lumbar vertebrae.
HIGH-lying umbilical arterial catheter found outside the desired T6-T9 position • Too high (above the sixth thoracic vertebra) or • Too low (below the ninth thoracic vertebra)	Adjust or replace the catheter so the tip lies between the sixth and ninth thoracic vertebrae.
Umbilical venous catheter too high or too low	Adjust or replace the catheter so the tip lies in the junction of the right atrium and the inferior vena cava.

Sample Case

This sample case will give you practice testing your knowledge, as well as provide experience in considering the multiple factors that go into the care of at-risk and sick women and newborns.

Use the material within this unit to help answer the questions.

Ms Hurt is in preterm labor with her fourth child and is admitted to your hospital. Her physical examination and vital signs are within reference ranges. She reports that her membranes ruptured the previous day, but labor did not start until shortly before she came to the hospital. Less than an hour after admission, a female baby weighing 2,015 g (4 lb 7 oz), with Apgar scores of 7 at 1 minute and 9 at 5 minutes, is born. Baby Hurt's initial vital signs are

Temperature: 36.6°C (98.0°F)	Pulse: 132 beats/min
Respirations: 52 breaths per minute	Blood pressure: 45/34 mm Hg

You obtain a Ballard score and determine that Baby Hurt is at 35 weeks' estimated gestational age and appropriate size for gestational age. You maintain the baby in skin-to-skin contact with the mother during the first hour after birth. She latches onto the breast and suckles briefly.

1. Is the baby _____ Well? _____ At risk? _____ Sick?

The baby is now 1 hour old, pink, and active. You recheck her vital signs.

2. Indicate which value(s) is (are) outside reference range.

Reference   Outside Reference

_____   _____   Pulse: 140 beats/min

_____   _____   Respirations: 50 breaths per minute and unlabored

_____   _____   Blood pressure: 48/30 mm Hg

You perform a blood glucose screening test and find that the result is 45 to 90 mg/dL.

3. Does this test result mean you should perform any of the following actions?

Yes   No

____   ____   Start an intravenous line with 10% glucose.

____   ____   Start early feedings (within 4 hours of birth).

____   ____   Repeat glucose screening test in an hour.

Next, you obtain a venous blood sample for a hematocrit value check. Shortly after the blood sample is sent, the laboratory technician calls and says the baby's hematocrit value is 49%.

4. Is the value _____ Within reference range? _____ High? _____ Low?

At 2½ hours of age, the baby remains pink but is less active. Her vital signs are now

Temperature: 36.7°C (98.0°F)   Pulse: 140 beats/min
Respirations: 68 breaths per minute,   Blood pressure: 50/34 mm Hg
occasional grunting and nasal flaring
Blood glucose level: 45 mg/dL

5. Is the baby now _____ Well? _____ At risk? _____ Sick?

The baby's lips remain pink, and the grunting and nasal flaring have not increased.

6. What would you do for this baby now? _____

Shortly after obtaining a radiograph at 3 hours of age, the baby begins retracting and has bluish lips. You give her 30% oxygen. The cyanosis does not disappear until you increase the oxygen level to 45%. She becomes pink when breathing 45% oxygen, and her oxygen saturation stabilizes at approximately 90%.

The chest radiograph findings indicate pneumonia. The baby is now 3 hours 15 minutes old. Her vital signs are

Temperature: 36.4°C (97.6°F)   Pulse: 150 beats/min
Respirations: 70 breaths per minute   Blood pressure: 52/34 mm Hg
with marked grunting and retracting
Blood glucose level: 25 to 45 mg/dL   Oxygen saturation: 88%

7. Which of the following is (are) now the most likely cause(s) for this baby's respiratory distress?

_____ Respiratory distress syndrome

_____ Transient tachypnea

_____ Pneumothorax

_____ Sepsis

_____ Pneumonia

8. What else should be done for this baby?

Yes   No

____ ____ Begin antibiotics. (Do so after obtaining a blood culture.)

____ ____ Obtain a serum sodium level.

____ ____ Administer sodium bicarbonate.

____ ____ Start a peripheral intravenous line.

9. If you selected "Begin antibiotics" in question 8, which of the following choices would be appropriate?

_____ Penicillin

_____ Gentamicin

_____ Penicillin and ampicillin

_____ Ampicillin and gentamicin

_____ None of the above

By 3½ hours of age, a peripheral intravenous line has been inserted, with an infusion of 10% dextrose in water (D10W) started and an umbilical arterial catheter inserted and connected to a heparin lock. After insertion of the umbilical arterial catheter, a radiograph is obtained to determine the catheter tip location and whether it should be repositioned.

At 4 hours of age, Baby Hurt is pink and receiving 45% oxygen. She has good muscle tone but is no longer active. Vital signs are

Temperature: 36.8°C (98.2°F)   Pulse: 145 beats/min
Respirations: 72 breaths per minute, Blood pressure: 56/36 mm Hg
grunting, nasal flaring, retractions
Blood glucose level: 45 to 90 mg/dL   Oximeter reading: 85% to 90%

Baby has received 6 mL of D10W and has had 1.3 mL of blood removed (1.0 mL for a blood culture and 0.3 mL for an arterial blood gas analysis). Arterial blood gas results (drawn when the baby was breathing 45% oxygen) are

Pao_2: 42 mm Hg   pH level: 7.32
$Paco_2$: 42 mm Hg HCO_3-: 20 mEq/L

10. **How would you interpret the arterial blood gas results?**

Pao_2 is _____ low.   pH level is _____ low.

_____ within reference range.   _____ within reference range.

_____ high.   _____ high.

$Paco_2$ is _____ low. HCO_3- is _____ low.

_____ within reference range.   _____ within reference range.

_____ high.   _____ high.

11. **How would you respond to these results?** _____

Check your answers with the list near the end of the unit, immediately following the Self-test Answers.

Self-test Answers

These are the answers to the Self-test questions and Sample Case. Please check them with the answers you gave and review the information in the unit wherever necessary.

Self-test A

A1. Well baby
At-risk baby
Sick baby

A2. Vital signs, color, activity, feeding pattern within reference ranges
No risk factors in prenatal and natal history
Passes meconium and urinates in the first 24 hours after birth

A3. Abnormal prenatal or natal history
Large for gestational age or small for gestational age
Preterm or post-term
Previously sick baby

A4. Any 6 of the following characteristics:
- Abnormal activity (tremors, irritability, seizures, decreased muscle tone, or little response to stimulation)
- Heart rate outside reference range (fast, slow, or irregular)
- Respiratory rate outside reference range (fast or slow) or pattern (episodes of apnea or difficulty breathing)
- Abnormal color (cyanotic; pale, gray, or mottled; red; jaundiced)
- Temperature outside reference range (high, low, unstable)
- Blood pressure outside reference range (low blood pressure, poor capillary refill time, weak pulses)
- Abnormal feeding pattern (poor feeding, abdominal distension, or recurrent vomiting)

Self-test B

B1. A. Airway: Make sure air is moving freely into the baby's lungs.
B. Breathing: Provide oxygen or assist the baby's ventilation as necessary.
C. Circulation: Correct a heart rate or blood pressure value outside of reference range.
S. Stabilize
— Check
  - Vital signs
  - Hematocrit value
  - Blood glucose level
— Restore them to reference range or as close as possible.
— Connect baby to a cardiorespiratory monitor and (usually) a pulse oximeter.
— Decide what other problems or risk factors the baby has; evaluate and treat.

B2. Do not feed a sick baby by mouth or feeding tube until vital signs are stable.
Do not bathe a sick or at-risk baby until the vital signs are stable. (Even then, a bath is unnecessary.)
Do not administer oxygen until you have determined a baby needs it.
Do not remove a baby from oxygen, once you have determined the baby needs oxygen.
Do not perform an extensive examination until all vital signs are stable; then conduct a gentle gestational aging and sizing examination.
Do not forget thorough hand cleansing before and after handling every baby.

B3. Risk factors
Vital signs and observations
Laboratory tests

Sample Case Answers

1. At risk. Review her history and physical examination findings. You know from your assessment of the baby that she has vital signs within reference ranges, is preterm, and is an appropriate size for gestational age. Therefore, this baby is not sick (vital signs within reference ranges), but she is at risk because she is preterm. The baby is also at risk because membranes were ruptured for longer than 18 hours.

2.
Reference	Outside Reference	
X	_____	Pulse: 140 beats/min
X	_____	Respirations: 50 breaths per minute and unlabored
X	_____	Blood pressure: 48/30 mm Hg

   (Review Subsection: Vital Signs and Observations.)

3.
Yes	No	
___	X	Start an intravenous line with 10% glucose.
X	___	Start early feedings (within 4 hours of birth).
X	___	Repeat the glucose screening test in an hour.

   (Review Subsection: Tests and Results.)

4. Within reference range (Review Subsection: Tests and Results.)

5. Sick. One of the vital signs (respirations) is outside reference range (tachypnea, grunting, and nasal flaring). You realize a baby in respiratory distress cannot be fed safely via nipple, so you withhold early feeding and plan to start an intravenous line. Remember the ABCS (*a*irway, *b*reathing, *c*irculation, *s*tabilize). Further evaluation of the baby's breathing is now important. (Airway is OK because the baby is not in acute respiratory distress, and circulation is OK as indicated by pulse and blood pressure within reference ranges.) Possible causes for the respiratory distress include (Review Subsection: Vital Signs and Observations.)

   * Respiratory distress syndrome—possible (preterm)
   * Transient tachypnea—possible
   * Meconium aspiration—unlikely (no meconium)
   * Pneumonia—possible (prolonged rupture of membranes)
   * Pneumothorax—possible
   * Airway obstruction—unlikely, given the clinical course
   * Sepsis—possible (prolonged rupture of membranes)
   * Shock—unlikely (blood pressure within reference range)
   * Hypoglycemia—unlikely (blood glucose within reference range)
   * Polycythemia or anemia—unlikely (hematocrit value within reference range)
   * Cold or overheated baby—unlikely (temperature within reference range)
   * Diaphragmatic hernia—unlikely, but possible
   * Tracheoesophageal fistula—unlikely, but possible
   * Congenital heart disease—unlikely, but possible

   You sort through these and are left with 5 likely reasons for the baby's illness.
   * Respiratory distress syndrome
   * Transient tachypnea
   * Pneumonia
   * Pneumothorax
   * Sepsis

6. Obtain
   - Chest radiograph
   - Arterial blood gas measurement
   - White blood cell count with differential

   Attach (unless already done)
   - Cardiorespiratory monitor
   - Pulse oximeter

   (Review Subsection: Vital Signs and Observations.)

7. ____ Respiratory distress syndrome
   ____ Transient tachypnea
   ____ Pneumothorax
   _X_ Sepsis
   _X_ Pneumonia

   The chest radiograph findings indicate pneumonia. Considering the prolonged rupture of amniotic membranes, bacterial pneumonia and sepsis are the most likely causes for the baby's respiratory distress.

8. Yes   No
   _X_   ____   Begin antibiotics. (Do so after obtaining a blood culture.)
   __   _X_   Obtain a serum sodium level.
   __   _X_   Administer sodium bicarbonate.
   _X_   ____   Start a peripheral intravenous line.

9. ____ Penicillin
   ____ Gentamicin
   ____ Penicillin and ampicillin
   _X_ Ampicillin and gentamicin
   ____ None of the above

   Antibiotics that are effective against gram-positive and gram-negative organisms should be administered. The combination of ampicillin and gentamicin is an appropriate choice.

10. Pao_2 is low.   pH level is within reference range.
    $Paco_2$ is within reference range. HCO_3- is within reference range.
    (Review Subsection: Tests and Results.)

11. Increase the baby's oxygen Fio_2 immediately, while monitoring oxygen saturation continuously. Recheck arterial blood gas values again in 10 to 30 minutes.

    At 4 hours of age, this baby is already quite sick. This baby will very likely become sicker before beginning to recover and will require several days of intensive care and several more days of convalescent care before she is ready to go home. Consultation with the regional perinatal center should be sought about appropriate respiratory support, further monitoring, and interventions.

Unit 9 Posttest

After completion of each unit there is a free online posttest available at www.cmevillage.com to test your understanding. Navigate to the PCEP pages on www.cmevillage.com and register to take the free posttests.

Once registered on the website and after completing all the unit posttests, pay the book exam fee ($15) and pass the test at 80% or greater to earn continuing education credits. Only start the PCEP book exam if you have time to complete it. If you take the book exam and are not connected to a printer, either print your certificate to a .pdf file and save it to print later or come back to www.cmevillage.com at any time and print a copy of your educational transcript.

Credits are only available by book, not by individual unit within the books. Available credits for completion of each book exam are as follows: Book 1: 14.5 credits; Book 2: 16 credits; Book 3: 17 credits; Book 4: 9 credits.

For more details, navigate to the PCEP webpages at www.cmevillage.com.

Unit 10: Preparation for Neonatal Transport

Objectives

In this unit, you will learn

A. Which newborns may benefit from transport

B. The primary goal for preparing a baby for transport

C. The minimum transport preparation needed for every baby

D. The transport preparation needed for babies with special problems

E. How to support parents of transported babies

Unit 10 Pretest

Before reading the unit, please answer the following questions. Select the *one best* answer to each question (unless otherwise instructed). Record your answers on the test and check them with the answers at the end of the book.

1A. A 1,500-g (3 lb 5 oz) baby is born with Apgar scores of 5 at 1 minute and 9 at 5 minutes, and the decision is made to transport her to a regional perinatal center. While you are waiting for the regional center transport team to arrive, she develops severe respiratory distress with retractions and cyanosis. Which of the following actions should happen within the next several minutes?

Yes	No	
____	____	Begin oxygen therapy.
____	____	Transport the baby to the radiology department for chest radiography.
____	____	Begin hourly tube feedings.
____	____	Obtain an arterial blood gas measurement.
____	____	Conduct a blood glucose screening test.
____	____	Attach a pulse oximeter to the baby.

1B. The baby continues to retract with respirations. Arterial blood gas results show PaO_2 below 35 mm Hg, $PaCO_2$ of 70 mm Hg, pH level below 7.15, and HCO_3- of 22 mEq/L. Which of the following actions is most appropriate?

A. Increase inspired oxygen concentration to 100%.

B. Transport the baby immediately to a regional perinatal center.

C. Intubate the baby's trachea and assist ventilation with a resuscitation bag.

D. Administer 8 mEq of sodium bicarbonate intravenously, slowly.

2. A baby is born with choanal atresia. An oral airway was immediately inserted, and the baby's vital signs are now within reference ranges and stable. Before transfer to a regional perinatal center, which of the following actions should be taken for this baby?

Yes	No	
____	____	Insert a peripheral intravenous line.
____	____	Obtain a blood culture.
____	____	Perform a blood glucose screening test.
____	____	Check the baby's blood pressure.
____	____	Obtain an electrocardiogram.

3. You suspect a baby has sepsis. You have obtained blood cultures and started the baby on antibiotics. Which of the following actions should also occur for this baby?

A. Restrict fluids.

B. Obtain an electrocardiogram.

C. Check the serum calcium level.

D. Conduct a blood gas analysis.

(continued)

Unit 10 Pretest (*continued*)

4. A 1,200-g (2 lb 10½ oz) baby is born in your delivery room. Apgar scores are 8 at 1 minute and 9 at 5 minutes, vital signs and color are within reference ranges, and there is no evidence of respiratory distress. Because of the baby's small size, plans are made to have the baby transported to a regional perinatal center. Which of these actions should be taken in your hospital by your staff, before the transport team arrives?

Yes	No	
____	____	Administer oxygen.
____	____	Perform a blood glucose screening test.
____	____	Obtain a chest radiograph.
____	____	Insert an umbilical arterial catheter.
____	____	Start a peripheral intravenous line.
____	____	Feed the baby by mouth.

5. The arterial blood gas analysis in a baby receiving 40% inspired oxygen shows $Paco_2$ of 30 mm Hg, Pao_2 of 42 mm Hg, pH level of 7.18, and HCO_3- of 11 mEq/L. What should be done for this baby?

Yes	No	
____	____	Investigate the cause of metabolic acidosis.
____	____	Provide bag-and-mask ventilation.
____	____	Intubate and use the bag to breathe for the baby.
____	____	Increase the baby's oxygen concentration.

6. A preterm baby is born after the amniotic membranes have been ruptured for 30 hours. At the time of rupture, amniotic fluid was foul smelling. The baby has Apgar scores of 5 at 1 minute and 7 at 5 minutes. At 30 minutes of age, the baby has a severe apneic episode that requires resuscitation. A decision is made to transport the baby to a regional perinatal center. Which of the following steps should be done now, before the regional center transport team arrives?

Yes	No	
____	____	Begin antibiotics, and then obtain a blood culture.
____	____	Insert an intravenous line.
____	____	Obtain a hematocrit value.
____	____	Perform a blood glucose screening test.
____	____	Give the baby a tube feeding.
____	____	Obtain a blood gas measurement.
____	____	Weigh the baby.
____	____	Draw a blood culture; start antibiotics.

(*continued*)

Unit 10 Pretest (*continued*)

7. A 4,500-g (9 lb 15 oz) baby is born to a woman with glucose tolerance outside reference range. He has Apgar scores of 9 at 1 minute and 10 at 5 minutes. At 45 minutes of age, the baby has a blood glucose screening test result of 0 to 25 mg/dL. A peripheral intravenous infusion of 10% dextrose is started, with improvement in the baby's condition. Plans are made to have the baby transported to a regional perinatal center. Which of the following actions should take place prior to arrival of the transport team?

Yes	No	
____	____	Check the baby's blood pressure.
____	____	Repeat a blood glucose screening test.
____	____	Give the baby oxygen.
____	____	Obtain a chest radiograph.

8. **True   False**   Babies who have experienced severe perinatal compromise require large amounts of fluid.

1. Why are maternal/fetal and neonatal transport important?

If maternal/fetal or neonatal intensive care is anticipated, referral to a regional perinatal center may be desirable for several reasons.

- Women or fetuses with certain conditions may require intensive care with highly specialized monitoring and evaluation techniques for extended periods.
- Improved maternal and neonatal outcomes have been demonstrated when high-risk pregnant women give birth in regional perinatal centers. Intrauterine transport is often less stressful for a baby than neonatal transport would be.
- Maternal/fetal transport allows a mother and baby to be close to each other soon after delivery.
- Maternal/fetal and neonatal transport to a regional perinatal center provides cost-effective use of highly sophisticated, expensive medical equipment and resources for patients who also require high staff to patient ratios.

2. What is neonatal transport?

Neonatal transport occurs when an at-risk or a sick newborn is transported to a regional perinatal center. Neonatal transport is most often accomplished by a team from a regional center that travels to the hospital of birth to transport a baby back to the regional center.

3. What is the goal of preparing any baby for transport?

The primary goal of preparing a baby for transport is to stabilize the baby's condition. It is more important to stabilize a baby and wait for a regional center transport team than to rush an unstable baby to a regional perinatal center.

 The stability of a baby's condition is far more important than the speed of transport.

4. Which babies require transport to a regional perinatal center?

This depends on the facilities and resources in your hospital. The medical and nursing staff of each hospital should meet and decide which neonatal conditions can be managed locally and which need to be referred. The pediatric and obstetric staff, in conjunction with the regional perinatal center, should develop policies to address the gestational age and birth weight requirements for a baby to remain in their hospital. Additionally, state regulations may dictate these policies, depending on the designated care level of the nursery.

In general, babies with the following conditions will need care provided by a regional perinatal center:

- Extremely preterm
- Extremely or very low birth weight
- Malformation(s)
- Surgical conditions
- Severe, acute medical illnesses
- Complex, long-term medical needs

5. What is the minimum preparation for *every* baby for transport?

A. Check vital signs
  - Temperature
  - Respiratory rate
  - Heart rate
  - Blood pressure
  - Oxygen saturation (SpO_2)

B. Perform laboratory tests
  - *Blood glucose screening test:* Important for nearly all babies.
  - *Hematocrit value:* Important for most babies.
  - *Blood gas levels:* At least one blood gas measurement is essential to determine how effectively the baby is ventilating. Oximetry can be used to monitor oxygenation.
  - *Other tests:* According to the baby's condition and the reason transport is needed.

C. Stabilize ventilation and oxygenation
  The degree of respiratory support provided should be adjusted according to pulse oximetry, clinical assessment of the degree of respiratory distress, and arterial blood gases.

D. Establish a fluid line
  This may be a peripheral intravenous line (PIV), an umbilical venous catheter (UVC), or an umbilical arterial catheter (UAC), depending on the baby's condition. A fluid line is important for 3 reasons:
  - Infusion of fluids during transport (via PIV or UVC)
  - Emergency medications that may be needed (via PIV or UVC)
  - Frequent blood sampling and/or continuous blood pressure monitoring (via UAC)

E. Determine the baby's gestational age and weight, unless the baby is too unstable, in which case an approximate weight can be used.

F. Call the regional perinatal center and discuss the baby's condition
  - *History:* Pregnancy complications, risk factors, findings at prenatal ultrasonography, Apgar scores, baby's weight and gestational age, delivery room/early neonatal course, etc
  - *Present status:* Physical examination, including a description of, for example, any malformations, vital signs, and oxygen and ventilation requirements
  - *Laboratory values:* Blood glucose screening test results, hematocrit values, blood gases, or chest radiographs
  - *Need for further special treatment*

  There will be some babies you recognize immediately as requiring transport; they may even be identified prior to birth (but a maternal transport could not have been arranged). It is reasonable to call the regional center to activate the transport process before all information is available. When additional information becomes available, a follow-up telephone call is usually helpful, to have a detailed discussion about the baby's condition. Regional centers vary in their policies of deploying their transport team prior to the birth of an infant. It is important to understand the regional center's policy so that both hospitals have consistent expectations of each other.

G. Discuss the baby's condition with the parents
  Document this conversation, obtain a signed permit for transport, and complete forms required to be compliant with the Health Insurance Portability and Accountability Act.

H. Obtain complete copies of the mother's and baby's charts.

I. Obtain copies of any radiographs of the baby (or make them electronically available to the regional perinatal center).

J. Continue optimum supportive care

Once a transport has been arranged, optimum care must be delivered while waiting for the transport team to arrive. It is your responsibility to ensure that the baby maintains adequate oxygenation, temperature, blood pressure, and stable metabolic status during this time.

Continuous updates on changes in the baby's condition should be relayed to the medical control officer from the regional perinatal center. The regional center should remain available for questions and guidance until the transport team arrives at the outlying hospital.

To provide optimum supportive care means you should check the baby's vital signs and certain laboratory tests repeatedly—often at an increased frequency. Chest radiographs or other tests may also need to be repeated, depending on the baby's condition.

 The care given during the first few hours after birth is every bit as important to a baby's outcome as the care given during the days or weeks spent at a regional perinatal center.

Some sick babies may need additional tests and procedures to be stabilized and prepared for transport. These have been discussed in the previous units. The material in this book will help you to decide which specific tests and procedures each individual baby requires.

Self-test

Now answer these questions to test yourself on the information in the last section.

1. What is the minimum preparation needed for every baby who will be transported?

_____
_____
_____
_____
_____
_____
_____
_____
_____
_____

2. What is the primary goal in preparing a baby for transport?

_____

3. List at least 3 groups of babies that are likely to need care at a regional perinatal center.

_____
_____
_____

Check your answers with the list near the end of the unit. Correct any incorrect answers and review the appropriate section in the unit.

6. How should you prepare babies with special problems for transport?

Some of the following information is *only* in this section. It is found nowhere else in the Perinatal Continuing Education Program books. Use the information you learned in previous units and the information in the following tables to help you stabilize babies with these particular problems. Ongoing discussion with the medical control officer from the regional center should take place if you are considering some of these interventions before the arrival of the transport team.

A. Respiratory Distress		
Perform These Tests or Procedures	**Look Particularly for These**	**Do This Before Transport**
Chest radiography	Pneumothorax	• Perform needle aspiration if the baby is in significant respiratory distress or if blood gas levels or oxygen saturation is outside the reference range. • For ongoing air leaks, a chest tube may be needed but should only be placed by a health professional who is experienced in the procedure.
Arterial blood gas analyses	Low Pao_2	• Increase the baby's inspired oxygen concentration. • Consider that the baby may have a pneumothorax. • Consider other causes (eg, persistent pulmonary hypertension of the newborn, meconium aspiration, cyanotic congenital heart disease).
	High $Paco_2$	• Consider bag-and-mask ventilation or endotracheal intubation and assisted ventilation. • Consider that the baby may have a pneumothorax.
	Low pH level	• If $Paco_2$ is high, consider providing assisted ventilation. • If $Paco_2$ and bicarbonate levels are low, determine and treat the cause of the acidosis and consider administering sodium bicarbonate after discussion with the regional referral center.
Blood cultures	Any baby with respiratory distress may be infected, with the infection being a cause of respiratory distress.	Consider obtaining blood cultures and beginning antibiotics.
Consider giving surfactant	Respiratory distress syndrome identified on radiographs and the baby has an endotracheal tube in place	Whether to give surfactant before transport depends on many factors. Lung compliance changes rapidly after surfactant administration, requiring close attention to ventilator management. Discuss with regional perinatal center staff.

B. Severe Perinatal Compromise

Perform These Tests or Procedures	Look Particularly for These	Do This Before Transport
Umbilical cord gas analyses	• Base deficit • pH level • Apgar scores	Thorough neurological assessment and discussion with the regional center if the infant may benefit from therapeutic hypothermia for treatment of hypoxic-ischemic encephalopathy.
Arterial blood gas analyses	• Low Pao_2 • Low pH level	• Increase inspired oxygen concentration. • If $Paco_2$ and bicarbonate level are low, consider administering sodium bicarbonate (discuss the appropriateness of this measure with your regional perinatal center staff).
Note: The kidneys and heart of a baby who experienced an episode of hypoxia or acidosis may not be able to handle a large amount of fluid.		• Restrict IV fluids, but beware the possible development of hypoglycemia. Use normal saline boluses as needed if there is evidence of hypovolemia (eg, low blood pressure and/or poor perfusion). • Consider that you may need to increase glucose concentration in the IV fluid.

Abbreviation: IV, intravenous.

C. Shock

Perform These Tests or Procedures	Look Particularly for These	Do This Before Transport
Blood pressure check	Low blood pressure	• Look for the cause of shock and treat it appropriately. • If no cause is apparent or if you suspect blood loss, administer physiological (normal) saline solution (10 mL/kg over 15–20 minutes) or O Rh-negative blood, if available.
Blood gas analyses	Low pH level	• Venous blood gas may be used to check pH level. • If there is any evidence of respiratory distress, however, obtain an arterial blood gas measurement.

D. Suspected Sepsis		
Perform These Tests or Procedures	**Look Particularly for These**	**Do This Before Transport**
Blood cultures		• Start antibiotics immediately after obtaining cultures. Do not wait for culture results. • Use antibiotics that combat gram-positive and gram-negative organisms. Ampicillin and gentamicin are the most common antibiotics used and provide good coverage for the most frequent causes of neonatal sepsis.
Blood gas analyses	Low pH level	• Venous blood gas measurement may be used to check the baby's pH level. • If there is any evidence of respiratory distress, however, obtain oximetry or an arterial blood gas measurement.
Consider a complete blood cell count.	Very low white blood cell count or ratio of immature to total polymorphs of > 0.2	Obtain cultures and start antibiotics, if not done earlier.

E. Seizures[a]		
Perform These Tests or Procedures	**Look Particularly for These**	**Do This Before Transport**
Blood glucose level check	Low blood glucose level	Administer glucose to the baby.
Blood calcium level check	Low blood calcium level	Intravenous Ca^{2+} administration may be indicated, but if given to the baby in an incorrect dose or concentration, serious adverse effects on cardiac function can result (discuss with regional perinatal center staff).
Consider lumbar puncture (based on the skill level of the health professionals at your institution).	High white blood cell count	• Culture the spinal fluid and treat the baby with antibiotics. DO NOT delay the start of antibiotics until after lumbar puncture. • If infection with a gram-negative organism is suspected, consider administering cephalosporin or other antibiotics that cross into the CSF. • If a viral infection is suspected (eg, human herpesvirus [herpes simplex]), send CSF for viral titer or polymerase chain reaction. • Use meningitis doses of ampicillin.
	Bloody	• Suspect birth trauma. • Blood may be introduced into the CSF at the time of lumbar puncture, if a small blood vessel is injured during the procedure (ie, a "traumatic tap"); interpret the results with caution.

Abbreviation: CSF, cerebrospinal fluid.

[a] If recommended after discussion with the medical control officer at the regional center, administer an anticonvulsant. Phenobarbital, 20 mg/kg delivered intravenously, is the most commonly recommend anticonvulsant in this situation. The dose may be repeated to achieve suppression of seizures, but be prepared to ventilate the baby if respiratory depression occurs. Also, if birth asphyxia is suspected, discuss with the regional center whether the infant is a candidate for therapeutic hypothermia. Maintain normothermia until the baby can be evaluated by a qualified examiner. Do not overheat the infant.

F. Suspected Congenital Heart Disease (CHD)		
Perform These Tests or Procedures	**Look Particularly for These**	**Do This Before Transport**
Blood pressure check (in all 4 extremities) *Hypotension* may be present due to poor cardiac output.	Hypotension	Babies with CHD may have hypotension or hypertension, depending on the type and severity of the defect.
	Hypertension	*Hypertension* may be present from obstructed blood flow that can occur with certain defects.
	Differences among extremities (right arm to legs)	Blood pressure may vary in different extremities. If blood pressure measurements from all 4 extremities vary significantly (5–8 mm Hg), that information may help establish a diagnosis and determine therapy.
Arterial blood gas analysis	Acidosis	*Metabolic acidosis* may be present because of poor cardiac output, in which case treatment with dopamine or sodium bicarbonate may be indicated. *Respiratory acidosis* may be present due to hypoventilation, in which case intubation and assisted ventilation may be indicated.
	Hypoxemia	Certain cardiac abnormalities cause *cyanotic* CHD. Other defects cause *acyanotic* heart disease (no cyanosis due to the defect itself). With cyanotic CHD, a baby's Pao_2 will rarely be > 50–60 mm Hg, even if the baby is breathing 100% oxygen. For these babies, an IV infusion of PGE_1 may be recommended. There are few situations in which PGE_1 therapy will make a baby's CHD symptoms worse for the few hours that may be required to establish a definitive diagnosis. For some unstable babies, PGE_1 therapy may dramatically improve their condition by dilating the ductus arteriosus, thereby permitting blood to flow to the lungs or allowing systemic circulation (depending on the nature of the cardiac lesion). *Consult with regional perinatal center experts when CHD is suspected.* If PGE_1 therapy is recommended, follow these guidelines: • *Route:* Administer via continuous IV infusion. Use a large central vein. Infuse into the umbilical vein, with the catheter tip located above the diaphragm. If that is not available, infusion through a peripheral vein is acceptable but may cause cutaneous flushing around the infusion site. Watch for side effects, including apnea, hyperthermia, hypotension, and flushing. • *Dose and rate:* Administer 0.05–0.10 mcg/kg/min. Usually 0.05 mcg/kg/min is adequate and is associated with fewer side effects. • *Preparation:* This drug is supplied in 500-mcg/mL vials. Dilute 1 ampule with 49 mL D5W. This equals 10 mcg/mL. Infuse at 0.6 mL/kg/min to equal 0.1 mcg/kg/min or at a different rate to achieve a different dose, as discussed with regional perinatal center staff. • *Side effects:* Fever and apnea are commonly seen soon after the initiation of PGE_1 therapy. *Be prepared, before the infusion of PGE_1 is started, to assist the baby's ventilation if apnea occurs.*

Abbreviations: CHD, congenital heart disease; D5W, 5% dextrose in water; IV, intravenous; PGE_1, prostaglandin E_1.

369

G. Congenital Malformations	
Condition	**Do This Before Transport**
For all conditions listed herein, follow steps 1 and 2 in the right-hand column.	1. Do not feed the baby. 2. Maintain hydration with IV fluids.
Choanal atresia	Place an oral airway. Intubate the baby if respiratory distress does not resolve with airway placement.
Diaphragmatic hernia	• Insert a nasogastric tube (8F) and suction it intermittently *or*, if a Replogle tube (double-lumen or sump) is available, use it and suction it continuously. • Place a decompression tube immediately, at the time of delivery. • Keep the baby positioned at a 45° angle (head up). • If the baby requires assisted ventilation, intubate. Do *not* use bag-and-mask ventilation.
Intestinal obstruction	Insert a nasogastric tube (8F) and apply intermittent suction *or*, if a Replogle tube (double lumen) is available, use it and apply continuous suction.
Meningomyelocele	• Place the baby on their abdomen. • If the meningomyelocele sac is ruptured, keep it covered with warm, sterile saline dressings. Use smooth, non-adhering dressing material; do *not* use gauze. • Place the baby in a sterile plastic bag or cover the lesion with a sterile plastic drape. • Avoid using latex products because they may cause sensitization.
Pierre Robin sequence (small mandible with respiratory distress)	• Insert a 10F or 12F catheter through the nose and into the posterior pharynx. This will break the suction that pulls the tongue into the airway, causing respiratory distress. • Place the baby on their abdomen. • If the baby requires further respiratory support, consider the use of a laryngeal mask airway, as intubation may be difficult.
Ruptured omphalocele or gastroschisis	• Administer IV fluids (D10W ½ NS) at a rate of 150 mL/kg/d. May need NS bolus for blood pressure instability with large fluid losses. • Place the baby's lower body in a bowel bag to keep urine and meconium away from the defect; place the baby and first bowel bag into another sterile bowel bag to enclose the defect and baby up to the axilla. This minimizes heat loss and trauma to the exposed organs and allows visualization of the defect. A small quantity (about 5–10 mL) of NS may be put in the second bowel bag to keep the intestines moist. If a bowel bag is not available, another sterile plastic bag or loose wrap may be used. • Do *not* wrap the intestines with gauze. Gauze, even if it seems soft, can damage the delicate surface of the organs. It may also act as a wick to draw away fluid and protein that may weep from the exposed surface of the organs. • Insert a nasogastric tube (8F) and suction it intermittently *or*, if a Replogle tube (double lumen) is available, use it and suction it continuously. • Position the baby on their side. To avoid decreased perfusion to the intestines, gently lift the intestines off the abdominal wall, suspending the intestines over the baby or off the bed.
Tracheoesophageal fistula	• Suction the pouch with a size 8F feeding tube. • Keep the baby positioned at a 45° angle (head up). The distal esophagus to the stomach may be connected to the trachea, which could result in the reflux of gastric acid into the lungs.

Abbreviations: D10W, 10% dextrose in water; IV, intravenous; NS, physiological (normal) saline solution.

Sample Case 1

Use the material in this unit *and in the previous unit* to help you respond to the questions in these sample cases.

Baby John is born at 32 weeks according to maternal dates, weighing 1,360 g (3 lb). He begins grunting and retracting almost from the moment of birth. He has a 1-minute Apgar score of 9 but, by 5 minutes, requires oxygen via a mask held to his face to stay pink. He is transferred in a warm incubator to the nursery while receiving 30% inspired oxygen concentration. Nothing else is known about the baby's history.

1. How would you classify this baby?

   ____ Well   ____ At risk   ____ Sick

2. What would you do immediately for this baby?

   _____

   _____

You find that the blood glucose screening level is 45 mg/dL, the blood pressure is 22/18 mm Hg, the hematocrit value is 31%, and the oxygen saturation is 92%.

3. What should be done now for this baby?

   _____

   _____

4. What 2 things would you do next?

   _____

   _____

Blood pressure is now 36/28 mm Hg, and the blood glucose screening level is now 90 mg/dL. The chest radiographic findings are consistent with respiratory distress syndrome. The arterial blood gas result with 60% inspired oxygen is

Pao_2:   62 mm Hg   pH level: 7.27

$Paco_2$: 45 mm Hg HCO_3-:   20 mEq/L

5. What would you do now for Baby John?

   Yes   No

   ____   ____   Increase the baby's inspired oxygen concentration.

   ____   ____   Decrease the baby's inspired oxygen concentration.

   ____   ____   Administer physiological (normal) saline solution.

   ____   ____   Administer a 25% glucose intravenous push.

At 40 minutes of age, the baby's vital signs are

   Temperature: 37.0°C (98.6°F) (radiant warmer servo control)

   Pulse: 152 beats per minute

   Respirations: 72 breaths per minute

   Blood pressure: 38/30 mm Hg

It has been decided that Baby John needs to be transferred to the regional perinatal center.

6. What else should be done to prepare this baby for transport?

_____

_____

_____

_____

_____

You continue this optimal supportive care (ie, frequent blood glucose screening tests, temperature control, frequent blood pressure measurements, arterial blood gas analyses, and assisting of the baby's ventilation, as necessary) and consult with regional perinatal center staff until the transport team arrives.

Check your answers with the list near the end of the unit.

Sample Case 2

Full-term Baby George, who is an appropriate size for gestational age, is born after an uncomplicated pregnancy and is pink, active, and irritable at 18 hours of age. His vital signs have been stable. The baby has breastfed well and has urinated, but he has not passed meconium since birth. His abdomen has become distended and slightly tense. He vomited after the last feeding.

1. How would you classify this baby?

    ____ Well   ____ At risk   ____ Sick

2. What would you think of as possible causes for the abdominal distension?

_____

_____

3. Of these things, which one is the most likely cause?

_____

_____

4. What should be done to evaluate this baby?

_____

_____

_____

_____

_____

The baby's vital signs are

Temperature: 37.0°C (98.6°F)

Pulse: 156 beats per minute

Respirations: 48 breaths per minute, unlabored

Blood pressure: 66/38 mm Hg

Blood glucose screening level: 90 mg/dL

5. How should this baby be fed?

_____

The laboratory calls and says that Baby George's hematocrit value is 52%.

6. How should this be treated?

_____

20 mL of gastric fluid have been suctioned through the nasogastric tube.

7. What should be done with this?

_____

The baby remains pink and active. The abdomen remains distended but is less tense. The mother and father come into the nursery and rock their baby. Vital signs are now

Temperature: 37.0°C (98.6°F)

Pulse: 148 beats per minute

Respirations: 48 breaths per minute

Blood pressure: 71/40 mm Hg

Blood glucose screening level: 90 mg/dL

An abdominal radiograph shows dilated loops of bowel consistent with an intestinal obstruction.

The decision is made to transfer this baby to the regional perinatal center. Regional center staff are contacted to arrange transport for Baby George.

8. What else should be done to prepare this baby for transport?

_____

_____

_____

_____

Check your answers with the list near the end of the unit.

Subsection: Caring for Parents of Transported Babies

Objectives

In this section you will learn

A. Why it is important for parents to be involved in the care of their sick or at-risk baby

B. Some ways to encourage emotional attachment of parents to their sick or at-risk baby

C. Special considerations when providing information to parents about their baby's condition

D. Special considerations for the hospitalized mother after the transport of her baby

Involving the parents is an essential aspect of caring for a sick or at-risk baby. Early, frequent, and close parental contact with a sick newborn is essential for developing a strong, healthy bond between parents and their baby. There are several things you can do for the family of every transported baby that will aid this attachment process.

1. How do you encourage emotional attachment with the baby?

Allow and encourage parents to enter the nursery to visit their baby before the transport team arrives. This can be done without interruption in the care given to the baby. In fact, it is important not to change a baby's care (unless the baby's condition changes) during parental visits.

A few simple techniques can be used to help foster the development of emotional ties between parents and their baby prior to transport.

- *Seeing and touching the baby:* All the equipment should be explained, but lengthy details are rarely needed at this time. Most parents immediately focus on their baby; some parents need more help. Have them stroke the baby's palm. Even the smallest and sickest babies can usually grasp a parent's finger.
- *Obtaining a photograph of the baby:* Discuss this and obtain permission from the parents before taking a photograph. All equipment should remain attached to the baby when the picture is taken. Most parents can see past the apparatus and focus on their baby. Alternatively, if permitted by your institutional policies, allow parents to take photos or videos with their own devices.
- *Obtaining handprint(s) or footprint(s) of the baby for the parents to keep.*

Whether a baby is perfectly formed but preterm or is full-term with a malformation, the baby is not the "ideal" healthy baby every parent imagines.

Parents need to establish strong bonds of affection and commitment to their baby during the stressful, rocky period of illness.

Parents of a baby with a malformation should be encouraged to see and touch their baby. What a parent imagines is almost always far worse than the baby's real condition. Parents need an honest and accurate understanding of their baby's condition so they can begin to deal with the real problems that confront their baby and themselves. Efforts to protect parents by restricting contact with the baby are not helpful.

The attitude of "Don't get involved because the baby will probably die" is also not realistic or helpful. Most sick babies do not die. Many preterm babies, given proper care, live and have few to no residual problems. Most term, sick babies also live and do well. Even if a baby dies, grieving is more easily accomplished and resolved when parents have close and caring ties with their baby than when they feel distant from, isolated from, or unimportant to their baby.

Regardless of the medical condition, parents need help as they begin the process of getting to know the unique characteristics, needs, and personality of their baby. Even parents who have long planned and waited for the birth of this baby are often fearful of undertaking the process of emotional attachment when confronted with a sick baby. Your understanding and assistance can be of tremendous value to parents at this time.

In addition, many fears and misunderstandings typically accompany the birth of a sick baby. Family members and parents may be inappropriately judgmental about whose "fault" it is that the baby is sick. It is the responsibility of the medical and nursing staff to explore with parents their feelings, correct misunderstandings, and facilitate the process of parents becoming acquainted with their newborn.

2. What should you tell the family about the baby's condition?

Parents should have a clear understanding of their baby's condition. Frequently, providing repeated discussions and explanations are necessary for parents to gain this understanding.

Serious conditions should be presented honestly and realistically. It is not necessary, however, to discuss all the *possible* complications. Many of these problems will not develop, but, once the possibility has been raised, it is difficult to erase it from a parent's mind. Doubts may linger long after danger has passed. For example, once parents have been told a preterm baby may have brain damage or an intellectual/developmental disability without any real evidence of this, it is not uncommon for parents, years later, to treat their child as if they have an intellectual disability or to watch anxiously for any sign the child is intellectually disabled. This may be because parents of even mildly ill babies often believe their baby will die or have a significantly adverse outcome. In other words, parents often expect the worst and may need to receive repeated reassurance about their baby's actual condition. Additionally, many parents think, but do not verbalize, that their baby will die, even if we as providers do not.

When a baby is being transported, it is helpful for the referring hospital staff to accompany the regional perinatal center transport team members when they discuss the baby's condition with the parents. The referring hospital staff can then reinforce what the transport team has said and correct any misunderstanding that may develop after the team has left.

3. How do you provide for parents' special needs?

Ideally, a mother should be transported to the regional perinatal center to which the baby is being transferred. If maternal transport is not possible, it may be helpful for the mother to have a private room so she is not confronted by roommates who are feeding and cuddling healthy newborns.

Visiting hours should be relaxed so parents can spend as much time together as they wish. Between employment, family responsibilities, and visiting the regional center to see their sick baby, it is often impractical, if not impossible, for the other parent to comply with visiting regulations. Close communication between parents is important for their relationship during this stressful time; it is also important for the other parent to relay accurate information about the baby to the mother. Often, the mother's partner will want to "protect" her from hearing about worsening illnesses or complications that have occurred. While this protective feeling is understandable, the mother should be fully informed. Additionally, the other parent may delay their bonding with the infant until it is guaranteed that the mother is safe. This is normal and expected.

After babies have been transferred to a regional perinatal center, mothers often need reassurance at unpredictable times about their baby's condition, such as when seeing a baby product advertisement on television or having a sleepless night. Talking with someone or calling the regional center may be helpful at these times.

In summary,

- Encourage parents to see and touch their baby. If needed, help them make this contact.
- Provide pictures or footprints of their baby, according to parents' wishes and available resources.
- Provide repeated, realistic explanations of the baby's condition.
- Give "bad news" only if, and when, complications develop. If by telephone, ensure there is another person immediately available to support the recipient of the news.
- Know what information the transport team has given the parents.
- Attempt to transfer the mother to the regional perinatal center to be closer to her baby.
- Consider providing the mother with a private room.
- Relax visitation policies.
- Provide emotional support to parents and other family members.

4. How do you arrange for transport of a baby?

A. Call the regional perinatal center

In the space below, write the hospital name, telephone number, and any special instructions you would use to make a neonatal referral and arrange for transport of a newborn.

_____

_____

_____

_____

_____

B. Discuss the baby's history and condition with regional center staff.

C. Prepare the baby (sections 5A–5I for all babies; sections 6A–6G for babies with special problems).

D. Continue to deliver optimum supportive care.

Self-test Answers

These are the answers to the Self-test questions and the Sample Cases. Please check them with the answers you gave and review the information in the unit wherever necessary.

1. Check the baby's vital signs.

   Obtain a blood glucose screening level, hematocrit value, and blood gas measurement and perform other tests, as indicated by the baby's condition.

   Stabilize ventilation and oxygenation.

   Establish a fluid line.

   Determine the baby's gestational age and approximate birth weight.

   Call the regional perinatal center and discuss the baby's condition.

   Obtain complete copies of the mother's and baby's charts.

   Obtain copies of any radiographs of the baby.

   Talk with the parents, document the discussion, and have a transport permit and other necessary forms signed.

   Continue to deliver optimum supportive care.

2. Stabilize the baby's condition and vital signs.

3. Babies with any of the following conditions:
   - Extreme prematurity
   - Malformation(s)
   - Surgical conditions
   - Severe, acute medical illnesses
   - Complex, long-term medical needs

   Note: Referral is often indicated for other babies too.

Sample Case 1

1. Sick. Baby John has respirations outside reference range and is therefore sick.
2. Check vital signs, blood glucose screening level, hematocrit value, and arterial blood gas measurements. Attach a pulse oximeter to the baby.
3. Insert an umbilical venous catheter. Administer 15 mL (10 mL/kg) of physiological (normal) saline solution, slowly, at a rate no faster than 1 to 2 mL/min. Send a blood sample for typing and crossmatching.

   (Review Unit 9, Identifying and Caring for Sick and At-Risk Babies, Subsection: Vital Signs and Observations, in this book as well as Section 6, How should you prepare babies with special problems for transport?, in this unit.)
4. Recheck the baby's blood pressure.

   Obtain a chest radiograph.
5. Yes No

Yes	No	
__	X	Increase the baby's inspired oxygen concentration (Review Unit 9, Identifying and Caring for Sick and At-Risk Babies, Subsection: Tests and Results, in this book).
__	X	Decrease the baby's inspired oxygen concentration.
__	X	Administer physiological (normal) saline solution. (Review Unit 9, Identifying and Caring for Sick and At-Risk Babies, Subsection: Vital Signs and Observations, in this book.)
__	X	Administer a 25% glucose intravenous push. (Review Unit 9, Identifying and Caring for Sick and At-Risk Babies, Subsection: Tests and Results, in this book.)

6. Obtain complete copies of the mother's and baby's charts.

Obtain copies of the baby's radiographs.

Discuss the baby's condition with the parents, document this discussion, and have a permit for transport and any other necessary forms signed. Answer any questions the parents have and encourage them to see and touch their baby.

(Review Section 5, What is the minimum preparation for *every* baby for transport?, in this unit.)

Continue to monitor the baby's vital signs, blood glucose screening levels, arterial blood gas measurements, and oximeter readings; provide supportive care; and respond to any changes in the baby's condition while you await the arrival of the transport team.

Sample Case 2

1. Sick. Baby George has an abnormal feeding pattern and is therefore sick.
2. Sepsis

Gastrointestinal obstruction

Necrotizing enterocolitis

(Review Unit 9, Identifying and Caring for Sick and At-Risk Babies, Subsection: Vital Signs and Observations, in this book.)

3. Gastrointestinal obstruction (The baby is pink and active, has vital signs within reference ranges, has breastfed well, and has no risk factors for sepsis. Sepsis is a possibility but is less likely than gastrointestinal obstruction in this baby. Necrotizing enterocolitis occurs most often in sick, preterm babies. This baby is term and was not previously sick, making gastrointestinal obstruction a more likely cause.)

4. Check the baby's vital signs.

Check the baby's blood glucose screening level and hematocrit value.

Check arterial or venous blood gas measurements (to look for a low pH level due to metabolic acidosis).

Consider obtaining cultures and beginning antibiotics.

Place a size 8F or larger nasogastric tube and connect it to low, constant suction, or leave the tube open to the air and, at frequent intervals, use a syringe to aspirate the stomach contents.

Obtain chest and abdominal radiographs.

(Continue to review Unit 9, Identifying and Caring for Sick and At-Risk Babies, Subsection: Vital Signs and Observations, in this book.)

5. This baby should not be fed by mouth or tube but should have a peripheral intravenous line started.

6. The hematocrit value is within reference range and therefore requires no treatment.

7. The gastric fluid may be discarded, but the volume should be recorded. Electrolytes are contained within the gastric juices. If significant volumes continue to be aspirated, the baby's serum electrolytes will need to be checked and sodium chloride may need to be added to the intravenous fluids to keep the baby's serum electrolyte levels within reference ranges.

(Review Unit 9, Identifying and Caring for Sick and At-Risk Babies, Subsection: Tests and Results, in this book.)

8. Obtain complete copies of the mother's and baby's charts.

Obtain copies of the baby's radiographs.

Discuss the baby's condition with the parents, document this discussion, and have a permit for transport and any other necessary forms signed. Answer any questions the parents have and encourage them to see and touch their baby.

(Review Section 5, What is the minimum preparation for *every* baby for transport?, in this unit.) You have already made the specific preparations necessary for transport of a baby with an intestinal obstruction (see Section 6G of this unit). Be sure to continue to suction intermittently from the gastric tube. Continue to monitor vital signs, provide supportive care, and respond to any changes in the baby's condition while you await the arrival of the transport team.

Unit 10 Posttest

After completion of each unit there is a free online posttest available at www.cmevillage.com to test your understanding. Navigate to the PCEP pages on www.cmevillage.com and register to take the free posttests.

Once registered on the website and after completing all the unit posttests, pay the book exam fee ($15) and pass the test at 80% or greater to earn continuing education credits. Only start the PCEP book exam if you have time to complete it. If you take the book exam and are not connected to a printer, either print your certificate to a .pdf file and save it to print later or come back to www.cmevillage.com at any time and print a copy of your educational transcript.

Credits are only available by book, not by individual unit within the books. Available credits for completion of each book exam are as follows: Book 1: 14.5 credits; Book 2: 16 credits; Book 3: 17 credits; Book 4: 9 credits.

For more details, navigate to the PCEP webpages at www.cmevillage.com.

Unit 11: Neonatal Abstinence Syndrome (Neonatal Opioid Withdrawal Syndrome)

Objectives

In this unit you will learn to

A. Identify neonatal abstinence syndrome (NAS)/neonatal opioid withdrawal syndrome (NOWS)

B. Recognize how newborns with NAS/NOWS present

C. Conduct a toxicology screening

D. Monitor newborns at risk for NAS/NOWS by using the Eat, Sleep, Console methodology

E. Manage neonates with NAS/NOWS

F. Conduct discharge planning for neonates with NAS/NOWS

G. Understand the outcomes of children with NAS/NOWS

Unit 11 Pretest

Before reading the unit, please answer the following questions. Select the *one best* answer to each question (unless otherwise instructed). Record your answers on the test and check them with the answers at the end of the book.

1. Neonatal opioid withdrawal syndrome (NOWS), also known as *neonatal abstinence syndrome* (NAS), is a multisystem disorder caused by the abrupt discontinuation of chronic fetal exposure to substances used by the mother during pregnancy. Which of the following statements describes a sign or symptom shown to be specific for NAS/NOWS?
    A. Irritability
    B. Sneezing
    C. Undisturbed tremors
    D. Uncoordinated suck
    E. High-pitched cry

2. The risk, timing, and duration of NAS/NOWS depends on the type of substance used by the mother. Which of the following exposures is most likely to result in withdrawal signs and symptoms in the first 24 hours after birth?
    A. Heroin
    B. Methadone
    C. Buprenorphine
    D. Oxycodone
    E. Naltrexone

3. How long should a healthy term neonate who is at risk for NAS/NOWS be monitored in the hospital after birth?
    A. 24 hours
    B. 48 hours
    C. 72 hours
    D. 96 hours
    E. 120 hours

4. Which of the following increases the risk and/or severity of developing NAS/NOWS in newborns exposed to in utero opioids?
    A. Female sex
    B. Co-exposure to benzodiazepines
    C. Prematurity
    D. Exposure to buprenorphine
    E. Lower birth weight

(*continued*)

Unit 11 Pretest (*continued*)

5. While NAS is a clinical diagnosis, toxicological confirmation is necessary to be able to identify the exact type of substance used, as well as confirm and/or rule out exposure to other licit and illicit substances. Which of the following statements regarding toxicology screening in the newborn is correct?

   A. Meconium toxicology screening has a long detection window, starting from the beginning of the second trimester of pregnancy.

   B. Urine toxicology screenings have a detection window of 5 to 7 days.

   C. The umbilical cord is a good screening biomatrix because of the high concentration of drugs in the cord.

   D. A negative toxicology screening result rules out NAS/NOWS.

   E. Toxicology screening is helpful in providing additional information on the frequency and patterns of drug use.

6. The Eat, Sleep, Console (ESC) approach was developed to assist in the monitoring and management of neonates with NAS. Which of the following statements regarding ESC is incorrect?

   A. A bottle-feeding newborn able to ingest 1 ounce per feeding is considered to be feeding well.

   B. A newborn able to sleep for 90 minutes undisturbed is considered to be sleeping well.

   C. A newborn able to be consoled in 10 minutes or less is considered consolable.

   D. The use of the ESC approach has led to a decrease in pharmacological treatment needs.

   E. The use of the ESC approach has led to a decreased length of stay.

7. **True   False**   The use of the ESC approach to manage newborns with NAS/NOWS is associated with an increased risk of hospital readmission for NAS symptoms.

8. Nonpharmacological interventions are the preferred first-line treatment for NAS/NOWS and should be optimized prior to considerations of pharmacological treatment. Which of the following statements regarding nonpharmacological management approaches is incorrect?

   A. Admission to the neonatal intensive care unit should be avoided whenever possible.

   B. Routine care should be clustered and should follow the newborn's schedule.

   C. Feeding the newborn every 3 hours is recommended to assist with establishing a routine.

   D. Rooming-in with the mother has been shown to be an effective way to reduce the length of hospital stay.

   E. Slow and rhythmic vertical rocking may be helpful in newborns with NAS/NOWS who are difficult to console.

9. **True   False**   Breastfeeding is contraindicated in neonates with NAS/NOWS.

10. **True   False**   Establishing a safe care plan for neonates with NAS/NOWS is a federal mandate.

1. What are neonatal abstinence syndrome (NAS) and neonatal opioid withdrawal syndrome (NOWS)?

Neonatal abstinence syndrome (NAS) is a multisystem disorder caused by the abrupt discontinuation of chronic fetal exposure to substances used by the mother during pregnancy. In most cases, NAS is caused by exposure to opioids, and this type of NAS is called *neonatal opioid withdrawal syndrome* (NOWS).

Other non-opioid substances used or abused by the mother during pregnancy can exacerbate NAS.

Over the past several decades there has been a dramatic increase in NAS cases as a result of increased maternal opioid use disorder in the United States. A 5-fold increase in NAS was observed between 2004 and 2014, with 1 affected neonate being born every 15 minutes. This increase in NAS cases has been associated with growing hospital costs. Of note, NAS affects rural and suburban areas disproportionately, with rural areas being more greatly affected.

2. How does NAS/NOWS present?

With NAS/NOWS, newborns have a constellation of behavioral and physiological signs and symptoms that are similar, despite marked differences in the properties of the causative agent. A generalized multisystem disorder, NAS/NOWS affects the baby's central nervous system, autonomic nervous system, and gastrointestinal system (Box 11.1). The most common signs and symptoms include irritability, excessive crying, undisturbed tremors, and exaggerated Moro reflex (https://med.stanford.edu/newborns/professional-education/drug-exposed-infants/neonatal-abstinence-syndrome.html).

Box 11.1. Neonatal Abstinence Syndrome Signs and Symptoms		
Central Nervous System	**Autonomic Nervous System**	**Gastrointestinal System**
Irritability	Sweating	Excessive/uncoordinated sucking
Tremors (undisturbed)[a]	Low-grade fever	Poor feeding
Sleep disturbances	Rhinorrhea	Vomiting
Excessive crying	Nasal stuffiness	Loose stools/diarrhea
High-pitched cry	Sneezing	Diaper rash
Hypertonia[a]	Yawning	Skin excoriation
Hyperreflexia	Skin mottling	Poor swallowing
Exaggerated Moro reflex[a]	Lacrimation	Dehydration
Restlessness	Mydriasis (dilated pupils)	Poor weight gain
Seizures (2%–11%)	Tachypnea	

[a] Signs and symptoms shown to be specific for neonatal abstinence syndrome.

Adapted from Kocherlakota P. Neonatal abstinence syndrome. *Pediatrics.* 2014;134(2):e547–e561.

The type of agent the neonate was exposed to in utero directly affects the symptoms and the severity of NAS. For example, compared with neonates exposed to buprenorphine, methadone-exposed neonates are more likely to experience tremors and a hyperactive Moro reflex. In contrast, buprenorphine-exposed neonates are more likely than methadone-exposed neonates to experience loose stools, nasal stuffiness, and sneezing. In addition, studies indicate that buprenorphine-exposed newborns have less severe NAS, including less severe symptoms with a decreased need for pharmacological interventions, as well as shorter length of stay. However, adherence to medication-assisted treatment (MAT) is lower for mothers taking buprenorphine than it is for those taking methadone.

The risk, timing, and duration of NAS depends on the type of opioids used by the mother (Table 11.1). Withdrawal from heroin typically occurs early in neonates, most often within the first 24 hours after birth. In contrast, neonates exposed to methadone or buprenorphine have delayed NAS manifestations, at 48 to 72 hours and 36 to 60 hours after birth, respectively.

It is important to recognize that NAS symptoms may be delayed for up to 4 weeks after birth and can therefore occur after hospital discharge. This emphasizes the importance of developing a plan for safe discharge that includes

- A minimum of 72 to 96 hours of observation in the hospital. Hospital discharge at 72 hours may be reasonable in neonates born to mothers taking opioids with a short half-life and who do not have NAS symptoms.
- Closed-loop communication with outpatient providers.

Table 11.1. Onset, Duration, and Frequency of Neonatal Abstinence Syndrome Caused by Various Substances			
Drug	Onset (hours)	Frequency (%)	Duration (days)
Opioids			
Heroin	24–48	40–80	8–10
Methadone	48–72	13–94	Up to 30 or more
Buprenorphine	36–60	22–67	Up to 28 or more
Prescription opioids	36–72	5–20	10–30
Non-opioids			
SSRIs	24–48	20–30	2–6
TCAs	24–48	20–50	2–6
Methamphetamines	24	2–49	7–10
Inhalants	24–48	48	2–7
Short-acting benzodiazepines	<24		3–5
Short-acting benzodiazepines	48–72		15–45

Abbreviations: SSRIs, selective serotonin reuptake inhibitors; TCAs, tricyclic antidepressants.

Adapted from Kocherlakota P. Neonatal abstinence syndrome. *Pediatrics*. 2014;134(2):e547–e561.

Not all neonates exposed to opioids in utero develop NAS. Risk factors have been identified that place a neonate at increased risk for developing NAS after chronic exposure to opioids in utero (*Pediatrics*. 2012;129[2]:e540–e560).

Maternal factors include

- The type of agent used
  — The incidence of NAS varies between opioids and is highest for newborns exposed to methadone (Table 11.1).
  — Whether the maternal dose of opioid affects the severity of withdrawal remains controversial. Some studies indicate that neonates exposed to lower doses of methadone (<30–40 mg/day) are less likely to develop severe NAS.
- Polysubstance use
  — Polysubstance exposures, particularly to benzodiazepines, increase the severity of NAS.
  — Tobacco exposure is also linked to more severe NAS in the neonate.

Newborn factors include

- Gestational age and birth weight
  — Prematurity and low birth weight are associated with decreased risk of NAS. The incidence and severity of withdrawal are less extensive in preterm neonates for multiple reasons: (1) the transmission of opioids across the placenta increases with advancing gestation; (2) preterm neonates have decreased amounts of fatty tissues, which limits drug accumulation; and (3) preterm neonates have decreased receptor development and sensitivity. This finding may also be due in part to the lack of assessment tools specifically designed for preterm infants.
  — Higher birth weight is associated with increased need for pharmacological treatment.
- Sex: Male newborns have more severe NAS symptoms.
- Genetic polymorphism (variation in the genes). *Polymorphism* is a term used in genetics to describe multiple forms of a single gene that exists in an individual or among a group of individuals. Polymorphisms in the opioid receptor mu 1 gene (*OPRM1*) and the catechol-O-methyltransferase (*COMT*) gene have been linked to decreased severity of NAS in exposed newborns.

3. How is a toxicology screening conducted?

While NAS is a clinical diagnosis, toxicological confirmation is necessary to

- Identify the exact type of substance used.
- Confirm and/or rule out exposure to other licit and illicit substances.

Toxicology screening involves the use of urine, meconium, umbilical cord, hair, or breast milk (human milk). Because of their long detection windows, the use of meconium or umbilical cord for drug screening is typically preferred (*Pediatr Clin North Am*. 2019;66[2]:353–367). The most commonly used screening methods are listed in Table 11.2.

Table 11.2. Most Commonly Used Specimens for Toxicology Screening			
Factor	**Urine**	**Meconium**	**Cord**
Detection window	Short (24–72 h) May be longer for chronic THC use and benzodiazepine	Long From the beginning of the second trimester	Long
Drug concentration	Moderate	High	Low
Advantages	Ease of collection Rapid results	Long window of detection	Long window of detection Easy and immediate collection
Disadvantages	Short window of detection First void often missed More false-negative findings than with meconium or cord	Lengthy collection Missed sample (in utero passage) Light and temperature sensitive Contamination with urine and/or transitional stool decreases sensitivity Does not reflect abstinence closer to term	Requires specific laboratory technique because of lower drug concentration Does not reflect abstinence closer to term

Abbreviation: THC, tetrahydrocannabinol.

Toxicology results should be interpreted within the clinical context. In addition, several limitations should be recognized.

- Toxicology screening does not provide information on frequency and patterns of use.
- Toxicology screening does not allow the differentiation between short-term and long-term use or between prescribed and illegal drug use.
- A negative toxicology screen result does not rule out NAS because of the potential for a false-negative finding.
- Health professionals should be aware of the possibility of false-positive results. For example, cold medicines can lead to false-positive results for amphetamines.

4. How should neonates at risk for NAS be monitored?

All neonates with the following risk factors should be closely monitored for the development of NAS:

- Known or suspected maternal opioid dependence or abuse
- Positive maternal drug screen result
- Positive newborn drug screen result

Assessments should begin within 3 to 4 hours after birth and should occur every 3 to 4 hours at the time of other routine care and **according to the newborn's schedule.** Continued monitoring in the hospital is recommended for a minimum of 96 hours for neonates who were exposed to methadone or buprenorphine (*Pediatrics*. 2012;129[2]:e540–e560).

While the use of standardized assessment tools is critical to improve the care of neonates with NAS (*Pediatrics.* 2014;134(2):e547–e561; *Pediatrics.* 2012;129[2]:e540–e560), there are currently no good data to compare the different tools. In addition, these scales were developed to assess symptoms of opioid (specifically heroin and methadone) withdrawal in term infants. As a result, they may be less sensitive in preterm infants and for other types of exposures.

Multiple assessment tools, based on observation of the newborn, are available (Table 11.3). The most widely used scale, the modified Finnegan neonatal abstinence severity score, has not been validated in its utility to improve outcomes. Other criticisms of these scoring systems include

- Overemphasis of minor symptoms that do not have a significant clinical impact on the newborn.
- Wide interobserver variability and need for rater training.
- Lack of validation studies to support the use of rigid cut-off for initiation of pharmacological therapy.

Table 11.3. Selected Assessment Tools for the Monitoring of Neonates With Neonatal Abstinence Syndrome	
Assessment Tool	**Description**
Finnegan Neonatal Abstinence Scoring System (FNASS)	32 items Pharmacological treatment initiated if the score is ≥ 8 on 3 consecutive scorings
The MOTHER NAS Scale[a] (modified FNASS)	21 items Pharmacological treatment initiated if the score is ≥ 8 on 3 consecutive scorings
Finnegan Neonatal Abstinence Scale–Short Form	7 items Inadequate to assess escalating symptoms
Simplified Finnegan Neonatal Abstinence Scoring System (sFNAS)	10 items Scores ≥ 6 and ≥ 10 have excellent specificity and negative predictive values for identifying newborns with Finnegan Neonatal Abstinence Scores ≥ 8 and ≥ 12
Neonatal Drug-Withdrawal Scoring System (Lipsitz)	11 items A score > 4 indicates clinically significant signs of withdrawal
Eat, Sleep, Console (ESC)	Simplified approach focusing on 3 **"functional"** criteria 1. **Eat.** Is the newborn feeding well? Tolerates feedings (appropriate amount for gestational and postnatal age) 2. **Sleep.** Is the newborn sleeping well? Able to sleep for at least 1 hour undisturbed 3. **Console.** Is the newborn consolable? Can be consoled in ≤ 10 minutes

[a] Used in the Maternal Opioid Treatment: Human Experimental Research (MOTHER) study.

To address some of these concerns, the Eat, Sleep, Console (ESC) approach was developed (Figure 11.1) (*Pediatrics*. 2017;139[6]:e20163360). ESC focuses on the overall well-being of the newborn by assessing 3 basic domains:

- **Eat:** Is the newborn feeding well? A newborn is considered to be feeding well if
  — Breastfeeding 8 to 12 times per day with effective latch and milk transfer.
  — Bottle-feeding an expected volume for age when showing hunger cues. The feeding volume average over a 3-hour period is more helpful than feeding volumes alone, particularly if cluster feeding is occurring.
- **Sleep:** Is the newborn sleeping well? A newborn who is able to sleep for 1 hour undisturbed is considered to be sleeping well.
- **Console:** Is the newborn consolable? A newborn who is able to be consoled in 10 minutes or less is considered consolable.

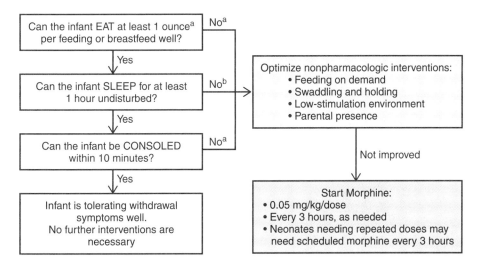

Figure 11.1. Using the Eat, Sleep, Console Approach to Monitor and Manage Neonates With Neonatal Abstinence Syndrome
[a] Bottle feeding an expected volume for age when showing hunger cues.
[b] If ANY one of the criteria indicate the answer "NO," a discussion amongst the interdisciplinary team is necessary to develop a plan of care for the neonate.
Adapted from Grossman MR, Berkwitt AK, Osborn RR, et al. An initiative to improve the quality of care of infants with neonatal abstinence syndrome. *Pediatrics*. 2017.

By using the ESC method, a newborn who is able to eat, sleep, and be consoled would be considered not to have clinically significant symptoms of NAS. If the answer is "no" to any one of these assessment points, however, the effect of NAS is clinically significant, and it may be necessary to consider pharmacological measures. Studies have shown that the use of the ESC method leads to improvements in NAS outcomes, including a decreased need for pharmacological interventions and decreased length of stay.

5. How should neonates with NAS be managed?

The care of newborns with NAS should be family centered and incorporate a low-stimulation environment, as well as feeding on demand. Focusing on the overall well-being of the newborn by using the ESC approach is recommended (see below). Nonpharmacological interventions are the preferred first-line treatment for NAS and should be optimized before considering pharmacological treatment.

Nonpharmacological Treatment

The goal of therapy is to allow the neonate with NAS to function as a normal neonate—feed well, sleep well, and be easily consoled. Nonpharmacological care, beginning at birth, is the first-line therapy in all cases. The cornerstone of nonpharmacological care includes

A. **Decreasing noxious stimuli**

It is important to provide a quiet, dark, and soothing environment for neonates with NAS. Thus, if medically appropriate, admission to a neonatal intensive care unit should be avoided.

Additionally, the following strategies may be used to support the neonate:

- Clustering of care to follow the newborn's schedule
- No disruption when sleeping
- Education of staff and families on effective comforting techniques, including
  — The 5 S's: swaddle, shush, sway, suck, sideline or C-position.
  — For babies that are difficult to calm, holding firmly in a "C-swaddle" (with the head and legs curled), slow and rhythmic head-to-toe swaying, vertical rocking, as well as firm patting or clapping, may be helpful. The clapping helps promote self-regulation and is a comforting technique that decreases signs of neurobehavioral dysregulation.

B. **Feeding on demand**

Newborns with NAS typically do better with frequent, small-volume feedings on demand. Cluster feeding patterns are common in this population.

- Breastfeeding
  — Women in a stable opioid substitution program should be encouraged to breastfeed, if not contraindicated.
  — Breastfeeding allows for increased maternal participation. In addition, it may decrease withdrawal symptoms and lead to reduced length of hospital stay.
  — Because of often poorly coordinated suck in these neonates, a lactation consultation is strongly recommended to support these mothers.
  — Health professionals should reassure the mother that the amount of methadone or buprenorphine in breast milk is small and that discontinuation of breastfeeding does not lead to an increase in NAS symptoms.

- Bottle feeding: When breast milk is not an option (for women who have an ongoing addiction, were not treated for drug addiction, are not in a MAT program, or received no prenatal care [which may affect follow-up compliance]), low-lactose or lactose-free formulas are recommended by experts to alleviate the gastrointestinal symptoms these babies experience.

Newborns with NAS are at increased risk of inadequate weight gain because of increased metabolic demand, and they require close weight monitoring. High-calorie feedings (24 cal/oz) should be considered early and—when required—are typically only needed for the first 2 weeks after birth. Alternatively, the use of a nasogastric tube for supplementation may also be considered in some neonates.

C. **Providing family-centered care**

Newborns should be kept with their mother or their family, whenever possible. Rooming-in can empower families and can lead to greater comfort in caring for the newborn. Parents who room-in with their babies can readily assess their newborn and provide immediate nonpharmacological interventions, including skin-to-skin care, swaddling, and feeding on demand (Table 11.4). In fact, rooming-in with the family is one of the most effective factors in reducing length of stay and pharmacological treatment needs. In addition to decreasing length of hospital stay, the presence of mothers at the bedside has been shown to decrease the severity of NAS. Based on these data, rooming-in is the preferred inpatient care model for neonates with NAS. Other benefits of forming a therapeutic alliance and engaging mothers and their families include

- Improved long-term outcomes of neonates with NAS.
- Increased maternal adherence to a maintenance program. While having a baby is often the motivation these mothers need to continue to strive for recovery or enter a treatment program, health professionals must recognize that attitude and stigma can have a profound negative effect and represent a substantial barrier to maternal recovery.

Despite these benefits, engaging these mothers can be challenging and requires a multidisciplinary approach that includes the involvement of social services.

Table 11.4. Summary of Nonpharmacological Measures in the Care of Newborns With Neonatal Abstinence Syndrome	
Intervention	**Purpose/Use**
Decrease external stimulation	
• Dim lights and cover the isolette or crib, if appropriate. Ideally, a crib canopy will be used when infants are in an open crib. • Decrease noise and ensure a quiet and soothing environment. • Use slow infant handling. • Avoid circumcision until NAS resolves.	The room should be as quiet as possible and dimly lit, and movements should be slow to minimize environmental stimulation that can be especially noxious during withdrawal.
Promote infant self-regulation	
• Nonnutritive sucking • Pacifier use • Swaddling/modified swaddling with a sleep sac when appropriate to prevent the infant from overheating • Prone, therapeutic sleep positioning	Nonnutritive sucking helps organize a dysregulated infant and prevents disorganization. Swaddling may help the infant with motor or muscle tone dysregulation. Infants who have poor motor control (thrashing or exaggerated rooting) respond to gentle head/limb restraint to help them regulate.
Supplemental comfort care measures • Holding (skin to skin with parent is optimal) • Rocking • Rubbing • Containment • Movement (ie, use of a swing and/or stroller) • Use of warm blanket • Soothing music	Gentle containment or pressure supports motor and muscle tone control. Rubbing is often better than patting when burping during feedings to avoid triggering the Moro reflex. Rocking helps to facilitate relaxation and eye contact. When rocking is vertical, it is thought to be more soothing than "regular" rocking or side-to-side rocking. Soothing music may be effective.

Abbreviation: NAS, neonatal abstinence syndrome.

Adapted from Pediatric Newborn Medicine Clinical Practice Guidelines: Care of the Neonate with Neonatal Abstinence Syndrome (NAS). Brigham and Women's Hospital; 2015. https://www.brighamandwomens.org/assets/BWH/pediatric-newborn-medicine/pdfs/dpnm-care-of-the-neonate-with-neonatal-abstinence-syndrome-(nas)-10.27.16.pdf. Accessed April 7, 2020.

Pharmacological Treatment

Pharmacological treatment may be required for newborns with severe NAS and for whom supportive care cannot be escalated further. Thresholds for treatment vary, based on the clinical assessment tools used to monitor these patients. Recommendations for initiation of pharmacological treatment based on the assessment tool selected are summarized below.

- ESC method (recommended): Consider pharmacological treatment if the neonate is
  — Not feeding well due to NAS symptoms such as irritability, uncoordinated suck, and/or tremors. Newborns with severe NAS may be unable to effectively feed within 10 minutes of showing hunger cues, may be unable to breastfeed for 10 minutes, or may be unable to bottle-feed 10 mL.
  — Not sleeping well due to NAS symptoms, such as tremors, increased startle, and/or irritability. Newborns with severe NAS may be unable to sleep for at least 1 hour after feeding.
  — Difficult to console. Newborns with severe NAS may not be able to be consoled in 10 minutes or less.
- Simplified Finnegan Neonatal Abstinence Severity Score:
  — Consider pharmacological treatment for 2 consecutive scores ≥ 8 or one score ≥ 12.
  — Strict adherence to scores alone, without overall assessment of the newborn's well-being, is not recommended.

Available therapeutic agents for the treatment of neonates with severe NAS are listed in Table 11.5 (*Pediatrics*. 2014;134[2]:e547–e561).

Table 11.5. Pharmacological Agents for the Treatment of Neonatal Abstinence Syndrome				
Agent	**Initial Dose**	**Interval**	**Titration**	**Maximum Dose**
First-Line Agents				
Morphine	0.05 mg/kg	As needed[a] every 3 hours for neonates needing repeated dosing	0.01 mg/kg/dose every 12 hours Until NAS symptoms are controlled	0.3 mg/kg per dose 1.3 mg/kg/day
	[a] For most neonates Morphine is the recommended agent when using the ESC method because of the short half-life of 9 hours (compared to a half-life of 25–32 hours for methadone). **Weaning** (if applicable): • Wean by 10% of the dose at the start of the wean. • Weaning interval: every 24 hours. More frequent weans may be tolerated in some neonates (maximum of 3 times daily). (For example, for a baby who is due for a dose of morphine but is eating, sleeping, and consoling well, the dose should not be given.) • Discontinue morphine when a single dose is 0.02 mg/kg • Hold or discontinue morphine if the baby shows signs of oversedation at any time. • Observe for 48 hours off morphine prior to discharge.			
Methadone	0.05–0.10 mg/kg	Every 6–12 hours	0.02 mg/kg	1 mg/kg/day
Buprenorphine[b]	4–5 µg/kg	Every 8 hours	0.8 µg/kg or 10%–25%	60 µg/kg/day
	[b] Sublingual administration			
Second-Line Agents				
Clonidine[c]	0.5–1.0 µg/kg	Every 6 hours[d]	0.5 µg/kg/dose	6 µg/kg/day
	[c] Can be considered a first-line therapy for neonatal withdrawal not caused by an opioid [d] Hold if systolic blood pressure < 55 mm Hg or heart rate < 80 beats/min **Weaning:** • If patient is receiving > 1 µg/kg/dose, decrease dose by 0.5 µg/kg/dose every 24 hours until 1 µg/kg/dose is reached. • Once receiving a 1 µg/kg/dose every 6 hours, decrease by a dosing interval (ie, to every 8 hours then every 12 hours, then every 24 hours, then off).			
Phenobarbital[e]	Loading: 10–16 mg/kg Maintenance: 2.5 mg/kg	Every 12 hours		
	[e] Monitor phenobarbital levels. *Note:* The use of phenobarbital is not recommended for the treatment of neonates with NOWS/NAS because of growing concerns about its adverse effects on long-term neurodevelopmental outcomes.			

Abbreviations: ESC, Eat, Sleep, Console; NAS, neonatal abstinence syndrome; NOWS, neonatal opioid withdrawal syndrome.

Self-test B

Now answer these questions to test yourself on the information in the last section.

B1. The Eat, Sleep, Console method focuses on the overall well-being of the neonate based on the assessment of 3 basic areas. By using this method, when would a baby be considered to be sleeping well?

_____

_____

B2. List 3 non-pharmacological measures that should be instituted as the first-line therapy for all newborns with neonatal abstinence syndrome/neonatal opioid withdrawal syndrome (NAS/NOWS).

_____

_____

_____

B3. When should pharmacological treatment be considered in neonates with NAS/NOWS?

_____

_____

_____

_____

B4. What is the recommended second-line pharmacological agent for neonates whose NAS/NOWS is not well controlled with opioids alone?

_____

Check your answers with the list that follows the Recommended Routines. Correct any incorrect answers and review the appropriate section in the unit.

---

6. How is discharge planning conducted for neonates with NAS/NOWS?

The establishment of a safe care plan for neonates with NAS is a federal mandate. The goal of the safe care plan is to ensure the safety as well as improve the outcomes for these patients and as such should include a safety plan for the newborn, as well as treatment and support resources for the mother (*Pediatr Clin North Am*. 2019;66[2]:353–367).

The safe care plan should ideally be established prior to discharge from the hospital and continued after discharge. To be successful, a coordinated multidisciplinary team approach is necessary, as well as collaboration with community providers.

The creation of a discharge checklist is recommended to guide health professionals through this process. The following elements should be included as part of the discharge checklist:

- The newborn has been monitored in the hospital for a minimum of 4 days, or until 48 hours after the last dose of medication.
- The newborn is feeding well.
- Caregivers have been educated on
  - How to recognize signs of NAS and how to respond to their newborn in a safe manner
  - How to soothe their baby
  - How to contact a health professional in case of concerns or emergency
  - Follow-up plans, including early pediatric follow-up appointments and home visits

- Healthy home environment (discussion points include securing the home from safety hazards, food safety, and exposure to violence)
        - Safe sleep (https://www.aap.org/en-us/advocacy-and-policy/aap-health-initiatives/child_death_review/Pages/Safe-Sleep.aspx)
- Plans for routine and acute pediatric care are in place, including
    - Discussion of the importance of attending post-discharge follow-up visits to
        - Monitor the baby for signs of NAS, recognizing that they may appear after hospital discharge
        - Monitor growth and development
        - Provide preventive care and immunizations
    - A plan for transportation
    - Discussion on when to contact health professionals for an acute visit
        - Trouble eating or sleeping
        - Crying more than expected
        - Loose stools and diaper rash
    - Discussion of the benefit of home nursing programs if available
    - Information on the role of early childhood intervention services
- Activation of community resources
    - Trauma-informed care services
    - Mentoring resources
- Involvement of child welfare services, if applicable

An example of a discharge checklist is shown in Table 11.6. Hospitals are encouraged to develop their own discharge checklist to incorporate local community agencies and mentoring resources.

For more information, please refer to the comprehensive guideline created by the Center for Substance Abuse Treatment, the Substance Abuse and Mental Health Services Administration, and the US Department of Health and Human Services.

Table 11.6. Discharge Checklist for Neonates With Neonatal Abstinence Syndrome	
Newborn	
Monitored in the hospital A MINIMUM of: • 96 hours (72 hours may be appropriate if the mother is taking an opioid with a short half-life—ie, heroin) • 24–48 hours after the last dose of medication • 24–48 hours after a wean if discharging home with medication	☐
Feeding well	☐
No NAS symptoms *or* symptoms easily managed with non-pharmacological measures	☐
Caregiver	
Able to recognize the signs of NAS	☐
Aware that the signs of NAS may persist for weeks after discharge	☐
Educated on how to intervene by using calming strategies (a low-stimulus environment, skin-to-skin, pacifier, swaddling, feeding on demand)	☐
Has demonstrated the ability to respond to newborn needs in a safe manner	☐
Educated on safe sleep practices	☐
Aware of follow-up requirements	☐
Has a transportation plan in place	☐
Knows how to contact a health care professional for questions or concerns	☐
Educated on the importance of maintaining recovery (if applicable)	☐
Outpatient Follow-Up	
Follow-up with a health care professional knowledgeable about NAS as soon as possible after discharge (and no longer than 5 days after discharge)	☐
Plan for continued lactation support of breastfeeding mothers	☐
The outpatient health care professionals have been notified by the inpatient team	☐
A plan is in place to contact the family if the appointment is missed	☐
Early intervention referral in place	☐
Home nursing visit in place if available	☐
Child Protective Services contacted if appropriate	☐

Abbreviation: NAS, neonatal abstinence syndrome.

Derived from Substance Abuse and Mental Health Services Administration. Clinical Guidance for Treating Pregnant and Parenting Women with Opioid Use Disorder and Their Infants. Substance Abuse and Mental Health Services Administration; 2018.

7. What are the outcomes of babies with NAS/NOWS?

While exposure to opioids in utero has a strong effect on short-term outcomes (NAS), there is debate as to whether or not it negatively affects long-term neurodevelopmental outcomes. This is largely secondary to the lack of prospective studies that adequately account for family characteristics and environmental factors. Regardless, compared with their peers, children with a history of NAS are at higher risk for hospital admission owing to abuse or neglect. In addition, children with a history of NAS also are at increased risk for the development of later substance use disorder (see below). After discharge from the hospital, a multidisciplinary approach to support these families may help mitigate the long-term effects of NAS.

Neurodevelopmental Outcomes

The long-term neurocognitive effects of NAS are difficult to ascertain because of the complex interplay of prenatal and environmental factors, such as family characteristics, exposure to substances other than opioids, adverse childhood experiences (ACEs), and other health or psychosocial factors. In addition, there is a lack of prospective studies that adequately control for prenatal exposures, NAS management needs, and parental sociodemographic factors. Despite these important limitations, significant concerns exist about the long-term effects of opioid exposure in utero.

Studies on the effects of heroin exposure have demonstrated that while cognitive and fine-motor performance at 17 to 21 years of age are within normal range, they are significantly worse than performance in control subjects who were matched for sex, age at testing, and caregiver education. Because of the high rate of polydrug exposure, as well as placement of children in the foster care system by 1 year of age, the effects of heroin on these outcomes cannot be fully ascertained. Children of heroin-dependent parents also have an 8-fold increased risk of depression, a 3-fold increased risk of attention disorder, and a 16-fold increased risk of substance use disorder when evaluated at ages 6 to 18 years. However, all of these outcomes are improved with programs that aim to decrease exposure to ACEs and foster resilience in the individual and family, which also calls into question the role of heroin exposure itself.

The effect of MAT is less clear, and data on the long-term effects on outcomes of such programs remain limited. The American College of Obstetricians and Gynecologists Committee on Healthcare for Underserved Women and the American Society of Addiction Medicine concluded that there is no significant difference in cognitive outcomes up to age 5 years between children exposed to methadone or buprenorphine when controlling for socioeconomic status, instability in the home environment, and maternal psychological distress.

Other investigators continue to raise concerns that NAS adversely affects long-term neurodevelopmental outcomes. In a cohort of Australian children, a neonatal diagnosis of NAS was strongly associated with a lower level of school performance, including lower scores on the National Assessment Program: Literacy and Numeracy in grade 7 when compared with control subjects in grade 5. A meta-analysis of methadone MAT on long-term outcomes concluded that children born to mothers who were taking methadone MAT are at risk of impaired neurodevelopment, with lower Mental Development Index and Psychomotor Development Index at age 2. In addition, they were found to be at increased risk for strabismus and nystagmus. The interpretation of these results is tempered because of intermediate- to poor-quality evidence. Another meta-analysis also identified significant differences in mental and physical development in children exposed to NAS. Finally, neonates with NAS have been found to have a smaller head circumference at birth, which further raises the concern that chronic opioid use during pregnancy adversely affects brain development.

Based on these data, children with a history of NAS should

- Undergo routine developmental screening with a plan for early referral for specialized assessments if concerns arise (from either the health professional or the caregiver).
- Receive early intervention services.
- Undergo a visual screening at 6 months of age.

Risk of Readmission

Health professionals who care for infants with a history of NAS should be aware of the increased risk of hospital admission in childhood. Infants with NAS have been shown to be more likely to be hospitalized in childhood due to assault, maltreatment, poisoning, mental or behavioral disorders, and visual disorders. Therefore, health professionals who care for these children should be alert for signs of child abuse or neglect.

Risk of Later Substance Use Disorder

A history of NAS is a risk factor for the later development of alcohol and/or drug use disorder in adulthood. This may be caused in part by genetic factors, including polymorphisms in the opioid receptor genes, as well as epigenetic factors (external or environmental factors that can influence gene function and do not involve changes in the DNA sequence). Additionally, social factors, such as an unstable or unsafe home environment, have been shown to play a significant role, emphasizing the importance of a multidisciplinary approach to support these families and mitigate the effects of addiction for themselves and for future generations of children.

Self-test C

Now answer these questions to test yourself on the information in the last section.

C1. In the United States, the number of neonatal abstinence syndrome (NAS) cases
  A. Has reached a plateau over the past few years
  B. Is rapidly increasing
  C. Is slowly decreasing

C2. Affected newborns present mostly with symptoms involving the following systems:
  A. Renal and integumental
  B. Cardiovascular and musculoskeletal
  C. Central nervous and gastrointestinal

C3. Onset of signs and symptoms of withdrawal appear
  A. As early as 24 hours after birth or as delayed as several days after birth
  B. At 2 weeks of age
  C. Immediately at birth

C4. **True**   **False**   The duration of symptoms depends on the type of exposure but can be prolonged, lasting for several weeks to months after birth.

C5. Which of the following is not true?
  A. The care of newborns with NAS should be family-centered and incorporate a low stimulation environment as well as feeding on demand.
  B. Focusing on the overall well-being of the newborn using the Eat, Sleep, Console approach is recommended.
  C. Nonpharmacological interventions are the preferred first-line treatment for NAS and should be optimized prior to considerations of pharmacologic treatment.
  D. Removal of the child from the home should be pursued.

Check your answers with the list that follows the Recommended Routines. Correct any incorrect answers and review the appropriate section in the unit.

NEONATAL ABSTINENCE SYNDROME (NEONATAL OPIOID WITHDRAWAL SYNDROME)

Recommended Routines

All the routines listed below are based on the principles of perinatal care presented in the unit you have just finished. They are recommended as part of routine perinatal care.

Read each routine carefully and decide whether it is standard operating procedure in your hospital. Check the appropriate blank next to each routine.

Procedure Standard in My Hospital	Needs Discussion by Our Staff	Recommended Routine
_____	_____	1. Establish a mechanism to promptly identify neonates at risk for neonatal abstinence syndrome/ neonatal opioid withdrawal syndrome (NAS/ NOWS) in your center.

- Ideally, this should start prenatally in close collaboration with obstetric providers.
- At birth, identify at-risk newborns by
  — Inquiring about the history of maternal substance use disorder with obstetrics providers
  — Reviewing maternal drug screening data, if available
- Discuss indications for sending a meconium or umbilical sample for drug screening.
  — Positive screening result according to the history or toxicology result in the mother
  — Newborn exhibiting signs of withdrawal
  — Other indications, such as history of abruption or small-for-gestational-age head circumference
- Clearly communicate the findings and the need for standardized monitoring to all pediatric providers.

(continued)

2. Develop a guideline for the monitoring of neonates at risk for NAS/NOWS that includes
   - When to initiate monitoring: Recommendations are to start monitoring within 4 to 6 hours of birth.
   - How to monitor at-risk newborns
     — Use the Eat, Sleep, Console method.
     — Use scoring tools, such as the modified Finnegan Neonatal Abstinence Scoring System score.
     — It is important that assessments occur on the baby's schedule, regardless of the monitoring method your center is using.
   - How long to monitor the baby in the hospital based on exposure
     — A minimum of 72 hours for short-acting opioids.
     — A minimum of 96 hours for longer-acting opioids.

3. Develop a guideline for the management of neonates with NAS/NOWS.
   - Emphasize the use of nonpharmacological care as a first-line therapy for all newborns with NAS.
     — Decrease stimuli.
     — Feed on demand.
     — Provide family-centered care.
   - Have clear recommendations on when pharmacological intervention is indicated and when to consider transfer, if applicable.
   - Ensure that social work personnel are involved in the care of the family from the time of admission to facilitate
     — Discharge planning.
     — Engagement of resources for the family after discharge.

_____ _____ 4. Develop a breastfeeding guideline for neonates born to mothers with a substance use disorder.
- Involve lactation consultant support in developing your guideline.
- Discuss the benefits of breastfeeding for mothers in a stable medication-assisted program who have no contraindications.
- Define when breastfeeding is contraindicated.
  — HIV infection
  — Active history of polysubstance drug use
  — Drug screen result indicating the use of non-prescribed medications
  — Your hospital's policy with regard to active marijuana use

_____ _____ 5. Create a discharge checklist for newborns with NAS/NOWS.

_____ _____ 6. Develop a curriculum to educate health professionals who are caring for families affected by substance use disorders:
- Include how, when, and where monitoring of at-risk newborns should occur.
- Include a recommendation for toxicology screening.
- Include education on nonpharmacological care and the role of pharmacological treatment.
- Discuss the steps involved in discharge planning for these patients.

Self-test Answers

These are the answers to the Self-test questions. Please check them with the answers you gave and review the information in the unit wherever necessary.

Self-test A

A1. Any 3 of the following signs or symptoms:
Irritability
Undisturbed tremors
Sleep disturbances
Excessive crying
High-pitched cry
Hypertonia
Hyperreflexia
Exaggerated Moro reflex
Restlessness
Seizures

A2. Any 3 of the following factors:
Term gestation
Good birth weight
Polysubstance exposure
Exposure to benzodiazepines
Genetic polymorphisms

A3. A minimum of 72 to 96 hours, based on the opioid type.

A4. A. A neonate born to a mother using heroin during pregnancy.

Self-test B

B1. A newborn able to sleep for 1 hour undisturbed is considered to be sleeping well.

B2. Any 3 of the following measures:
Decrease noxious stimuli
Cluster care on the baby's schedule
Do not disturb a sleeping baby
Use comforting techniques, such as the 5 S's (swaddle, shush, sway, suck, sideline or C-position)
Feed on demand
Provide family-centered care

B3. When the baby is not able to eat, sleep, or console, despite receiving optimized nonpharmacological care; or, for centers using the modified Finnegan Neonatal Abstinence Scoring System, when the baby has 2 consecutive scores ≥ 8 or one score ≥ 12

B4. Clonidine

Self-test C

C1. B. Is rapidly increasing

C2. C. Central nervous and gastrointestinal

C3. A. As early as 24 hours after birth or as delayed as several days after birth

C4. True. The duration of symptoms depends on the type of exposure but can be prolonged, lasting for several weeks to months after birth.

C5. D. Removal of the child from the home should be pursued.

Unit 11 Posttest

After completion of each unit, there is a free online posttest available at www.cmevillage.com to test your understanding. Navigate to the PCEP pages on www.cmevillage.com and register to take the free posttests.

Once registered on the website and after completing all the unit posttests, pay the book exam fee ($15) and pass the test at 80% or greater to earn continuing education credits. Only start the PCEP book examination if you have time to complete it. If you take the book examination and are not connected to a printer, either print your certificate to a .pdf file and save it to print later, or come back to www.cmevillage.com at any time and print a copy of your educational transcript.

Credits are only available by book, not by individual unit within the books. Available credits for completion of each book examination are as follows: Book 1: 14.5 credits; Book 2: 16 credits; Book 3: 17 credits; and Book 4: 9 credits.

For more details, navigate to the PCEP webpages at www.cmevillage.com.

PCEP

Perinatal Continuing Education Program

Pretest Answer Key
Book 3: Neonatal Care

Unit 1: Oxygen

1. B. From an arterial blood gas sample
2. B. Change the inspired oxygen to 40%
3. C. Oxygen in the blood
4. A. Arterial blood gas measurements
5. D. A preterm baby with an arterial blood oxygen tension (Pao_2) of 60 mm Hg
6. D. Use an oxygen blender

7. True
8. False
9. True
10. False
11. False
12. True
13. True

Unit 2: Respiratory Distress

1. C. Lips
2. B. Tachypnea
3. D. Surfactant deficiency
4. C. A 38-week, appropriate-for-gestational-age baby whose mother's membranes had been ruptured for 6 hours before delivery
5. B. Obtain a chest radiograph
6. A. Expected, unless accompanied by brady-cardia or cyanosis
7. D. 1, 2, 3, 4
8. B. Apnea shows the baby is getting worse quickly

9. D. >90%
10. A. decrease
11. False
12. True
13. True
14. C. Preterm baby with respiratory distress syndrome
15. A. High blood pressure
16. C. Anemia
17. B. 1.0%
18. True

Unit 3: Umbilical Catheters

1. A. Umbilical artery
2. A. Umbilical venous catheter
3. B. Umbilical arterial catheter
4.

Yes	No	
X	___	Thrombosis
X	___	Blood infection
___	X	Brain damage
___	X	Kidney damage
___	X	Loss of toe from embolus

5. False
6. True
7. A. Administration of emergency medications
8. C. Remove the catheter

409

Unit 4: Low Blood Pressure (Hypotension)

1. D. All of the above
2. C. Systolic blood pressure
3. B. 20 mL
4. A. 180 mL (6 oz)
5. C. 45 mL (1½ oz)
6. D. Physiological (normal) saline solution
7. E. A, B, and C
8. False
9. B. Polycythemia
10. C. Hypotensive

Unit 5: Intravenous Therapy

1. Yes	No	
X	___	A 1,590-g (3 lb 8 oz), vigorous baby on the first day after birth
___	X	A 3,175-g (7 lb) baby with Apgar scores of 6 at 1 minute and 9 at 5 minutes
X	___	A 3,620-g (8 lb) baby with suspected sepsis who has ingested 120 mL (4 oz) of formula during the past 24 hours
___	X	A 2,720-g (6 lb), vigorous baby whose mother was hospitalized with bacterial pneumonia at 20 weeks of gestation

2. B. An exchange transfusion
3. D. 10% dextrose in water
4. C. 120 mL/kg per 24 hours
5. False
6. A. Blood electrolyte values
7. B. 100 mL
8. C. 325 mL per 24 hours

Unit 6: Feeding

1. B. When there was excess amniotic fluid
2. A. A 3-day-old, term baby who has not produced stool
3. D. All of the above
4. C. Peripheral intravenous fluids
5. True
6. True
7. True
8. A. Babies born at 30 weeks' gestational age who are appropriate for gestational age with a strong suck reflex
9. B. Check for a soft, nondistended abdomen
10. True
11. False
12. True

Unit 7: Hyperbilirubinemia

1. C. Bilirubin level of 9 mg/dL at 10 hours of age in a full-term baby
2. D. A baby with hypertension
3. B. Obtain blood samples for laboratory tests
4. C. Caused by bilirubin levels outside of reference range
5. A. They have decreased removal of bilirubin by the liver
6. A. a lower

7. B. Anemia
8. A. Platelet count
9. Yes   No

Yes	No	
___	X	Cover the baby's eyes only for the first 8 hours of phototherapy.
___	X	Discontinue phototherapy immediately if a rash appears.
X	___	Completely undress the baby down to the diaper.
___	X	Restrict the baby's fluid intake.
___	X	Restrict the baby's feedings.

10. False
11. False
12. True

Unit 8: Infections

1. A. A low body temperature
2. C. An infected baby may develop metabolic acidosis
3. C. Obtain blood cultures
4. B. Require handwashing between handling babies
5. D. Their immune system is immature
6. True
7. True
8. False
9. True
10. False
11. True
12. True
13. Yes   No

Yes	No	
X	___	Rupture of membranes 24 hours prior to delivery
X	___	Active labor for 24 hours
___	X	Father's skin colonized with staphylococcal epidermidis

14. Yes   No

Yes	No	
X	___	The baby was at risk for infection at the time of birth.
X	___	Reduced temperature is a clinical sign of infection in babies.
___	X	This baby probably has a localized infection.
X	___	The first actions to take are to begin supportive care and obtain cultures from this baby.
X	___	You should obtain blood cultures and promptly begin antibiotics.
___	X	Ampicillin alone is an appropriate treatment for this baby.

Unit 9: Identifying and Caring for Sick and At-Risk Babies

1A. Yes No

___ _X_ Give the baby supplemental oxygen.

_X_ ___ Do a gestational age and size examination.

_X_ ___ Perform a blood glucose screening test.

___ _X_ Start an intravenous line and administer 8 mL of 10% glucose.

_X_ ___ Repeat vital sign checks frequently.

1B. Yes No

___ _X_ Small for gestational age

_X_ ___ Preterm

_X_ ___ Large for gestational age

___ _X_ Post-term

1C. Yes No

_X_ ___ Hypoglycemia

___ _X_ Diarrhea

___ _X_ Meconium aspiration

_X_ ___ Respiratory distress syndrome

___ _X_ Neonatal diabetes mellitus

1D. Yes No

_X_ ___ Start oral feedings (breast or bottle).

___ _X_ Begin antibiotic therapy.

___ _X_ Place the baby under photo-therapy lights.

_X_ ___ Repeat blood glucose screening tests.

___ _X_ Give the baby supplemental oxygen.

___ _X_ Treat this baby like she is a healthy baby.

2A.

Do Immediately	Do in Next Several Minutes	Not Indicated	
	X		Perform a blood glucose screening test.
		X	Administer epinephrine 0.5 mL (1:10,000).
	X		Connect an oximeter to the baby.
X			Assist ventilation with bag and mask.
		X	Stimulate the baby with warm water.
	X		Obtain a hematocrit value.
	X		Check the baby's blood pressure.
	X		Perform a blood gas analysis.
	X		Take the baby's temperature.

2B. Yes No

_X_ ___ Common problem of preterm birth

_X_ ___ Sepsis

_X_ ___ Hypoglycemia

_X_ ___ Aspirated formula

___ _X_ Blood oxygen level too high

Unit 10: Preparation for Neonatal Transport

1A. Yes No

  X   Begin oxygen therapy.

      X Transport the baby to the radiology department for chest radiography.

      X Begin hourly tube feedings.

  X   Obtain an arterial blood gas measurement.

  X   Conduct a blood glucose screening test.

  X   Attach a pulse oximeter to the baby.

1B. C. Intubate the baby's trachea and assist ventilation with a resuscitation bag

2. Yes No

  X   Insert a peripheral intravenous line.

      X Obtain a blood culture.

  X   Perform a blood glucose screening test.

  X   Check the baby's blood pressure.

      X Obtain an electrocardiogram.

3. D. Conduct a blood gas analysis

4. Yes No

      X Administer oxygen.

  X   Perform a blood glucose screening test.

      X Obtain a chest radiograph.

      X Insert an umbilical arterial catheter.

  X   Start a peripheral intravenous line.

      X Feed the baby by mouth.

5. Yes No

  X   Investigate the cause of metabolic acidosis.

      X Provide bag-and-mask ventilation.

      X Intubate and use the bag to breathe for the baby.

  X   Increase the baby's oxygen concentration.

6. Yes No

      X Begin antibiotics, and then obtain a blood culture.

  X   Insert an intravenous line.

  X   Obtain a hematocrit value.

  X   Perform a blood glucose screening test.

      X Give the baby a tube feeding.

  X   Obtain a blood gas measurement.

      X Weigh the baby.

  X   Draw a blood culture; start antibiotics.

7. Yes No

  X   Check the baby's blood pressure.

  X   Repeat a blood glucose screening test.

      X Give the baby oxygen.

      X Obtain a chest radiograph.

8. False

413

Unit 11: Neonatal Abstinence Syndrome (Neonatal Opioid Withdrawal Syndrome)

1. C. Undisturbed tremors
2. A. Heroin
3. D. 96 hours
4. B. Co-exposure to benzodiazepines
5. A. Meconium toxicology screening has a long detection window, starting from the beginning of the second trimester of pregnancy
6. B. A newborn able to sleep for 90 minutes undisturbed is considered to be sleeping well
7. True
8. C. Feeding the newborn every 3 hours is recommended to assist with establishing a routine
9. False
10. True

Glossary

ABO incompatibility: A condition that may lead to neonatal hemolytic disease. The pregnant woman has group O red blood cells and antibodies to group A and B red blood cells. These antibodies are transferred to the fetus and cause destruction of fetal red blood cells. While this process is similar to Rh incompatibility, the hemolytic disease resulting from ABO incompatibility is less severe than the disease caused by Rh incompatibility. Unlike Rh incompatibility, ABO incompatibility cannot be prevented by giving the mother Rh immune globulin.

Acidosis: Abnormally *low* pH of the blood. The range of blood pH in a healthy neonate is between 7.25 and 7.35. A blood pH of 7.20 or lower is considered severe acidosis. Acidosis may result from metabolic disturbances in which the serum bicarbonate is low or inadequate respiratory efforts in which serum carbon dioxide is high. Often metabolic and respiratory factors simultaneously influence the blood pH. Acidotic babies are usually lethargic and may have mottled or grayish colored skin. If extremely acidotic, babies typically take deep, regular gasping breaths. If a baby is gasping, the pH is probably 7.00 or less. Acidosis should be corrected promptly, most commonly with assisted ventilation when due to inadequate respiratory effort or occasionally by administration of sodium bicarbonate if due to metabolic factors.

Acoustic stimulation: A test in which fetal response to a sound when produced by a device placed against the maternal abdomen and triggered to give a loud, 1-second buzz is used as an estimate of fetal well-being. This test may be used during a nonstress test or labor.

Adrenaline: Official British Pharmacopoeia name for epinephrine. The trademark name for epinephrine preparations is *Adrenalin.*

AGA: *See* Appropriate for gestational age.

Age, adjusted: *See* Age, corrected.

Age, chronological: Number of days, weeks, months, or years that have elapsed since birth.

Age, conceptional: Time elapsed between the day of conception and day of delivery. *Note:* The term *conceptual age* is incorrect and should not be used. *Conceptional age* may be used when conception occurred as a result of assisted reproductive technology, but should *not* be used to indicate the age of a fetus or newborn. *See also* Age, gestational.

Age, corrected: Chronologic age in weeks or months reduced by the number of weeks born before 40 weeks of gestation. It is used only for children up to 3 years of age who were born preterm. It is the preferred term to use after neonatal hospitalization, and should be used instead of *adjusted age.* *Example:* A 24-month-old child born at 28 weeks' gestation has a corrected age of 21 months.

Age, gestational: Number of completed weeks between the first day of the woman's last menstrual period and the day of delivery (or the date an assessment is performed if the woman has not yet delivered). If pregnancy was achieved using assisted reproductive technology and, therefore, the date of fertilization or implantation is defined, gestational age may be calculated by adding 2 weeks to the conceptional age.

Age, postmenstrual: Weeks of gestational age plus chronologic age. It is the preferred term to describe the age of preterm infants during neonatal hospitalization. *Note: Postconceptional age* should *not* be used. *Example:* A baby born at $33^{1/7}$ weeks with a chronologic age of $5^{4/7}$ weeks has a postmenstrual age of $38^{5/7}$ weeks.

AIDS: Symptomatic stage of the illness caused by HIV.

Albumin: The major protein in blood.

Alkalosis: Abnormally *high* pH of the blood. Range of blood pH in a healthy neonate is between 7.25 and 7.35. Alkalosis may result from a high serum bicarbonate or, more commonly, when the carbon dioxide concentration in a baby's blood is lowered by hyperventilation (assisting the baby's breathing at an excessively fast rate). Babies who are alkalotic may not respond to stimulation intended to increase their breathing efforts until their blood carbon dioxide level rises toward the reference range.

Alpha fetoprotein: A normal fetal serum protein. When a fetus has an open neural tube defect, such as anencephaly or meningomyelocele, increased amounts of this protein pass into the amniotic fluid and the pregnant woman's blood, thus providing the basis for an antenatal screening test. Low or high maternal serum alpha fetoprotein levels may also indicate certain other fetal chromosomal defects or congenital malformations.

ALT: Alanine transaminase. The serum level of this enzyme is used as a measure of liver function. When liver cells are destroyed by disease or trauma, transaminases are released into the bloodstream. The higher the ALT, the greater the number of destroyed or damaged liver cells.

Alveoli: The numerous, small, saclike structures in the lungs where the exchange of oxygen and carbon dioxide between the lungs and blood takes place.

Amniocentesis: A procedure used to obtain amniotic fluid for tests to determine genetic makeup, health, or maturity of the fetus. Using ultrasound guidance, a needle is inserted through a pregnant woman's abdominal wall and into the uterus where a sample of amniotic fluid is withdrawn, usually at 16 to 20 weeks' gestation. If done earlier (11–13 weeks), there is often insufficient amniotic fluid and the complication rate is higher.

Amnioinfusion: Infusion of fluid into the amniotic cavity. Amnioinfusion may be done by either of the following procedures: after membranes have ruptured, by passing a catheter through the cervix and into the uterus and infusing physiologic (normal) saline solution or otherwise by infusing saline through an amniocentesis needle placed through the maternal abdominal wall and into the uterus. Amnioinfusion may be used to reduce cord compression (as indicated by variable fetal heart rate decelerations) during labor when oligohydramnios is present.

Amnion: The inner membrane surrounding the fetus. The amnion lines the chorion but is separate from it. Together these membranes contain the fetus and amniotic fluid.

Amniotic fluid: Fluid that surrounds the fetus and makes up the "water" in the "bag of waters." It provides a liquid environment in which the fetus can grow freely and serves as insulation, protecting the fetus from temperature changes. It also protects the fetus from a blow to the uterus by distributing equally in all directions any force applied to the uterus. Amniotic fluid is composed mainly of fetal urine, but also contains cells from the fetus's skin and chemical compounds from the fetus's respiratory passages.

Amniotic fluid analysis: Evaluation of various compounds in the amniotic fluid that relate to fetal lung maturity and fetal health. Fetal skin cells that normally float in the amniotic fluid may also be obtained with amniocentesis and grown in a culture to allow determination of fetal chromosomal status.

Amniotic fluid embolism: Amniotic fluid that escapes into the maternal circulation, usually late in labor or immediately postpartum. Rather than causing a mechanical blockage in the circulation as emboli of other origin might do, amniotic fluid embolism is thought to cause an anaphylactic-type response in susceptible women. This response is dramatic and severe, with sudden onset of hypoxia and hypotension. Seizures or cardiac arrest may occur. If a woman survives the initial phase, disseminated intravascular coagulation often follows. Although rare, it is associated with a high maternal mortality rate.

Analgesia: Relative relief of pain without loss of consciousness. Administration of specific medications is the most common way to provide analgesia.

Anemia: Abnormally low number of red blood cells. The red blood cells may be lost because of bleeding, destroyed because of disease process, or produced in insufficient numbers. Anemia is determined by measuring the hemoglobin or hematocrit.

Anencephaly: A lethal congenital defect of neural tube development in which there is partial or complete absence of the skull and brain.

Anesthesia: Total relief of pain, with or without loss of consciousness. Usually requires more invasive techniques than that required for analgesia. General inhalation anesthesia produces loss of consciousness, while major conduction anesthesia, such as spinal or epidural injection of long-lasting local anesthetics, produces total loss of pain in a specific area of the body without loss of consciousness.

Anomaly, congenital: Malformation resulting from abnormal development during embryonic or fetal growth. For example, a cleft lip is a congenital anomaly, as is gastroschisis, anencephaly, and countless others. Used synonymously with *congenital malformation.*

Antenatal: Period during pregnancy before birth. Synonymous with *prenatal.*

Antenatal testing: Techniques used to evaluate fetal growth and well-being prior to the onset of labor. Examples include nonstress test, biophysical profile, and ultrasonography.

Antepartum: Period of pregnancy before delivery. Most often used for period of pregnancy preceding the onset of labor. (*Intrapartum* is used to refer to the time during labor.) Used in reference to the woman.

Antibody: A type of blood protein produced by the body's lymph tissue in response to an antigen (a protein that is foreign to the bloodstream). Each specific antibody is formed as a defense mechanism against a specific antigen.

Antibody screening test: A test of maternal serum against a large variety of blood group antigens as a screening test for possible blood group incompatibility between a pregnant woman and her fetus. If the antibody screening test result is positive, the individual blood group incompatibility should be identified. *See also* Coombs test.

Antibody titers: A test used to indicate the relative concentration of a particular antibody present in a person's blood. *Example:* A high rubella titer indicates a person has been exposed to rubella (German measles) and formed a significant amount of antibody against the rubella virus and, therefore, will most likely be able to ward off another attack of the virus without becoming ill.

Anticonvulsants: Drugs given to prevent the occurrence of seizures (convulsions). The most common anticonvulsants used in infants are phenobarbital and phenytoin (Dilantin). Anticonvulsant therapy, with certain medications, for a pregnant woman with a seizure disorder may affect health of the fetus.

Antiphospholipid antibody syndrome (APS): Development of antibodies to naturally occurring phospholipids in the blood, causing abnormal phospholipid function. Antiphospholipid antibodies may be present in healthy women but are more commonly associated with a generalized disease (eg, lupus erythematosus). They have a strong association with recurrent miscarriage, fetal growth restriction, preeclampsia, and other factors adversely affecting fetal or maternal health.

Aorta: Main artery leaving the heart and feeding the systemic circulation. It passes through the chest and abdomen, where it branches into smaller arteries. In a newborn, an umbilical arterial catheter passes through one of the arteries in the umbilical cord and into the abdominal section of the aorta.

Apgar score: A score given to newborns and based on heart rate, respiratory effort, muscle tone, reflex irritability, and color. The score is given 1 minute after the baby's head and feet are delivered (not from the time the cord is cut) and again when the baby is 5 minutes of age. If the 5-minute score is less than 7, additional scores are given every 5 minutes for a total of 20 minutes. The 1-minute Apgar score indicates a baby's immediate condition; the 5-minute score reflects the baby's condition and effectiveness of resuscitative efforts. A low 5-minute score is a worrisome sign. It is not, however, a certain indicator of damage. Likewise, a high score is not a guarantee of a healthy baby. The score is named for Dr Virginia Apgar, who developed it. The 5 letters of her name may also be used to signify the 5 components of the score: A = appearance (color), P = pulse (heart rate), G = grimace (reflex irritability), A = activity (muscle tone), and R = respirations.

Apnea: Stoppage of breathing for 15 seconds or longer, or stoppage of breathing for less than 15 seconds if also accompanied by bradycardia or cyanosis.

Appropriate for gestational age (AGA): Refers to a baby whose weight is above the 10th percentile and below the 90th percentile for babies of that gestational age.

APS: *See* Antiphospholipid antibody syndrome.

Arrhythmia: Abnormal rhythm of the heartbeat. *Fetal* arrhythmias are rare. One of the more common ones is congenital heart block, which occurs almost exclusively with maternal systemic lupus erythematosus, although it is uncommon even in that situation. With a *maternal* arrhythmia, the more persistent the arrhythmia and farther the rate is from normal (either faster or slower), the more likely it is there will be a deleterious effect on maternal cardiac output and, thus, on blood flow to the uterus.

Artery: Any blood vessel that carries blood away from the heart.

Asphyxia: A condition resulting from inadequate oxygenation or blood flow and characterized by low blood oxygen concentration, high blood carbon dioxide concentration, metabolic acidosis, and organ injury.

Aspiration: (1) Breathing in or inhaling of a fluid (eg, formula, meconium, or amniotic fluid) into the lungs. Aspiration usually interferes with lung function and oxygenation. If inhaled, meconium is irritating as well as obstructing, resulting in meconium aspiration syndrome, which often causes serious and sometimes fatal lung disease. (2) Removal of fluids or gases from a cavity, such as the stomach, by suction. *Example:* A nasogastric tube is inserted and an empty syringe is attached to the tube and used to suck out or aspirate air and gastric juices from the stomach.

Assisted ventilation: Use of mechanical devices to help a person breathe. Bag and mask with bag breathing, endotracheal tube with bag breathing, or a respirator machine may each be used to assist ventilation.

AST: Aspartate transaminase. The serum level of this enzyme is used as a measure of liver function. As with alanine aminotransaminase, liver damage causes transaminases to be released into the bloodstream.

Atelectasis: Condition in which lung alveoli have collapsed and remain shut.

Atony: Loss of muscle tone or strength. Uterine atony is a leading cause of postpartum hemorrhage.

Axillary: Refers to the axilla, or armpit.

Bacteriuria: Presence of bacteria in the urine.

Bag breathing: Artificially breathing for a person by inflating the lungs with a resuscitation bag and mask or resuscitation bag and endotracheal tube.

Ballooning of lower uterine segment: A sign of impending labor, either term or preterm. The process leading to labor produces thinning of the lower uterine segment of myometrium, so that the lower segment "balloons out" into the anterior fornix of the vagina. The ballooned segment may be seen during speculum examination or palpated during digital examination.

BCG: Bacille Calmette-Guérin. Vaccine made from the Calmette-Guérin strain of *Mycobacterium bovis* for immunization against tuberculosis.

Beneficence: Acting for the benefit of a patient.

β-human chorionic gonadotropin (β-hCG): A hormone produced by trophoblastic cells of the chorionic villi. It is the first biochemical marker of pregnancy and produced in increasing amounts until maximal levels are reached at 8 to 10 weeks. When β-hCG is present in the blood or urine of a woman, she is pregnant. High titers are found with multifetal gestation and erythroblastosis fetalis; extremely high titers may be seen with hydatidiform mole and choriocarcinoma, while declining or low levels are found with spontaneous abortion and ectopic pregnancy.

Betamimetic: A drug that stimulates β-adrenergic receptors of smooth muscle, such as the myometrium (uterine muscle), causing decreased contractions. Used to suppress the onset of premature labor. A betamimetic drug is also called a *β-adrenergic receptor agonist*. An example is terbutaline.

Bilirubin: A substance produced from the breakdown of red blood cells. High blood bilirubin level causes the yellow coloring of the skin (and sclera) that is termed *jaundice*.

Biophysical profile (BPP): A combination of measures used to evaluate fetal well-being. Each of the 5 components (nonstress test, ultrasound evaluation of amniotic fluid volume, fetal body movements, muscle tone, and respirations) is scored. Each measure is given 2 points if present, zero if absent (there is no score of 1). The scores are added together for the final BPP score.

Biparietal diameter (BPD): Diameter of the skull, measured as the distance between the parietal bones, which lie just above each ear. Ultrasonography is used to determine BPD of the fetal skull. Serial BPD measurements are used to assess fetal growth and estimate fetal gestational age.

Bishop score: A system that scores cervical dilation, effacement, consistency, and position, as well as station of the presenting part to assess the "readiness" of a cervix for labor. Scores correlate with the likelihood that an attempt at induction of labor will be successful.

Blood gas measurement: Determination of the pH and concentration of oxygen, carbon dioxide, and bicarbonate in the blood.

Blood glucose screening test: Any of several commercially available, small, thin, plastic reagent strips designed to estimate blood glucose level with a single drop of blood. A color change caused by a drop of blood placed on the reagent pad provides an estimate of the blood glucose level. In addition, several handheld devices are designed to draw in a tiny amount of blood and give a digital readout of the glucose level.

Blood group: Numerous blood groups are in humans, each defined by their antigenic responses. The major blood groups are A, B, AB, and O, which are then further defined by their Rh type, positive or negative, as well as various other minor antigens. *Note:* Every person is exposed to the major blood group antigens (A and B) soon after birth, because the antigens are found in air, food, and water. Each person who lacks one or both of the major blood group genes (A or B) will make antibodies against the antigens they lack. Thus, persons with blood group O develop anti-A and anti-B antibodies and keep them throughout life. If given a blood transfusion with group A or B blood, a person with group O blood will have a transfusion reaction, which may in some cases be fatal. Similar reactions occur when a person with group B blood is given group A blood, or vice versa. Group "AB" persons do not make antibodies against either A or B because they have both antigens on their red blood cells. Persons with group AB blood can receive blood from people with any major blood group, but AB blood should be transfused only into persons with AB blood. Persons with group O blood should receive only blood transfusions with O blood, but O blood may be used to transfuse a person with any major blood group. This is why a person with AB blood is called a *universal recipient* and a person with O blood is called a *universal donor.*

Blood pressure, diastolic: Lowest point of the blood pressure between heartbeats, when the heart is relaxed.

Blood pressure, mean: The diastolic blood pressure plus one-third of the difference between the systolic and diastolic blood pressure.

Blood pressure, systolic: Highest point of the blood pressure. The blood pressure during the heartbeat, when the heart is contracted.

Blood smear: A thin layer of blood spread across a glass slide and studied under a microscope to determine the types of blood cells present.

Blood type: *See* Blood group.

Bloody show: Bloody mucus passed from the vagina in late pregnancy, usually associated with cervical effacement. It often heralds the onset of labor and is a normal finding. Any bleeding in pregnancy, however, should be investigated.

BPD: *See* Biparietal diameter.

BPP: *See* Biophysical profile.

Brachial plexus nerve injury: Paralysis of the arm that results from injury to the upper brachial plexus. Is associated with shoulder dystocia or a difficult breech delivery when traction is applied to the shoulder, stretching the nerve trunks exiting from the cervical spinal cord (brachial plexus). However, about one-half of these injuries occur in children in whom there was no evidence of either shoulder dystocia or breech delivery. The injury, therefore, may be initiated before birth by deformation of the neck and shoulder by abnormal positioning of the fetus. Many such palsies will recover within the first few years after birth.

Bracht maneuver: A method of delivering breech presentations in cases in which delivery is imminent and neither a practitioner skilled in vaginal breech delivery nor cesarean delivery is immediately available.

Bradycardia: Slow heart rate. (1) *Fetal:* Considered to be a baseline heart rate of less than 110 beats/min for 2 minutes or longer. Bradycardia alone may or may not indicate fetal distress. (2) *Neonatal:* Considered to be a sustained heart rate less than 100 beats/min.

Breech presentation: The feet- or buttocks-first presentation of a fetus. (1) *Frank:* Buttocks presenting, with the fetus's legs extended upward alongside the body. (2) *Footling:* One foot can be felt below the buttocks. (3) *Double footling:* Both feet can be felt below the buttocks. (4) *Complete:* Buttocks presenting, with the knees flexed.

Bronchopulmonary dysplasia (BPD): Also called *chronic lung disease*. A form of chronic lung disease sometimes seen in infants who have required ventilator therapy for any of a variety of lung problems, including respiratory distress syndrome and meconium aspiration syndrome. Bronchopulmonary dysplasia is thought to result from the combined effects of oxygen free-radical injury of premature lungs and trauma to the lungs produced by high airway pressures generated by ventilators.

Brow presentation: The brow (forehead) of the fetus is the presenting part. On vaginal examination, the anterior fontanel can be felt, but the posterior fontanel cannot. Management depends on whether the presentation stays brow or changes to face or the baby's neck flexes and the presentation becomes vertex.

Caput succedaneum: Edema of the fetal scalp that develops during labor. This swelling crosses suture lines of the skull. Caput succedaneum may occur with a normal, spontaneous vaginal delivery, but a lengthy labor or delivery by vacuum extraction increases the risk of occurrence.

Cardiac massage: *See* Chest compressions.

Cardiac output: Output of the left ventricle in milliliters per minute.

Central nervous system depression: Condition in which the body is less reactive than normal to stimuli, such as a pinprick. Central nervous system depression may be characterized by delayed reflexes, lethargy, or coma. It may result from a variety of causes, including certain drugs, certain metabolic disorders, or asphyxia.

Cephalhematoma: Also called *cephalohematoma*. Hematoma under the periosteum of the skull and limited to one cranial bone (does not cross suture lines) of the newborn. It is usually seen following prolonged labor and difficult delivery, but may also occur with uncomplicated birth. Delivery with forceps or vacuum extraction increases the risk of occurrence.

Cephalopelvic disproportion (CPD): *See* Fetopelvic disproportion.

Cerclage of the cervix: The procedure of placing a suture around the cervix to prevent it from dilating prematurely. There are several different techniques for placing the suture. Cervical cerclage is used as a treatment for incompetent cervix.

Cervix: The lower, narrow end of the uterus, which opens into the vagina.

Cesarean delivery: Surgical delivery of the fetus through an abdominal incision. The uterine incision may be classical (vertical, cutting through both the contractile and non-contractile segments) or confined to the non-contractile lower uterine segment (either vertical or transverse incision).

Chest compressions: Artificial pumping of blood through the heart by a bellows effect created from intermittent compression of the sternum, over the heart, during resuscitation.

Chickenpox: *See* Varicella-zoster virus.

Chlamydia: A type of microorganism with several species. Capable of producing a variety of illnesses, including eye infection, pneumonia, and infection of the genitourinary tract.

Choanal atresia: Congenital blockage of the nasal airway. Because babies breathe mainly through their noses, a baby with choanal atresia will have severe respiratory distress at birth. The immediate treatment is insertion of an oral airway. Surgical repair when the baby is stable is required for permanent correction.

Chorioamnionitis: Inflammation of the fetal membranes, also known as *intra-amniotic infection,* or IAI. The fetus may also become infected.

Chorion: Fetal membrane that surrounds the amnion, but is separate from it, and lies against the decidual lining of the uterine cavity (endometrium). During embryonic development, the chorion gives rise to the placenta.

Chorionic villus sampling (CVS): A highly specialized technique in which a tiny portion of the chorionic villi, which contain the same genetic material as the fetus, is obtained in a manner similar to a needle biopsy. The cells obtained may be analyzed for chromosomal defects. Chorionic villus sampling may be done as early as 10 weeks' gestation, with preliminary results available within as little as 2 days, allowing earlier and more rapid detection of chromosomal disorders than is possible with amniocentesis. The incidence of complications is similar to the risks associated with amniocentesis.

Chromosome: The material (DNA protein) in each body cell that contains the genes, or information regarding hereditary factors. Each normal cell contains 46 chromosomes. Each chromosome contains numerous genes. A baby acquires one-half of chromosomes from the mother and one-half from the father. A chromosomal defect results from an abnormal number of chromosomes or structural damage to the chromosomes. *Example:* Each cell in the body of a baby with Down syndrome (trisomy 21) contains 47 instead of 46 chromosomes.

Chronic lung disease (CLD): *See* Bronchopulmonary dysplasia.

Circulatory system: The system that carries blood through the body and consists of the heart and blood vessels. The systemic circulatory system carries blood to and from the head, arms, legs, trunk, and all body organs except the lungs. The pulmonary circulatory system carries blood to the lungs, where carbon dioxide is released and oxygen is collected, and returns the oxygenated blood to the systemic circulatory system.

Cirrhosis: Chronic degeneration of the hepatic cells, replacing them with fibrosis and nodular tissue and resulting in liver failure. Chronic hepatitis and alcoholism are common causes.

CLD: Chronic lung disease. *See* Bronchopulmonary dysplasia.

CMV: *See* Cytomegalovirus.

Coagulation: The process of blood clot formation.

Colon: The large intestine, which is between the small intestine and rectum.

Colonization: Persistent, asymptomatic presence of bacteria in a particular area of the body. If symptoms develop, it becomes an infection. *Example:* Many women have vaginal or rectal colonization with group B β-hemolytic streptococci but are entirely without symptoms, although maternal group B β-hemolytic streptococci colonization poses a risk for life-threatening neonatal infection.

Compliance (of lung): Refers to elastic properties of the lungs. Babies with certain lung diseases have decreased compliance (stiff lungs) and thus cannot expand their lungs well during inhalation.

Comprehensive ultrasound: Detailed ultrasound examination designed to review all parts of fetal anatomy. Done when congenital malformations are suspected.

Condyloma: Warty growth of skin in the genital area caused by human papillomavirus.

Congenital: Refers to conditions that are present at birth, regardless of cause. Congenital defects may result from a variety of causes, including genetic factors, chromosomal factors, diseases affecting the pregnant woman, and drugs taken by the woman. The cause, however, of most congenital defects is unknown. *Note: Congenital* and *hereditary* are not synonymous. *Congenital* means present at birth. *Hereditary* means the genetic transmission from parent to child of a particular trait, which may be the trait for a specific inheritable disease and associated malformations. Some defects are congenital and hereditary, but many are simply congenital with no genetic link.

Congenital rubella syndrome: A group of congenital anomalies resulting from an intrauterine rubella infection. Anomalies commonly include cataracts, heart defects, deafness, microcephaly (abnormally small head), and intellectual disability.

Congestive heart failure: A condition that develops when the heart cannot pump as much blood as it receives. As a result, fluid backs up into the lungs and other tissues, causing edema and respiratory distress. Congestive heart failure may result from a diseased or malformed heart, severe lung disease, or too much fluid given to the patient.

Conjugation of bilirubin: Process that occurs in the liver and combines bilirubin with another chemical so it may be removed from the blood and pass out of the body in the feces. Failure of bilirubin conjugation is one cause of jaundice.

Conjunctivitis: Inflammation of the membrane that covers the eye and lines the eyelids. Certain genital tract infections, particularly *Chlamydia* and gonorrhea, in a pregnant woman can cause severe conjunctivitis and eye damage in a newborn, unless proper neonatal treatment is given.

Continuous positive airway pressure (CPAP): A steady pressure delivered to the lungs by means of a special apparatus or mechanical ventilator. Continuous positive airway pressure may be used for babies with respiratory distress syndrome to prevent alveoli from collapsing during expiration.

Contraction stress test (CST): Termed *oxytocin challenge test* when oxytocin is used to induce contractions. A brief period of uterine contractions (either spontaneous or induced with nipple stimulation or intravenous oxytocin administration) during which the fetal heart rate and uterine contractions are monitored with an external monitor. It is a test used in certain high-risk pregnancies to assess fetal well-being.

Coombs test: Test to determine the presence of antibodies in blood or on red blood cells. There are 2 forms of the test. The direct Coombs test detects antibodies attached to the red blood cells; the indirect Coombs test detects antibodies within the serum. *Example:* The direct test is used to detect antibodies present on the red blood cells of Rh-positive babies born to Rh-negative sensitized women. The indirect test is used on a woman's blood to detect antibodies to fetal Rh-positive cells. *See also* Antibody screening test.

Cord presentation: Also referred to as *funic presentation.* A situation in which the umbilical cord lies against the membranes over the cervix, beneath the fetal presenting part. This poses a risk for cord injury or prolapse when the membranes rupture.

Cordocentesis: *See* Percutaneous umbilical blood sampling.

Corticosteroids: Refers to any of the steroids of the adrenal cortex. Betamethasone and dexamethasone are artificially prepared steroids that may be given to a woman to speed up the process of lung maturation in her fetus when preterm delivery is unavoidable.

COVID-19: Coronavirus disease 2019, the clinical illness caused by infection with SARS-CoV-2 (severe acute respiratory syndrome coronavirus 2), a novel coronavirus that caused a global pandemic beginning in late 2019.

CPAP: *See* Continuous positive airway pressure.

CPD: Cephalopelvic disproportion. *See* Fetopelvic disproportion.

Creatinine: A chemical in the blood excreted in urine and used as an indication of renal function.

Cryoprecipitate: A concentrated form of plasma. In a much smaller volume, it contains fibrinogen, coagulation factor VIII, and some, but not all, of the other coagulation factors found in fresh frozen plasma. Used in the treatment of severe disseminated intravascular coagulation.

CST: *See* Contraction stress test.

CVS: *See* Chorionic villus sampling.

Cyanosis: Bluish coloration of the skin. (1) *Central cyanosis:* Bluish coloration of the skin and mucous membranes due to inadequate arterial blood oxygen concentration. Sometimes babies with central cyanosis are described as appearing dusky. (2) *Acrocyanosis:* Cyanosis of the hands and feet only, which is generally not associated with low blood oxygen concentration.

Cytomegalic inclusion disease: An infection with cytomegalovirus. Maternal infection may go unnoticed, but fetal infection, especially early in gestation, can damage every organ system. The disease commonly causes an enlarged liver and spleen, encephalitis, microcephaly, intracranial calcification, and visual or hearing defects.

Cytomegalovirus (CMV): The virus that causes cytomegalic inclusion disease.

Debridement: Removal of dead tissue and foreign matter from a wound.

Deceleration: *See* Fetal heart rate deceleration.

Decidua: Endometrium that has been modified by the hormonal effects of pregnancy; the endometrium during pregnancy.

Deflexed head: The fetal head is not round. It is longer from front to back (occipitomental diameter is approximately 13.5 cm at term) than it is from side to side (biparietal diameter is approximately 9.5 cm at term). When the fetal head is well flexed with the chin on the chest, the top of the head, with a maximum diameter of 9.5 to 10 cm, is presented to the pelvis. In most cases, the pelvis is larger than this, allowing the head (largest part of the fetus) to pass through it. When the head is deflexed, as it is in brow and face presentations, the farther the chin is from the chest, the larger the diameter is presented to the pelvis. These presentations make vaginal delivery difficult or impossible without risk of serious damage to the fetus or woman.

Deformation: Structural defect of a fetus caused by mechanical force, rather than abnormal embryonic development or an inherited disease. External factors, such as uterine fibroids or amniotic bands, may produce a deformity by compressing parts of the fetus. Prolonged oligohydramnios can also cause deformities, due to lack of the amniotic fluid cushion normally provided to a growing fetus. Sometimes these deformities, such as an angulated spine or flattened head, resolve spontaneously over time. In other cases, cosmetic surgery will be needed for correction. Malformation and deformation are not synonymous. *Malformation* is the term used when a congenital anomaly is due to *abnormal development* of the fetus. *Deformation* is the term used when a congenital anomaly is due to *external mechanical force* applied to a growing fetus.

Dehiscence: Separation of an incision that had been surgically united. The separation may be partial, involving only the outer layer, or complete through all tissue layers. In perinatal care, this term is most commonly applied to the postoperative separation of an abdominal incision or development of an opening in a uterine scar from a previous cesarean delivery.

Diabetes, gestational: Also called *glucose intolerance of pregnancy* or *gestational diabetes mellitus.* Disturbance of glucose metabolism that mimics diabetes mellitus and first appears during pregnancy and, in many cases, disappears after delivery. Women with this condition are more likely than the general population, however, to develop insulin-dependent diabetes later in life. Because normal control of blood glucose during pregnancy is important for fetal well-being, and because this metabolic problem is fairly common, screening tests for abnormal glucose tolerance are recommended for every prenatal patient.

Diabetes mellitus: A metabolic disorder in which the body's ability to use glucose is impaired because of a disturbance in normal production of or response to insulin. This leads to high blood glucose levels and other metabolic imbalances. Diabetes mellitus during pregnancy places the woman and fetus at risk for certain serious problems and may affect health of the newborn.

Diaphragm: The primary muscle of breathing that separates the chest cavity from the abdominal cavity.

Diaphragmatic hernia: A defect in the diaphragm through which abdominal organs slip and enter the chest, where they compress the lungs. If abdominal organs enter the chest cavity early in gestation, development of one or both of the lungs can be severely inhibited.

DIC: *See* Disseminated intravascular coagulation.

Digital examination: Examination of the cervix and, during labor, the presenting part of the fetus, with a gloved hand inserted in the vagina (examination is done using your fingers, or digits), as opposed to a speculum examination to view the cervix.

Digitalis: A drug that increases the contraction force of the heart while at the same time decreasing the rate at which the heart beats. Sometimes used to treat congestive heart failure.

Dilation: The condition of being stretched beyond normal dimensions. In perinatal care this most commonly refers to the degree of opening in the cervical os.

Dipstick: Thin, narrow paper or plastic strip (or "stick") with chemical reagents that change color in the presence of certain conditions in the liquid being tested. Different types of dipstick test for different substances, and some dipsticks have several reagent patches to test for several substances on the same stick. Dipsticks are used to test body fluids, such as vaginal secretions, gastric aspirate, and urine. Examples of their use in perinatal care include testing vaginal secretions for pH to help identify rupture of the membranes and urine for protein in women with hypertension.

Disseminated intravascular coagulation (DIC): An acquired disturbance of the body's blood coagulation processes in which coagulation factors are consumed, leaving the blood incapable of coagulating. Certain serious illnesses may trigger the onset of DIC in neonates or adults. Most commonly in neonates, DIC may accompany severe sepsis, hypoxia, acidosis, or hypotension. In pregnant women, DIC may accompany placental abruption, retained dead fetus syndrome, or sepsis. Blood platelets and coagulation factors are activated abnormally by the release of thromboplastic substances into the circulation. As a result, numerous fibrin clots are formed in the capillaries. Red blood cells may be broken down as blood flow pushes the cells through the clogged capillaries, which may lead to hemolytic anemia. In addition, oozing from puncture sites, surgical incisions or other wounds, and easy bruising may occur as the platelets and coagulation factors are consumed by the fibrin clots and are no longer available to maintain normal blood coagulation. Neonates with DIC, especially preterm babies, are also at risk for pulmonary or intracranial hemorrhage. Treatment, which is complex, is directed at correcting the underlying disease process and providing emergency management to correct the coagulation deficit.

Diuretics: Drugs (eg, furosemide, thiazides, spironolactone) given to prevent or decrease fluid buildup in the lungs and body by increasing urine output.

DNA testing: Also called *genetic testing*. Samples of tissues (eg, blood, urine, skin) are treated, using a highly technical process, to extract the DNA of chromosomes (and mitochondria). Tests can then reveal defective genes that cause specific diseases. Most disease-causing genes, however, have not yet been identified.

Dolichocephalic: Long headed; typically refers to the elongated head of a fetus in breech position when ultrasonography is used to measure the fetal skull biparietal diameter. This head shape reduces the accuracy of biparietal diameter measurements.

Doppler instrument: A device used to detect changes of blood flow through a blood vessel. A Doppler instrument may be used to detect fetal heartbeats.

Double setup: A vaginal examination performed in an operating room, with everything in readiness for either a vaginal or cesarean delivery. Used in cases of suspected placenta previa during labor, in which the examination itself may trigger such profuse hemorrhage that immediate surgery is required.

Down syndrome: Also called *trisomy 21*. A chromosomal abnormality resulting in a typical facial appearance, intellectual disability, and sometimes other congenital defects, particularly cardiac defects. Individuals with Down syndrome have 47 instead of the normal 46 chromosomes, with one additional copy of chromosome 21 in each cell.

Ductus arteriosus: A blood vessel in the fetus that connects the pulmonary artery and aorta. This allows less blood to go to the fetal lungs and more blood to go to the systemic and placental circulation. Normally this vessel closes shortly after birth, thus redirecting blood flow to the lungs. A *patent ductus arteriosus* means the ductus arteriosus persistently remains open after birth. As a result, and with changes in pressure that occur within the circulatory system once placental circulation is eliminated, blood may flow from the aorta into the pulmonary artery, resulting in too much blood directed to the lungs. This may cause congestive heart failure in the baby.

Dusky: *See* Cyanosis.

Dye test: In perinatal care, this usually refers to a test done to determine if the amniotic membranes are ruptured. There is no indication for a dye test unless there is reason to suspect that rupture of membranes has occurred, other tests are negative, *and* the diagnosis of ruptured membranes will affect clinical management. Amniocentesis is done under ultrasound guidance. If indicated, a sample of amniotic fluid is withdrawn for testing. A dye, usually indigo carmine, is then introduced through the amniocentesis needle. A sterile gauze pad (4 × 4 in) is placed high in the woman's vagina. If no dye appears on the pad after 20 to 30 minutes of sitting or walking, it is most likely that the membranes are intact and have not ruptured.

Dyspnea: Difficult breathing, labored. This may accompany any variety of disease states or be a result of physical exertion in a healthy person.

Dystocia: Difficult labor. (1) *Uterine:* Abnormal labor, particularly prolonged. Used to refer to weak or ineffective uterine contractions. Usually used to describe a labor that has ceased progressing such that a cesarean delivery is necessary. (2) *Shoulder:* Situation in which the shoulders of a baby in vertex presentation become trapped after delivery of the head. This is an emergency, requiring immediate intervention to avoid severe fetal hypoxia.

ECG: *See* electrocardiograph.

Eclampsia: Term used to describe the condition in which convulsions or coma develop in a pregnant or postpartum woman with pregnancy-related hypertension. The condition of preeclampsia becomes eclampsia whenever seizures or coma develop.

EDD: Estimated date of delivery. *See* Pregnancy due date.

Edema: Swelling due to an excessive amount of fluid in the tissues.

Effacement: The process of thinning of the cervix prior to and after the onset of labor.

Electrocardiograph: Also called *electrocardiogram, electronic cardiac monitor*. A device used for recording the heart's electrical activity.

Electrolyte: A substance that dissociates into ions when in solution (and thereby makes the solution capable of conducting electricity). Commonly refers to sodium, potassium, chloride, and bicarbonate in blood.

Embolus: A blood clot or other plug (eg, an air bubble) carried by the blood from a larger to smaller blood vessel, where it lodges and obstructs the blood flow. Plural: emboli.

Embryo: Term used for the product of conception, from the time a fertilized egg is implanted until all major structures and organs are defined. In humans, this is the first 8 weeks of development after conception (10 weeks after the last menstrual period). After 8 weeks and until birth, the term *fetus* is used.

Endocrine system: Refers to organs that release hormones into the blood.

Endometritis: Infection of inner lining of the uterine cavity, the endometrium.

Engagement, engaged: Term applied during late pregnancy or in labor that indicates that the largest diameter of the presenting part is at or below the smallest diameter of the pelvis. Usually the presenting part is the fetal head, which is said to be engaged when a vaginal examination reveals the head to be at or below the ischial spines.

Environmental oxygen: *See* Inspired oxygen.

Epidural: A technique for providing anesthesia during labor. A hollow needle is inserted between 2 vertebrae in the woman's spine, and a catheter is threaded through the needle and into the epidural space of the spinal column. A local anesthetic is then injected through the catheter into the epidural space. This eliminates all sensation for the nerve roots that the drug contacts. The greater the volume of anesthetic medication injected, the greater the number of nerve roots affected and, therefore, the larger the area of body that is anesthetized. By anesthetizing only some of the spinal nerve roots, epidural anesthesia provides pain relief during labor but, at the same time, may also permit walking. As with spinal anesthesia, the anesthetic medication also blocks the sympathetic nerves leaving the spinal cord. Because of this, blood pressure of the woman may decline and requires careful monitoring. (For this reason, a loading dose of 500–1,000 mL of physiologic [normal] saline solution may be given intravenously prior to introduction of the anesthetic.)

Epigastric: Area immediately below the tip of the sternum in the center of the upper abdomen. Pain felt here is usually related to liver or gallbladder disease. Of most importance in pregnant women with preeclampsia, the onset of epigastric pain indicates swelling of the liver capsule. This often precedes the onset of the first convulsion of eclampsia.

Epiglottis: The flap of cartilage that overlies the larynx. The epiglottis is open during breathing and closes over the larynx during swallowing to prevent food from entering the trachea.

Epinephrine: A natural body hormone that is released by adrenal glands into the blood during stress. It may also be used as a drug during resuscitation to constrict blood vessels and increase blood pressure, and to increase heart rate and volume of blood pumped.

Erb palsy: The most common form of brachial plexus nerve injury in newborns.

Erythema: Redness of the skin produced by dilation of the smallest blood vessels. *Example:* The redness that occurs around an infected wound.

Erythroblastosis fetalis: Hemolytic anemia resulting from the passage of antibodies between the pregnant woman and the fetus across the placenta during pregnancy. Red blood cell alloantibodies may develop in a woman when fetal red blood cells enter the maternal circulation during a prior pregnancy (most commonly at the time of delivery), or as a result of a blood transfusion (less common). The placenta transfers immunoglobulin G antibodies from mother to fetus during pregnancy. If the fetal red blood cells exhibit the specific antigen to which the mother has an alloantibody, the interaction between the antibody and antigen leads to breakdown (hemolysis) of the fetal red blood cells. As the fetal blood-forming organs produce red blood cells more rapidly than normal to replace those undergoing hemolysis, immature fetal red blood cells (erythroblasts) are released into the fetal circulation. The consequences of untreated fetal hemolytic anemia can include fetal hydrops and stillbirth.

Esophagus: The muscular tube that connects the throat and stomach.

Etiology: The cause of anything. *Example:* Sepsis may be the etiology of hyperbilirubinemia in a newborn.

Exchange transfusion: Process during which a baby's blood is removed and replaced with donor blood so that when the exchange transfusion is completed, most of the baby's blood has been replaced by donor blood. Most often, exchange transfusions are used as a treatment for severe hyperbilirubinemia.

Expiration: (1) Period during the breathing cycle when the person is breathing out or exhaling. (2) The end of a period of usefulness, validity, or effectiveness, such as the expiration date for a product or medication, after which time the item should not be used. (3) Death.

Face presentation: The face is the presenting part. The chin (mentum) is the reference point, and it may rotate either anteriorly (mentum anterior), in which case vaginal delivery is likely if the pelvis is normal in size, or posteriorly. When the chin rotates posteriorly into the hollow of the sacrum (mentum posterior), vaginal delivery is impossible unless the forces of labor or use of obstetric forceps are successful in rotating the chin to the anterior position. Cesarean delivery is usually performed for mentum posterior position.

FAD: *See* Fetal activity determination.

FAE: *See* Fetal alcohol effects.

Familial: Used to describe a disease or defect that affects more members of a family than would be expected by chance.

FAS: *See* Fetal alcohol syndrome.

Fat, brown: Fat tissue that has a rich blood and nerve supply. Babies have proportionally more brown fat than do adults and metabolize or "burn" it as their main source of heat production, while adults produce heat mainly by shivering. Extra oxygen and calories are used when brown fat is metabolized.

Fat, white: Type of fat that has few blood vessels and appears whitish. It is used mainly for insulation and as a reserve supply of energy and is not nearly as metabolically active as brown fat.

Fatty acids: Substances resulting from the breakdown of fat. Fatty acids decrease binding of bilirubin to albumin, thus increasing the chance of brain damage from hyperbilirubinemia.

Femoral pulse: Pulse felt in the groin, over the femoral artery.

Fern test: A test for amniotic fluid in the vagina, used when rupture of membranes is suspected. When there is a pool of fluid in the vagina, a drop of it is smeared on a glass slide and allowed to dry in the air. Salt content of the amniotic fluid will dry in a typical pattern, resembling a fern, while other fluids (eg, urine) will not. If a fern pattern is seen, the membranes are ruptured.

Fetal activity determination (FAD): A noninvasive means to monitor fetal well-being that may be used by either low- or high-risk pregnant women. Approximately 80% of gross fetal movements observed on ultrasound are felt by the pregnant woman. Beginning at approximately 28 weeks' gestation, a pregnant woman records fetal activity daily according to one of several accepted protocols. Any significant decrease in activity warrants prompt (the same day) investigation of fetal condition.

Fetal alcohol effects (FAE): The effects of maternal alcohol ingestion during pregnancy may be seen in a baby without the baby having all the findings typical of fetal alcohol syndrome.

Fetal alcohol syndrome (FAS): Constellation of findings, including intellectual disability, that may occur in fetuses of women who ingest alcohol during pregnancy, especially early in gestation.

Fetal echocardiogram: An ultrasonographic technique that shows movements of the walls and valves of the beating heart of a fetus. Certain valvular and other abnormalities of the fetal heart may be seen. Used only when there is some reason to suspect that the fetus may have an abnormal heart.

Fetal heart rate, baseline: Approximate average fetal heart rate during any 10-minute period that is free of accelerations, decelerations, and marked variability (>25 beats/min). The reference baseline range is between 110 and 160 beats/min.

Fetal heart rate acceleration: Abrupt increase (at least 15 beats/min) in fetal heart rate (onset to peak rate occurs in <30 seconds) that lasts at least 15 seconds but less than 2 minutes.

Fetal heart rate deceleration: A decrease in the fetal heart rate that then returns to baseline. There are 3 types of decelerations (early, late, and variable), which are defined by their shape and relationship to uterine contractions.

Fetal heart rate variability: Fluctuations in baseline fetal heart rate that are irregular in amplitude and frequency. Visual inspection is used to classify the peak-to-trough beats per minute difference as absent (no detectable change from baseline), minimal (fluctuation of ≤5 beats/min), moderate (fluctuation of 6–25 beats/min), or marked (fluctuation of ≥25 beats/min).

Fetal lung maturity: Analysis of a sample of amniotic fluid for the presence of surfactant components. The lecithin to sphingomyelin ratio is one such test. *See also* Pulmonary maturity.

Fetal membranes: The amnion and chorion.

Fetal monitoring, external: Refers to continuous electronic monitoring using a device strapped to the woman's abdomen to detect the fetal heart rate, periodic rate changes, and timing of the uterine contractions.

Fetal monitoring, internal: Refers to continuous electronic monitoring using a wire attached to the fetal presenting part to detect fetal heart rate and a pressure transducer placed inside the uterus to detect onset and intensity of uterine contractions.

Fetal pole: A term used to describe the appearance of either end of the fetal body when the fetus is so small the head cannot be distinguished from the breech.

Fetopelvic disproportion (FPD): Condition in which the internal size of the maternal pelvis is too small or the fetal head is too large to allow vaginal delivery. Because exact measurements of the fetal head and maternal pelvis cannot be made, this is a relative term.

Fetoscope: A specially constructed stethoscope used to listen to fetal heart rate.

Fetus: After development of organ systems (after the first 8 weeks from conception/10 weeks from the last menstrual period), an embryo is called a *fetus* until delivery.

F_{IO_2}: Fractional inspired oxygen. The percentage of oxygen being inhaled. An environmental oxygen concentration of 55% may also be written $F_{IO_2} = 55\%$. The F_{IO_2} of room air is 21%.

Flaccid: Limp.

Flexion: Bending of a body part. *Example:* Flexion of the arm occurs when the elbow is bent. By contrast, *extension* means the straightening of a body part.

Flip-flop phenomenon: Flip flop is caused by lowering the environmental oxygen concentration too rapidly, or allowing a baby requiring oxygen therapy to breathe room air for even a short period. In response, the arteries to the lungs constrict, thus limiting the amount of blood that can be oxygenated in the lungs. The baby then requires an environmental oxygen concentration even higher than that breathed previously to achieve the same arterial blood oxygen concentration.

Foramen ovale: The opening between the 2 upper chambers (atria) of the heart in the fetus. It consists of redundant tissue in the interatrial wall that results in a functional closure of the opening when left atrial pressure exceeds right atrial pressure shortly after birth.

Forceps: Obstetric forceps are 2 metal instruments, made in mirror image of each other, curved laterally to follow the shape of the fetal head and vertically to fit the curve of the maternal pelvis. Used to assist vaginal delivery of the fetal head and shorten the second stage of labor, for either maternal or fetal reasons. They are made in a variety of sizes and shapes, including forceps designed to help deliver the after-coming head in breech presentations. When forceps are used, the delivery is classified as *midforceps, low forceps,* or *outlet forceps,* depending on fetal station and position when the forceps are applied.

FPD: *See* Fetopelvic disproportion.

Fundal height: During pregnancy, the fundus of the uterus can be felt higher and higher in the maternal abdomen. The distance between the fundus and symphysis pubis (front pelvic bone) is the fundal height. It is used as an estimate of gestational age of the fetus. Consistency in the technique used (preferably by the same examiner) throughout pregnancy is important for accurate results.

Fundus: The broad top two-thirds of the uterus.

Gastroschisis: A defect of the abdominal wall during embryonic development, allowing abdominal organs to protrude into amniotic fluid. As opposed to omphalocele, no peritoneal sac covers the organs with gastroschisis.

GBS: *See* Group B β-hemolytic streptococcus.

GDM: Gestational diabetes mellitus. *See* Diabetes, gestational.

General inhalation anesthesia: An anesthetic technique that produces loss of consciousness. The patient is usually given barbiturates or narcotics to induce anesthesia, followed by paralyzing drugs, endotracheal intubation, and artificial ventilation. Anesthetic gases are used to continue the anesthetic state until the surgical procedure is completed. Because the gases are quickly cleared from the blood by the lungs, the patient "wakes up" within a few minutes after the anesthetic gases are stopped. With this type of anesthesia, the drugs and gases used can cross the placenta and may depress a fetus. Anesthesia provided to an obstetric patient must consider the unique physiological state of a pregnant woman as well as the potential effect drugs given to her may have on the fetus.

Geneticist: A physician who specializes in knowing how genes are inherited by children from their parents and the association between certain genetic abnormalities and specific physical characteristics.

Genitourinary tract: Pertaining to the reproductive organs and urinary organs.

Gestational diabetes mellitus (GDM): *See* Diabetes, gestational.

Glottis: The vocal cords and opening between them that leads to the trachea.

Glucose tolerance test (GTT): A test for abnormal glucose metabolism. A fasting patient is given a standard dose of glucose orally, with the blood level of glucose determined at standard intervals.

Glycogen: Main storage form of glucose in the body. It is changed to glucose and released to the bloodstream as needed.

Glycosylated hemoglobin (hemoglobin A_{1C}): Reflects circulating blood glucose for the previous 3 months. It is used as an indicator of long-term glucose control.

Gonorrheal ophthalmia, neonatal: Eye infection in newborns that results from gonorrhea bacteria acquired by a baby during the birth process, if the woman has gonorrhea. Silver nitrate drops or erythromycin ointment placed in the baby's eyes shortly after delivery prevents the development of this potentially damaging infection.

Gram stain: A specific stain for bacteria that separates gram-positive bacteria (which stain blue) from gram-negative bacteria (which stain red). These 2 categories of bacteria vary in the types of disease they cause and their antibiotic sensitivity. Gram stain of an infected body fluid (eg, urine, pus, amniotic fluid) may identify the type of organism causing the infection and
allow appropriate antibiotic therapy to begin before culture and sensitivity studies can be completed.

Gravidity: Number of pregnancies a woman has had, regardless of pregnancy outcome. With her first pregnancy, a woman is a *primigravida*. With her second pregnancy, a woman is, technically, a *secundigravida*, and with her third or subsequent pregnancies, a *multigravida*. In practice, however, *secundigravida* is rarely used and *multigravida* is used to refer to any woman with her second, or subsequent, pregnancy. *See also* Parity.

Group B β-hemolytic streptococcus (GBS): A type of streptococcal bacteria that can cause serious or fatal neonatal illness. Some women, without evidence of infection, have chronic GBS vaginal or rectal colonization, which may infect the fetus before delivery or the baby at the time of delivery.

Growth restriction: Describes fetuses that, on serial examination, are significantly smaller than would be expected, with their growth falling below the 10th percentile for their gestational age.

Grunting: A sign of respiratory distress in a neonate. The grunt or whine occurs during expiration as a result of the baby exhaling against a partially closed glottis. The baby grunts in an attempt to trap air in the lungs and hold open the alveoli. Grunting sometimes may be normal immediately following birth; after 1 to 2 hours it is always abnormal.

GTT: *See* Glucose tolerance test.

HBIG: Hepatitis B immune globulin. Administration of HBIG soon after delivery is part of the treatment for newborns whose mothers are hepatitis B surface antigen–positive (test for hepatitis B).

HBsAg: *See* Hepatitis B surface antigen.

HCT: *See* Hematocrit.

Heart murmur, functional: A heart murmur that does not result from disease or an abnormality of the heart. A functional heart murmur is *not* associated with abnormal functioning of the heart.

HELLP syndrome: Hemolysis, elevated liver enzymes, low platelet count occurring in association with preeclampsia. An uncommon and severe form of pregnancy-related hypertension.

Hematocrit (Hct): A blood test showing the percentage of red blood cells in whole blood. *Example:* An Hct of 40 means that 40% of the blood is red blood cells and 60% is plasma and other cells.

Hemoglobin (Hgb): (1) Blood test showing the concentration of Hgb in blood. (2) Oxygen-carrying part of red blood cells.

Hemoglobinopathy: A genetic disorder that causes a change in the molecular structure of hemoglobin in the red blood cells and results in certain typical laboratory and clinical changes, frequently including anemia. Sickle cell disease is one type of hemoglobinopathy.

Hemolysis: Breakdown of red blood cells. Hemolytic anemia, therefore, is anemia that results from the destruction of red blood cells, rather than loss of blood or inadequate production of red blood cells.

Hemorrhage: Bleeding; most often used to indicate severe bleeding.

Heparin lock: A technique used to prevent blood clot formation in an arterial or venous catheter, when a continuous infusion of fluids is not being used. A solution of intravenous fluids with a specific concentration of heparin is flushed through the catheter and then the stopcock is closed to the catheter.

Hepatitis: Serious inflammation of the liver usually caused by a viral infection. There are several forms of hepatitis, depending on the specific causative agent and mode of transmission. Infection may be acute or chronic.

Hepatitis B surface antigen (HBsAg): Term for protein on the surface of the hepatitis B virus. Screening all prenatal patients for this antigen identifies women who are carriers for hepatitis B, and therefore at risk for passing the virus to their fetuses before birth. Such newborns should be given hepatitis B immune globulin and hepatitis B vaccine soon after birth.

Hepatosplenomegaly: Enlargement of the liver and spleen.

Hereditary: Used to describe a condition that is transmitted by the genes, from parents to their children. *Example:* Cystic fibrosis is a hereditary disease, and eye color is a hereditary trait.

Heredity: Genetic transmission from parent to child of traits and characteristics. *Example:* A baby with brown eyes can be said to have that color of eyes as part of his or her heredity.

Herpes: Refers to diseases caused by herpesvirus. Maternal herpes may have serious consequences for the newborn.

Hgb: *See* Hemoglobin.

HIE: *See* Hypoxic-ischemic encephalopathy.

HIV: The virus that causes AIDS, which attacks and eventually overcomes the body's immune system.

HPV: Human papillomavirus.

Hyaline membrane disease: Older name for *neonatal respiratory distress syndrome*.

Hydatidiform mole: A pregnancy characterized by grossly abnormal development of the chorionic villi, which eventually form a mass of cysts. Usually, but not always, no fetus is present. Excessive secretion from the trophoblast cells leads to very high levels of β-human chorionic gonadotropin. Vaginal bleeding during the first trimester is common and may be the presenting sign. Uterine size does not usually correspond to expected size for the dates of a pregnancy: larger than expected in about 50% of cases and smaller than expected in about 30% of cases.

Hydramnios: Also called *polyhydramnios*. Abnormally large amount of amniotic fluid. It may be associated with fetal abnormalities (particularly gastrointestinal tract abnormalities that prevent amniotic fluid from being swallowed into the gastrointestinal tract of the fetus) or certain maternal medical illnesses; however, in most cases, the cause of hydramnios is unknown.

Hydrocephalus: Enlargement of the head due to abnormally large collection of cerebrospinal fluid in the brain. It may be congenital or acquired after birth. Accumulation of cerebrospinal fluid may be caused by a blockage in the normal flow of fluid around the brain and spinal cord or by a decrease in the normal absorption of the fluid.

Hydrops fetalis: Edema in the entire body of a fetus, accompanied by at least one effusion in a body cavity (pleural, pericardial, or peritoneal). Usually a result of severe hemolytic anemia caused by Rh disease or other alloimmunizations, but may (rarely) be caused by certain other serious in utero conditions or viral infections. In many cases the cause for hydrops is not clear.

Hyperbilirubinemia: Excess amount of bilirubin in the blood.

Hyperbilirubinemia, physiological: Hyperbilirubinemia due to a baby's immature liver, which has a limited ability to excrete bilirubin from the body, rather than hyperbilirubinemia due to a disease process such as ABO incompatibility.

Hyperkalemia: High blood potassium level.

Hypernatremia: High blood sodium level.

Hyperosmolar: Used to describe a liquid with a higher concentration of particles than found in a physiological fluid. For example, an intravenous solution may be hyperosmolar compared to blood, or formula may be hyperosmolar compared to human (breast) milk.

Hypertension: High blood pressure. In adults, generally defined as higher than 130/80 mm Hg.

Hyperthermia: High body temperature; fever. In adults, generally defined as greater than or equal to 38.0°C (100.4°F).

Hypertonic: Used to describe a solution that is more concentrated than body fluid and therefore will draw water out of the body's cells, causing the cells to shrink.

Hypocalcemia: Low blood calcium level.

Hypoglycemia: Low blood glucose level.

Hypotension: Low blood pressure.

Hypothermia: Low body temperature.

Hypovolemia: Low blood volume.

Hypoxemia: Low concentration of oxygen in the arterial blood.

Hypoxia: A deficiency of oxygen and perfusion in the body tissues resulting in compromised metabolism and injured tissue.

Hypoxic-ischemic encephalopathy (HIE): Neonatal brain injury that presents at birth and is caused by a newborn experiencing a hypoxic and/or ischemic event around the time of delivery.

IAI: *See* Intra-amniotic infection.

Icterus: *See* Jaundice.

Ileitis: Inflammation of the ileum, the distal portion of the small bowel (between the jejunum and cecum). Usually represents Crohn disease, a chronic inflammation of the intestinal tract, most often affecting the terminal ileum (may also involve the colon). Cause is unknown, complications are frequent (eg, abscess, obstruction, fistula formation), and recurrence after treatment is common.

Ileus: Obstruction of the intestines. Commonly used to refer to a dynamic or functional ileus in which there is an absence of peristalsis resulting from postsurgical inhibition of bowel motility but frequently not associated with a mechanical blockage of the intestines.

Immune thrombocytopenic purpura (ITP): A disease of unknown cause in which the body destroys its own platelets, causing thrombocytopenia and resulting in coagulation disorders and easy bruising. The fetus of a woman with ITP may also have thrombocytopenia. Formerly called *idiopathic thrombocytopenic purpura.*

In utero: Latin for "inside the uterus."

In utero resuscitation: Term applied to measures taken to improve fetal oxygenation when there is a non-reassuring fetal heart rate pattern during labor. These measures include provision of 100% oxygen by mask to the woman, correction of maternal hypotension (turn woman on her side or from one side to the other, give fluids, or elevate legs), and reduction of uterine activity (stop oxytocin; consider use of tocolytics).

Incompetent cervix: A condition in which the cervix (lower part of the uterus and entrance to the birth canal) dilates prematurely, causing a spontaneous abortion or preterm delivery. A woman with an incompetent cervix is at risk for a preterm delivery with each pregnancy. *See also* Cerclage of the cervix.

Infant death rate: Number of babies that die within the first year after birth (365 days) per 1,000 live births.

Infective endocarditis: An infectious inflammatory process in which the infecting bacteria form growths on the heart valves or endocardium. The process may have an acute or subacute course. Diagnosis is usually made during the subacute, longer-lasting stage. Heart tissue is permanently damaged, and the infection can be difficult or impossible to treat effectively. Patients with heart valve malformations are particularly prone to developing these infective growths on the abnormal valves and surrounding endocardium.

Inferior vena cava: The major vein returning blood from the lower body to the right side of the heart.

Infiltration of intravenous fluids: Occurs when an intravenous catheter or needle in a peripheral vein perforates the wall of the vein and the intravenous fluids infuse into the surrounding tissue instead of bloodstream. Swelling and tenderness develop near the tip of the catheter. An infiltrated intravenous catheter should be removed immediately because some intravenous fluids can cause severe tissue damage.

Infusion pump: A machine used to push fluid at a controlled, preset rate into an artery or vein. All neonatal infusions should use a pump so the volume infused can be controlled precisely. Some pumps infuse fluids by means of small, regular pulses, while other pumps, particularly syringe pumps, infuse continuously.

INH: Isoniazid hydrazide. Generic name for an antituberculosis medication.

Insensible water loss: Body fluid lost through the skin and respiratory passages.

Inspired oxygen: The oxygen concentration that is being inhaled (*not* the concentration in the blood). Also called *environmental oxygen.*

Intra-amniotic infection (IAI): Formerly known as *chorioamnionitis,* or infection of the fetal membranes, which puts the fetus at risk for also becoming infected with the same organism.

Intra-arterial infusion: An infusion of fluid into an artery (eg, via a peripheral or an umbilical arterial catheter).

Intracardiac: Inside the heart.

Intrapartum: Period of pregnancy during labor.

Intrauterine: Inside the uterus.

Intubation, endotracheal: Insertion of a hollow tube (endotracheal tube) into the trachea to suction foreign matter, such as meconium, from the trachea or deliver air or oxygen under pressure directly into the lungs by assisted ventilation.

Iron: A mineral important for the formation of red blood cells. Iron deficiency is a common cause of anemia.

Isosmolar: Of the same particle concentration as body fluid.

ITP: *See* Immune thrombocytopenic purpura.

IUGR: In utero growth restriction. *See* Growth restriction.

Jaundice: Also called *icterus*. Yellow coloration of the skin and mucous membranes resulting from hyperbilirubinemia.

Karyotype: The complete set of chromosomes of the nucleus of a cell. Also used to refer to the photomicrograph of the chromosomes arranged in a standard order. The process of identifying a karyotype uses a technique that stops cells in their reproductive cycle and causes the individual chromosomes to swell, thus allowing each chromosome to be identified and counted. This technique is used to identify conditions, such as Down syndrome (trisomy 21) or Turner syndrome (monosomy X), that are caused by an excess or deficiency of one or more chromosomes. The technique cannot identify individual genes that comprise each chromosome.

Lactic acid: A by-product from one of the body's metabolic pathways. During periods of poor oxygenation, metabolism may be incomplete and lactic acid may build up, thus resulting in low blood pH or acidosis.

Large for gestational age (LGA): Refers to an infant whose weight is above the 90th percentile for infants of that gestational age.

Laryngoscope: An instrument used to visualize the glottis during endotracheal intubation.

Larynx: The area containing the vocal cords and located between the base of the tongue and the trachea.

Leopold maneuvers: A method of systematically palpating the abdomen of a pregnant woman to determine fetal presentation and position.

Lethargy: Condition of diminished activity due to drowsiness, medication, or illness.

LGA: *See* Large for gestational age.

Lie: Relationship of the long axis of the fetus's body with that of the maternal spine (transverse, oblique, or longitudinal).

Lightening: The feeling of decreased abdominal distension a pregnant woman has as the fetus and uterus descend into the pelvic cavity during the last 4 weeks of a term pregnancy.

Macrosomia: Large body size. A newborn weighing more than 4,000 g (8 lb 13 oz) at birth is considered macrosomic.

Maladaptation: Failure to adapt to stresses of the environment.

Malformation, congenital: A defect that occurs during embryonic or fetal development. Used synonymously with *congenital anomaly* but not *deformation*. *See also* Deformation.

Maternal serum alpha fetoprotein (MSAFP): *See* Alpha fetoprotein.

Maternal-fetal medicine (MFM): The subspecialty of obstetrics and gynecology that deals specifically with the care of high-risk pregnancies.

Maximum vertical pocket (MVP): A way of estimating the relative volume of amniotic fluid using ultrasound identification and measurement of the single deepest pocket of amniotic fluid of at least 1 cm in width.

McRoberts maneuver: Used to relieve shoulder dystocia by elevating and flexing the woman's legs so her knees and thighs are held as closely as possible against her abdomen and chest. This extreme flexion of the maternal hips rotates the pelvis in such a way that there is more room for the anterior shoulder to slip under the symphysis pubis, allowing delivery.

Meconium: The dark green-brown sticky material that makes up a baby's first stools. It is formed by the fetus in utero from intestinal secretions and swallowed amniotic fluid. The rectum may relax and release meconium into the amniotic fluid in post-term gestations and during periods of fetal stress. Meconium-stained amniotic fluid may therefore be a worrisome sign but does not always indicate fetal jeopardy.

Meningitis: Inflammation of the membranes that surround the brain and spinal cord.

Meningomyelocele: Congenital defect of the spinal column. Part of the spinal cord and surrounding membranes protrude through an opening in the spine and form a sac on the baby's back. The sac may be large or small, and located anywhere along the baby's spine. There may be various degrees of neurologic impairment occurring below the level of the meningomyelocele. It may be detected in the fetus by assessment of maternal serum alpha fetoprotein.

Metabolism: All the physical and chemical processes that produce and maintain body tissue.

Methimazole: A mercaptol-imidazole compound used to treat hyperthyroidism.

MFM: *See* Maternal-fetal medicine.

Morbidity: Any complication or damage that results from an illness.

Mortality: Death.

Motility: Movement.

MSAFP: Maternal serum alpha fetoprotein. *See* Alpha fetoprotein.

Multifetal gestation: More than one fetus. Multifetal gestation may be used to describe a pregnancy involving twins, triplets, quadruplets, quintuplets, or more.

Multigravida: Precise term for a pregnant woman who has had 2 or more previous pregnancies. Commonly used, however, to refer to a pregnant woman who has had one or more previous pregnancies. (*Secundigravida* is the precise term for a woman in her second pregnancy.)

MVP: *See* Maximum vertical pocket.

Myometrium: The muscular wall of the uterus.

Naloxone hydrochloride (Narcan): A drug that counteracts the depressant effects of narcotics. Naloxone may be given to a depressed baby whose mother received narcotic pain medication shortly before delivery. Adequate oxygenation with assisted ventilation, as necessary, should be provided *before* time is taken to give this drug. Naloxone should be used with caution if maternal drug addiction is suspected.

Narcan: *See* Naloxone hydrochloride.

NAS: *See* Neonatal abstinence syndrome.

Nasal flaring: A sign of neonatal respiratory distress. Edges of the nostrils fan outward as the baby inhales.

Nasogastric tube: A pliable tube that is inserted through the baby's nose, down the esophagus, and into the stomach. It is used for feeding or to decompress the stomach by intermittent or constant suctioning of air or gastric juices out of the stomach.

NEC: *See* Necrotizing enterocolitis.

Necrotizing enterocolitis (NEC): A serious disease in which sections of the intestines are injured and may die. Medical treatment may result in complete resolution, but in some cases portions of the intestines must be surgically removed. It occurs more often in preterm infants, but the cause is unclear.

Neonatal: Refers to the time period from delivery through the first 28 days.

Neonatal abstinence syndrome (NAS): Constellation of findings, including jitteriness, irritability, hypertonia, seizures, sneezing, tachycardia, difficulty with feedings, or diarrhea, often occurring in babies born to women who used heroin or methadone during pregnancy. These findings result from the baby's sudden withdrawal from maternal drugs following delivery.

Neonate: Baby from birth through the first 28 days of age.

Neonatal opioid withdrawal syndrome (NOWS): A condition that results from newborns being exposed to opioids in the womb. NOWS symptoms can include tremors, excessive crying and irritability, and problems with sleeping, feeding, and breathing.

Neonatologist: A pediatrician who specializes in caring for newborns, particularly at-risk and sick babies.

Nephrosis: General term used for any noninfectious disease of the kidney.

Neural tube defect: Used to describe any congenital defect in the brain or spinal cord (structures that developed from the neural tube of the embryo), including anencephaly, encephalocele, and meningomyelocele.

Neutral thermal environment: The very narrow environmental temperature range that keeps a baby's body temperature normal, with the baby having to use the least amount of calories and oxygen to produce heat.

Nitrazine: Trade name for phenaphthazine.

Nonhemolytic jaundice: Hyperbilirubinemia not resulting from an excessive breakdown of red blood cells.

Nonmaleficence: Avoiding harm to a patient.

Nonstress test (NST): One of several measures used to assess fetal well-being in high-risk pregnancies, during which spontaneous fetal heart rate accelerations in relation to fetal activity are monitored with an external electronic monitor. The pregnant woman is resting during the procedure and receives no medication.

NOWS: *See* Neonatal opioid withdrawal syndrome.

NST: *See* Nonstress test.

OCT: Oxytocin challenge test. *See* Contraction stress test.

Oligohydramnios: An abnormally low amount of amniotic fluid. It may be associated with abnormalities of the fetal kidney, ureter, or urethra (fetal urine is the primary component of amniotic fluid); certain fetal chromosomal defects; fetal growth restriction; uteroplacental insufficiency; positional deformities (due to prolonged uterine pressure in the absence of a fluid cushion); and umbilical cord compression (particularly during labor). Oligohydramnios may also result from early, prolonged rupture of membranes.

Omphalocele: A congenital opening in the abdominal wall allowing the abdominal organs, covered with a peritoneal membrane, to protrude and form a sac outside the abdominal cavity. *See also* Gastroschisis.

Ophthalmia: General term for any disease of the eye.

Oral airway: A device that allows babies with blocked nasal passages to breathe through their mouths. It is inserted into the mouth and keeps the tongue forward, preventing it from obstructing the airway.

Orogastric tube: A pliable tube that is inserted through the baby's mouth, down the esophagus, and into the stomach. It is used for the same purposes as a nasogastric tube.

Orthopnea: Shortness of breath while lying down. It is usually caused by heart or lung failure and is characterized by the patient sitting up to sleep.

Osmolarity: Concentration of particles in a solution. Synonymous with *osmolality*.

Ovulation: Release of an egg, ready for fertilization, from an ovary.

Ovum: Female reproductive cell that, after fertilization and implantation, becomes an embryo.

Oximeter: A device that reads the color of blood and reports the percentage saturation of hemoglobin with oxygen (Spo_2). The probe of an oximeter emits a light that is sensed by a detector. *See also* Pulse oximetry.

Oxygen hood: Also called *oxyhood*. A small plastic box with a neck space designed to fit over a baby's head and allow precise control of a baby's inspired (environmental) oxygen concentration.

Oxyhemoglobin saturation: Hemoglobin is the oxygen-carrying component of red blood cells. The amount of oxygen attached to hemoglobin is measured as percent saturation and called *oxyhemoglobin saturation* (commonly shortened to "% sat" or "O_2 sat"). The degree of saturation can range from 0% to 100%.

Oxytocin: A hormone occurring naturally in the body and also used to induce labor, enhance weak labor contractions, and cause contraction of the uterus after delivery of the placenta.

Oxytocin challenge test (OCT): *See* Contraction stress test.

$Paco_2$ or Pco_2: Concentration of carbon dioxide in the blood (*a* specifies arterial blood).

Palate: Roof of the mouth. The structure that separates the oral and nasal passages. A cleft palate is one that is split from front to back, sometimes with an opening so deep that the mouth and nasal passages are connected.

Pao_2 or Po_2: Concentration of oxygen in the blood (*a* specifies arterial blood).

Parens patriae: The duty of the state to protect the vulnerable or incompetent.

Parenteral: Taking something into the body in a manner other than through the digestive canal (which is enteral).

Parity: The condition of a woman with respect to having had one or more pregnancies reach a gestational age of viability. Parity is determined by the number of pregnancies that reached viability, whether the fetuses were live-born or stillborn, and not the number of fetuses. Twins, triplets, or more do not increase a woman's parity. *Nulliparity* is the condition of having carried no pregnancies to an age of viability; *primiparity,* of having carried one pregnancy to an age of viability; *secundiparity,* of having 2 pregnancies reach viability; and *multiparity,* of having had 3 or more pregnancies reach viability. In practice, however, *secundiparity* is rarely used and *multiparity* is used for any woman who has had 2 or more pregnancies reach an age of viability. *Example:* A woman whose first pregnancy ended in stillborn twins at 30 weeks' gestation, second pregnancy ended in a single, healthy fetus born at 39 weeks, and third pregnancy ended in spontaneous abortion at 10 weeks has a parity of 2. She is now pregnant for the fourth time, at 32 weeks' gestation, and therefore has a gravidity of 4. She may be described as a gravida 4, para 2. When she delivers the current pregnancy, she will become a G4 P3.

Pelvis, contracted: Smaller than normal-sized pelvis. The pelvis may be too small to allow the vaginal birth of a baby.

Percutaneous umbilical blood sampling (PUBS): Also called *cordocentesis.* A highly specialized technique during which a needle is inserted through a pregnant woman's abdominal wall into the uterus and then directly into an artery or vein of the umbilical cord, usually near the base of the cord at the placenta. Ultrasound visualization of the fetus, placenta, and umbilical cord is used throughout the procedure. A sample of fetal blood is obtained. Percutaneous umbilical blood sampling may be used to detect congenital infections, isoimmune diseases, and chromosomal defects (for chromosomal defects, fetal blood can yield results in a few days, while amniotic fluid cell culture may take several weeks). Percutaneous umbilical blood sampling may also be used to give a direct blood transfusion to a fetus in cases of severe anemia.

Perfusion: The flow of blood through an organ or tissue.

Pericarditis: Inflammation of the pericardium, the sac of fibrous tissue surrounding the heart. Pericarditis is sometimes caused by infection and other times by an inflammatory, noninfectious disease such as systemic lupus erythematosus.

Perinatal: The time surrounding a baby's birth. The perinatal period begins at 22 completed weeks and ends 7 completed days after birth.

Perinatologist: Technically, a subspecialist physician who cares for the fetus and neonate. Often used, incorrectly, to refer to an obstetrician with subspecialty training in maternal-fetal medicine.

Perinatology: Now more commonly referred to as *maternal-fetal medicine*, perinatology is a subspecialty of obstetrics and gynecology that focuses on the care of patients with complicated pregnancies and the diagnosis and care of conditions that affect the fetus before birth.

Periodic heart rate changes: Fetal heart rate accelerations and decelerations. Their occurrence and relationship to fetal activity or uterine contractions is used as an estimate of fetal well-being, for antenatal testing, and during labor.

Peripheral: The outward and surface parts of the body. *Example:* Peripheral circulation is the blood flow in the skin, arms, and legs.

pH level: Refers to the acidity or alkalinity of a liquid. A blood pH level outside the reference range indicates metabolic or respiratory disturbance.

Pharynx: Throat above the esophagus and below the nasal passages.

Phenaphthazine (Nitrazine): A pH-sensitive dye embedded in paper that, when dipped into fluids, estimates pH of the fluid. Used primarily to distinguish amniotic fluid (which has an alkaline pH) from urine or vaginal secretions (which are acidic) in pregnant patients with symptoms of premature rupture of the membranes.

Phototherapy: Use of fluorescent, tungsten-halogen, or fiberoptic lights to treat hyperbilirubinemia in neonates by breaking down bilirubin accumulated in the skin. The color of phototherapy lights ranges from nearly white to deep blue, depending on the type and brand of lights.

Pierre Robin syndrome: A group of congenital anomalies that include a small jaw, a cleft palate, and backward displacement of the tongue. Babies with Pierre Robin syndrome may have great difficulty breathing or eating.

Placenta: Organ that joins the woman and fetus during pregnancy. The umbilical cord is implanted on one side, while the other side is attached to the uterus. Maternal and fetal blood does not mix directly, but nutrients and waste products are exchanged across a thin membrane that separates maternal and fetal blood.

Placenta accreta: Term used to describe a rare condition of implantation in which the implanting trophoblasts not only penetrate the endometrium but continue into the myometrium as well. This eliminates the normal cleavage plane in the decidua (endometrium during pregnancy) that allows normal spontaneous separation of the placenta following delivery. Attempts to remove a placenta accreta by manual separation usually result in excessive hemorrhage. Hysterectomy may be the only way to remove the placenta, as separation from the myometrium may be impossible, and emergency surgery may be required if heavy bleeding begins.

Placenta previa: Abnormally low implantation of the placenta in the lower segment of the uterus. As the placenta grows with pregnancy, it spreads so that it partially or completely covers the internal cervical os at term. The resultant position of the placenta is in front of the fetus. Thus, a vaginal delivery would require delivery of the placenta before the fetus. Painless vaginal bleeding during the third trimester is the most common sign of placenta previa. If not identified earlier, severe hemorrhage with maternal and fetal compromise may occur as the cervix dilates during labor. Whether placenta previa is identified prenatally or not until after labor has begun, cesarean delivery is required for the health of the woman and fetus. *Note:* Early in gestation a placenta may appear to be low lying, but not be later in pregnancy. A diagnosis of placenta previa cannot be made until after 20 weeks' gestation and should be reconfirmed at 26 to 28 weeks.

Placental abruption: Premature separation of a normally placed placenta. Placental separation can occur at any time during pregnancy, but is most likely to occur during late pregnancy and before the onset of labor. Several risk factors are associated with placental abruption, but usually the cause is unknown. Depending on the degree of separation, bleeding may be slight or severe. If severe, both the woman and fetus may go into shock. Bleeding, even severe bleeding, can be completely hidden behind the placenta. In the most severe cases, the uterus is tense, boardlike, and tender. The woman's blood pressure may fall, and symptoms of shock or disseminated intravascular coagulation may develop. Fetal distress is common, and fetal death may occur. Placental abruption requires an emergency response.

Placental perfusion: Blood from the uterine artery flows into the intervillous space, bathing the placental villi that protrude into this space with nutrients and oxygen. Flow of blood through the intervillous space allows perfusion of nutrients and oxygen into the fetus from the maternal blood and waste products of fetal metabolism to pass from the fetus to the maternal circulation. Fetal and maternal blood does not mix. Nutrients and waste are exchanged across the thin membrane of the placental villi.

Pneumonia: Inflammation of the lungs. Neonatal pneumonia has many possible causes, such as bacterial infection, aspiration of formula, or aspiration of meconium.

Pneumothorax: Rupture in the lung that allows air to leak outside the lung, form a collection of air between the lung and chest wall, and thereby compress the lung so it cannot expand fully. Often when a pneumothorax develops, a baby suddenly becomes cyanotic and shows signs of increased respiratory distress. There are decreased breath sounds over the affected lung. Insertion of a tube or needle into the chest is required to remove the air pocket and
allow the lung to re-expand. Plural: pneumothoraces (rupture in both lungs).

Polycythemia: Abnormally high number of red blood cells. It is more common in infants of diabetic mothers and in newborns small for gestational age.

Polyhydramnios: Synonymous with *hydramnios*, although *hydramnios* is now the preferred term for this condition.

Position, fetal: Relationship of the fetal-presenting part to the maternal pelvis. In vertex presentations, the posterior fontanel is the reference point. With breech presentations, it is the tip of the fetal sacrum; with face presentations, the chin; and with brow presentations, the anterior fontanel. Position is not the same as presentation. A fetus in vertex presentation may be in any of several positions. *Example:* Left occiput anterior position indicates that the fetal occiput, as determined by position of the posterior fontanel, is located on the left side of the anterior part of the woman's pelvis.

Positive-pressure ventilation: Artificial breathing for a person by forcing air or oxygen into the lungs under pressure by bag and mask, bag and endotracheal tube, T-piece resuscitator, or mechanical ventilator.

Post-term: Refers to a fetus or baby whose gestation has been longer than 42 completed weeks.

Postnatal: The time after delivery, used in reference to the baby.

Postpartum: The time after delivery, used in reference to the mother.

Potter syndrome: A rare, fatal congenital malformation with characteristic facial appearance and absent or hypoplastic kidneys. Oligohydramnios may be noted in the mother. These babies are often born at term, are frequently small for gestational age, and may have hypoplastic lungs.

Preconceptional: Before conception. Refers to counseling women or families *before* conception regarding the risks of various problems during pregnancy. This is particularly important when a woman has a disease known to affect pregnancy or fetal development or a family history of such problems or pregnancy carries increased risks for a woman because of an illness or condition she has.

Preeclampsia: New-onset hypertension in pregnancy with excretion of protein into the urine, with or without other laboratory abnormalities or symptoms.

Pregnancy due date: Expected date for the onset of labor. On average, the date of delivery will occur 280 days, or 40 weeks, after the first day of the last menstrual period. The reference range of variation is 2 weeks before or after the calculated due date. Babies delivered between 37 and 42 weeks' gestation are considered *term*. Babies delivered prior to the onset of the 37th week are designated *preterm*, and those delivered after $41^{6/7}$ weeks are considered *postterm*. Inaccuracies can occur with calculating the due date because the date of the menstrual period may not be recalled correctly or there are variations in the length of the preovulatory phase of a menstrual
cycle. In some women with irregular periods, the preovulatory phase may be prolonged several weeks or even months.

Premature rupture of membranes (PROM): Rupture of the membranes ("bag of waters") before the onset of labor.

Prenatal: The time during pregnancy and before birth of the baby. Synonymous with *antenatal*.

Presentation: Refers to that part of the fetus that is in the birth canal and will deliver first. The normal presentation, near term and during labor and delivery, is vertex (headfirst). Any other presentation at that time is considered abnormal.

Preterm: Refers to that part of pregnancy between $20^{0/7}$ weeks and $36^{6/7}$ weeks (eg, preterm labor, preterm rupture of the membranes, or an infant born before 37 weeks' gestation).

Primary infection: First episode of a given infection. Some infections, such as cytomegalovirus or herpes, remain latent, without symptoms, in a person but may recur from time to time. The primary infection, however, is the most severe and likely to be the most damaging to a fetus or newborn. Other infections, such as syphilis or gonorrhea, may be cured, but if reinfection occurs, it will be as severe as the first infection.

Primigravida: A woman pregnant for the first time. *See also* Gravidity.

Primipara: A woman who has had one pregnancy carried to viability. *See also* Parity.

Prodromal labor: Refers to a patient having contractions but without sufficient cervical changes to make the diagnosis of true labor.

Prodrome: The time before a disease or process reaches its full strength. *Example:* The prodrome of a herpes infection may be mild itching in the area where the vesicles will later appear. This could be described as prodromal itching.

Prognosis: A forecast of the most likely outcome of an illness.

Prolapse: Falling out of a viscus. For example, an umbilical cord that slips through the cervix ahead of the fetus is a prolapsed cord, or a uterus that falls partially or completely into the vagina has prolapsed.

Prolapsed cord: Premature expulsion of the umbilical cord during labor and before the fetus is delivered. This is an emergency situation because a prolapsed cord is likely to be compressed, which may cause severe fetal compromise.

PROM: *See* Premature rupture of membranes.

Propylthiouracil (PTU): An antithyroid agent used to treat hyperthyroidism during the first trimester of pregnancy.

Proteinuria: Condition in which proteins from the blood are present in the urine. Also called *albuminuria*.

Psychosis: Any major mental disorder in which the person loses contact with reality and is unable to process information rationally.

PTU: *See* Propylthiouracil.

PUBS: *See* Percutaneous umbilical blood sampling.

Pudendal block: Nerve block by injection of local anesthetic into the area of the pudendal nerve. Used primarily for anesthesia of the perineum for delivery.

Pulmonary: Refers to the lungs.

Pulmonary hypoplasia: Underdevelopment of the fetal lungs, usually related to in utero compression of the fetal chest or lungs that prevents appropriate growth. This is seen with diaphragmatic hernia and with severe oligohydramnios, such as may occur with Potter syndrome.

Pulmonary maturity: Refers to relative ability of the fetal lungs to function normally if the fetus were to be delivered at the time a test for pulmonary maturity is performed. As the lungs mature, various chemicals produced by the fetal lungs appear in the amniotic fluid. Lecithin to sphingomyelin ratio, phosphatidyl glycerol detection, or lamellar body count may be performed on a sample of amniotic fluid to assess fetal lung maturity.

Pulse oximetry: Uses a noninvasive device that allows continuous measurement of the saturation of hemoglobin with oxygen. Hemoglobin changes color from blue to red as it becomes increasingly saturated with oxygen. A pulse oximeter uses a tiny light to shine through the skin and a light detector to measure the color of light coming through the skin. The color of light coming through the skin is determined by the amount of oxygen carried by hemoglobin in the red blood cells. From this the percentage of saturation is calculated (SpO_2). The percentage of saturation is not the same as a PaO_2 value, which measures the amount of oxygen dissolved in plasma.

Quickening: The first time fetal movements can be felt by the pregnant woman. This usually occurs between 16 and 20 weeks of gestation. Quickening generally occurs later in pregnancy for a primigravida than a woman who has had a previous pregnancy.

Radiant warmer: A servo-controlled heating device that is placed over a baby and provides radiant heat to keep body temperature normal.

RDS: *See* Respiratory distress syndrome.

Respiratory distress syndrome (RDS): Formerly called *hyaline membrane disease*. A disease mainly affecting preterm infants, due to immaturity of the lungs and lack of surfactant. Without surfactant, the alveoli collapse during exhalation and are difficult to open with the next breath.

Resuscitation: The process of restoring or supporting cardiac function, blood pressure, and respiration so as to provide adequate oxygenation and perfusion to a baby, child, or adult who is apparently dead or near death. For newborns, resuscitation is needed most often in the delivery room; for adults, resuscitation may be needed after any of a number of life-threatening events.

Resuscitation team: This concept refers to the fact that more than one person is needed to provide resuscitation. At least 2, preferably 3, health care professionals, skilled in the techniques of resuscitation, are needed for each resuscitation.

Reticulocyte count: Estimation of the number of newly formed red blood cells (reticulocytes) in a blood sample.

Retinopathy of prematurity (ROP): Abnormal blood vessel growth in the eye that may lead to detachment of the retina and partial or complete blindness. Blood vessel changes may result from many factors, including excessively high arterial blood oxygen concentrations for a period that can be as short as a few hours. The more preterm a baby, the more likely the baby is to develop ROP. Often ROP resolves spontaneously, but if permitted to proceed unchecked, scarring may occur and the retina may detach. It is critical that babies with ROP be followed by an ophthalmologist trained in examining babies so that laser therapy may be used to check the progression.

Retractions: A sign of respiratory distress. These occur with each breath as the skin is pulled inward between the ribs as a baby tries to expand stiff lungs.

Retrolental fibroplasia (RLF): Scarring phase of retinopathy of prematurity.

Rh alloimmunization: Formerly referred to as Rh sensitization. (1) Development of antibodies by an Rh-negative woman pregnant with an Rh-positive fetus. The antibodies cross the placenta into the fetus's blood, thus causing hemolysis of the fetus's red blood cells. (2) Development of antibodies against the Rh-positive red blood cells following a transfusion of Rh-positive blood unintentionally given to an Rh-negative person.

Rh blood type: Besides the major blood groups of A, B, O, and AB, there are a number of minor groups, of which the Rh system is the most important for perinatal care. Prevalence of the Rh factor varies by ethnic and racial groups. In the white population, 85% have the Rh antigen and are said to be Rh positive, while 15% lack the Rh antigen and, therefore, are Rh negative. Regardless of ethnic or racial heritage, persons who lack a blood antigen can make antibodies against that blood group. This means that Rh-negative persons can make antibodies against Rh-positive blood, if their immune system has been exposed to that blood (from external transfusion or transplacental transfer). Persons who have developed such antibodies are said to be alloimmunized, or sensitized to that blood group. *See also* Rh alloimmunization and Erythroblastosis fetalis.

Rh disease: *See* Erythroblastosis fetalis.

RhIg: Rh immune globulin (RhoGAM is one commercial name for Rh immune globulin products). The antibodies from sensitized Rh-negative persons can be harvested, purified, and prepared for safe injection into another Rh-negative, but unsensitized, woman. The product is called Rh immune globulin, or RhIg. The injected antibodies contained in RhIg prevent alloimmunization by reacting with the antigens on the few Rh-positive blood cells that may have escaped from the fetus into the maternal circulation. Rh-negative, unsensitized women should receive RhIg at 28 weeks' gestation and again following delivery. Rh-negative, unsensitized women should also receive RhIg within 72 hours of an abortion or an episode of vaginal bleeding during pregnancy. Protection lasts for 12 weeks. Therefore, depending on the course of the pregnancy, subsequent doses may also be needed. Use of RhIg protects fetuses in future pregnancies from Rh disease.

Rhinitis: Inflammation of mucous membranes of the nasal passages, causing a characteristic runny or stuffy nose. Although generally uncommon in newborns, rhinitis is frequently found in babies with congenital syphilis.

RLF: *See* Retrolental fibroplasia and Retinopathy of prematurity.

ROP: *In neonatal care*, retinopathy of prematurity. *In obstetric care*, an abbreviation for a specific position (right occiput posterior) of a vertex presentation during labor. *See also* Retinopathy of prematurity.

Rotation (of the fetal head): Gradual turning of the fetus during labor for the fetal head to accommodate size and shape of the maternal pelvis as the fetus descends through it.

Rubella: A mild viral infection, also called *German measles*. A rubella infection in a pregnant woman during early pregnancy may result in infection of the fetus and cause rubella syndrome.

SARS-CoV-2: Severe acute respiratory syndrome coronavirus 2, a novel coronavirus that caused a global pandemic of COVID-19 (coronavirus disease 2019), beginning in late 2019.

Scalp stimulation test: Test in which fetal heart rate response to mechanical stimulation of the fetal scalp (by examiner's gloved finger or sterile instrument) is assessed. Used as an estimate of fetal well-being during labor.

Scaphoid abdomen: Sunken or hollow-looking abdomen, occurring when there is a diaphragmatic hernia, which allows the intestines to slip from the abdomen through a hole in the diaphragm and into the chest cavity.

Secondary infection: Recurrent infection. *See also* Primary infection.

Sepsis: Infection of the blood. Also referred to as *septicemia*.

Serum bicarbonate: Also called *blood* or *plasma bicarbonate*. Concentration of bicarbonate in the blood. Bicarbonate is the main body chemical responsible for the acid-base balance of the blood.

Serum urea nitrogen: A blood chemistry test of renal function. The higher the serum urea nitrogen, the more urinary excretion has been impaired.

Servo control: A mechanism that automatically maintains skin temperature at a preset temperature. A thermistor probe is taped to the baby, registers the skin temperature, and in turn activates a radiant warmer or incubator to continue to produce heat, or to stop heating.

Sexually transmitted infection (STI): An infection that is transmitted from one partner to another during sexual activity. Many infections can be transmitted in this way, but certain STIs can have significant effect on the fetus or newborn, including syphilis, gonorrhea, *Chlamydia*, and HIV.

SGA: *See* Small for gestational age.

Shock: Collapse of the circulatory system due to inadequate blood volume, cardiac function, or vasomotor tone. *In babies*, the causes are most often hypovolemia, sepsis, or severe acidosis. Symptoms are hypotension, rapid respirations, pallor, weak pulses, and slow refilling of blanched skin. *In pregnant women*, the cause is most often hemorrhage. Because of the expanded blood volume of pregnancy and vasoconstrictive capabilities of most (young, healthy) pregnant women, blood loss may be severe before symptoms of shock (hypotension, weak and rapid pulse, rapid respirations, anxiousness or confusion, and cold, clammy, pale skin) become evident.

Short bowel syndrome: A syndrome of weight loss and dehydration related to having less than the normal length of intestine. The less intestine a baby has, the less well nutrients can be absorbed. Short bowel syndrome may result from a baby being born with an abnormally short bowel or may be the result of a portion of the intestines having been removed for treatment of certain types of bowel disease.

Shoulder dystocia: Situation in which the baby's shoulders become wedged between the maternal symphysis and sacrum after delivery of the fetal head. The head may be pulled back against the perineum as the woman relaxes her push that delivered the head (the "turtle sign"). Various procedures may be tried to free the shoulders. Severe asphyxia or fetal death can occur if there is significant delay in delivery of the shoulders and trunk.

Shunt: A diversion of fluid from its normal pathway. (1) *Blood:* In some sick babies, blood will be shunted from the right side of the heart to the left (baby will be blue); in other babies, the shunt will be from the left side of the heart to the right (baby will be in congestive heart failure). Commonly seen in babies with congenital heart disease or severe lung disease in which the blood cannot be normally oxygenated. (2) *Cerebrospinal fluid:* An artificial pathway for the flow of cerebrospinal fluid when blockage is in the normal pathway, resulting in hydrocephalus. Typically, cerebrospinal fluid is shunted through a one-way valve from the ventricles into a small tube tunneled under the skin and empties into the abdominal cavity. This is called a *ventriculoperitoneal*, or V-P, shunt.

Sickle cell anemia: A genetic hemoglobinopathy causing chronic anemia. Crises, resulting from infarction of various body areas clogged by the sickled cells obstructing small blood vessels, may occur periodically. Management during pregnancy is particularly complicated.

Sickle cell–hemoglobin C disease: A hemoglobinopathy similar to sickle cell anemia.

Sickle cell–thalassemia disease: Sickle cell disease and thalassemia are genetically transmitted anemic diseases caused by abnormal hemoglobin. *See* Hemoglobinopathy.

Sims position: The patient rests on one side, with the upper leg drawn up so that the knee is close to the chest. Often used with an emergency delivery in bed or outside the hospital. This position does not allow for much assistance by an attendant but has the advantage of placing less tension on the perineum during delivery and, therefore, may result in fewer lacerations.

SLE: Systemic lupus erythematosus.

Small for gestational age (SGA): A baby whose weight is lower than the 10th percentile for infants of that gestational age.

"Sniffing" position: Proper position of a baby's head during bag-and-mask ventilation or endotracheal intubation. The head and back are in straight alignment, with the chin pulled forward as if sniffing. This position is different from the one used for endotracheal intubation of an adult because the relative size and relationship of anatomic structures is different between babies and adults. The neck is *not* hyperextended (bent backward to an extreme degree) during endotracheal intubation in babies.

Sodium bicarbonate: Drug used to counteract metabolic acidosis. After being given to a baby, it rapidly changes to carbon dioxide and water. Therefore, it should be given only to babies who are breathing adequately on their own or receiving adequate assisted ventilation. These babies can "blow off" the excess carbon dioxide formed. If sodium bicarbonate is given to a baby with a high $Paco_2$, it will make the $Paco_2$ go even higher and thereby worsen the acidosis.

Spinal (block): An anesthetic technique in which a local anesthetic is introduced into the subarachnoid space of the spinal canal through a hollow needle placed (temporarily) in the spine. It is technically easier to perform placement of an epidural catheter because spinal fluid in the subarachnoid space will flow out through the hollow needle and, thereby, identify proper placement of the needle before injection of the anesthetic. Because the anesthetic also blocks sympathetic nerves leaving the spinal cord, the blood pressure of the woman may decline. (For this reason, a loading dose of 500–1,000 mL of physiologic [normal] saline solution may be given intravenously prior to introduction of the anesthetic.) Spinal anesthetics are not ordinarily given until the second stage of labor has begun because the anesthetics used do not remain effective for longer than 2 hours.

Spo_2: The percentage of saturation of hemoglobin by oxygen as detected by a pulse oximeter, which reads and reports how red the blood is. Fully saturated hemoglobin appears bright red, while desaturated hemoglobin appears blue.

Sterile vaginal examination: Vaginal examination with a speculum, using sterile technique. In this situation, sterility obviously cannot be ensured. When a woman is pregnant and rupture of membranes is known or suspected, the goal is to minimize the risk of introducing bacteria during examination.

Sternum: The breastbone. The chest bone that joins the left and right ribs.

STI: *See* Sexually transmitted infection.

Stopcock: Small device with 3 openings and a lever to close any 1 of the 3 openings. One opening is designed to fit the hub of an intravenous catheter, umbilical catheter, or similar catheter. The other 2 are designed to connect with a syringe or intravenous fluid tubing.

Stylet: Slender metal probe with a blunt tip that may be inserted inside an endotracheal tube to make the tube stiffer during intubation. Also, the solid, removable center within certain needles.

Succenturiate lobe of placenta: A malformation of the placenta in which the placenta has a second lobe, with the umbilical blood vessels traversing membranes between the main placenta and accessory or succenturiate lobe. Umbilical vessels between the 2 lobes may lie over the cervical os (creating the condition known as vasa previa) and can be torn, particularly if the membranes are ruptured artificially. Also, the succenturiate lobe may produce a placenta previa if it lies over the os, even though a previous ultrasound may have reported a normally placed placenta, which may be accurate for the main portion of the placenta.

Superimposed preeclampsia: Development of preeclampsia in a woman who already has chronic hypertension. Sometimes it is difficult to tell if the increase in blood pressure is due to poor control of existing hypertension or development of preeclampsia. If the blood pressure increases and there is increasing proteinuria, superimposed preeclampsia is most likely. This complication increases the risk of development of eclampsia.

Supine: Position of a person when he or she is flat on his or her back.

Supine hypotension: In late pregnancy, the enlarged uterus may compress the vena cava when a woman lies on her back. This reduces return of blood to the heart and, thus, reduces cardiac output. This then causes a reduction in blood pressure and in the perfusion of body tissues. The woman may feel faint. Most pregnant women lie on their sides to sleep. During labor it may be helpful to have a woman lie on her side as much as possible. If supine hypotension develops with a woman resting on her back, uterine blood flow may be affected, which might result in a non-reassuring fetal heart rate pattern. One measure to take if a non-reassuring fetal heart pattern occurs during labor is to turn a woman onto her side (if on her back) or from one side to the other to relieve pressure on the vena cava.

Suprapubic puncture: A technique used to tap the bladder of a newborn. A needle is inserted into the center of the lower abdomen, above the pubic bone, and into the bladder to obtain a sterile urine specimen for culture.

Surfactant: A group of substances, including lecithin, that contributes to compliance (elasticity) of the lungs by coating the alveoli and allowing them to stay open during exhalation. Without surfactant, the alveoli collapse during expiration and are difficult to open with the next breath.

Symphysis pubis: Connection between the right and left hip bones in front of the body, in the pubic area.

Systemic: Refers to the whole body.

Tachycardia: Rapid heart rate. (1) *Fetal* tachycardia is considered to be a sustained heart rate faster than 160 beats/min. (2) *Neonatal* tachycardia is considered to be a sustained heart rate faster than 180 beats/min while a baby is quiet and at rest.

Tachypnea: Rapid respiratory rate. In a neonate, tachypnea is considered to be a sustained breathing rate faster than 60 breaths/min.

Tent: Small cone-shaped device made of material that can expand. Used to dilate an orifice or keep a wound open. In obstetrics, tents may be used for cervical ripening and may also be called osmotic dilators.

Teratogen: A substance that causes malformations in the developing embryo. Certain medications are known teratogens and should not be taken during pregnancy. Most congenital malformations, however, cannot be traced to a teratogen but are instead due to unknown factors (most common) or hereditary factors.

Thalassemia: Any one of several hereditary hemolytic anemias caused by abnormal hemoglobin.

Thermistor probe: A small sensing device that measures temperature continuously and is able to detect very small changes. Servo-control devices operate by a thermistor probe attached to the baby and then the radiant warmer or incubator.

Thrombocytopenia: Abnormally low number of blood platelets.

Thrombophlebitis: Inflammation of a vein associated with the formation of a thrombus. In a superficial blood vessel, a thin red streak will form in the skin directly over the path of the blood vessel and the area will feel warm to the touch. Thrombophlebitis may develop at the site of a peripheral intravenous catheter, in which case the catheter should be removed and the intravenous catheter restarted into another vein. Further treatment is rarely needed. If thrombophlebitis develops in deep veins, however, it is a serious condition, generally requiring treatment with intravenous heparin.

Thrombosis: The process involved in formation of a thrombus (blood clot in a vessel).

Thrombus: A blood clot that gradually forms inside a blood vessel and may become large enough to obstruct blood flow. If a thrombus separates from the blood vessel and is carried in the blood, it becomes an embolus. Plural: thrombi.

Thyroid storm: A sudden worsening of adult hyperthyroidism, usually triggered by trauma or surgery and characterized by marked tachycardia and fever.

Thyroid-stimulating hormone (TSH): A protein secreted by the anterior pituitary gland that stimulates thyroid function.

Thyroid-stimulating immunoglobulin (TSI): An antibody produced by lymphocytes that, for unknown reasons, stimulates the thyroid to release thyroxin. These antibodies may cross the placenta and cause hyperthyroidism in the fetus.

Tocolysis: Administration of a drug to stop uterine contractions.

Tonus: The amount of continuous contraction of muscle. *Uterine tonus* refers to how tightly the muscle of the uterus is contracted between labor contractions. With an internal monitor, it is measured as the resting pressure in the uterus between contractions. *Hypertonus* refers to a uterus that remains excessively tense and does not relax normally between labor contractions.

TORCH: Toxoplasmosis, other agents, rubella, cytomegalovirus, and herpes simplex. A specific group of infections that can cause in utero fetal infection (usually resulting in severe damage) or, in the case of herpes, life-threatening neonatal infection. The "other" category includes less common, serious infections such as varicella, coxsackievirus B, and syphilis.

Toxemia: Term formerly used to refer, collectively, to all forms of hypertensive disorders of pregnancy.

Toxoplasmosis: Disease caused by a type of protozoa (a type of microscopic one-cell organism). Toxoplasmosis in a woman may go unnoticed but may infect the fetus, thus causing congenital toxoplasmosis. Congenital toxoplasmosis damages the central nervous system of the fetus and may lead to blindness, brain defects, or death.

Trachea: The windpipe or tube of stacked cartilaginous rings that descends into the chest cavity from the larynx and branches into the right and left bronchi, which branch further into smaller bronchioles inside the lungs.

Transfusion, fetal-fetal: Situation that may occur, in utero, between fetuses of a multifetal gestation, when there is a connection between an artery of one fetus and a vein of the other in a monochorionic placenta. The fetus on the arterial side becomes a chronic blood donor to the fetus on the venous or recipient side. When born, the donor twin may be pale, severely anemic, and small for gestational age. The recipient twin may be red, polycythemic, and, occasionally, large for gestational age.

Transfusion, fetal-maternal: Situation that may occur in utero if an abnormal connection develops between the fetal and maternal circulation in the placenta. The reverse direction of maternal-fetal transfusion apparently does not occur. The newborn may present with findings similar to the "donor" fetus described in fetal-fetal transfusion. To diagnose this condition, the woman's blood can be tested for the presence of fetal cells with the Kleihauer-Betke test.

Transverse lie: The body of the fetus lies horizontally across the maternal pelvis and hence across the birth canal entrance. A cesarean delivery is required for safe delivery of a fetus in transverse lie.

Trendelenburg position: A position of the body that may be used for surgery or examination. The patient lies supine on an inclined surface, with the head lowered below the level of the feet.

Trimester: A period of 3 months. The time during pregnancy is often divided into the first trimester (first through third month), second trimester (fourth through sixth month), and third trimester (seventh through ninth month).

Trisomy: Chromosomal abnormality in which there is an extra (third) chromosome of one of a normal pair of chromosomes. The most common is trisomy 21 (three 21 chromosomes), which is also called Down syndrome. Other trisomies also occur, such as trisomy 13 (three 13 chromosomes) and trisomy 18 (three 18 chromosomes), both of which have a characteristic set of multiple congenital anomalies.

TSH: *See* Thyroid-stimulating hormone.

TSI: *See* Thyroid-stimulating immunoglobulin.

Turner syndrome: A chromosomal abnormality in which there are 45 chromosomes, with the absent chromosome being one sex chromosome (45,X) instead of the typical 46,XX (female) or 46,XY (male). These individuals are phenotypically female and may have physical abnormalities including webbed neck, low hairline, and certain skeletal, urinary tract, lymph system, and cardiac abnormalities. The baby will have female external genitalia, but the ovaries may be completely absent and sexual development will be severely impaired.

Twin-twin transfusion: *See* Transfusion, fetal-fetal.

Twins, conjoined: Twin fetuses joined together, usually at the chest or abdomen but may be at almost any site, and sharing one or more organs. This results from incomplete separation during the process of twinning of single ovum (which, if completely split, would have become identical twins). The greater the degree of organ sharing, the less likely one or both twins can survive surgical separation.

Twins, fraternal: Two fetuses created from the fertilization and implantation of 2 separate ova.

Twins, identical: Two fetuses created from the division of one fertilized ovum.

Ultrasonography (US): A technique used to visualize the fetus and placenta by means of sound waves, which bounce off of these structures and are turned into a picture outline. Used to assess fetal growth, fetal well-being, congenital abnormalities, multifetal gestation, placental location, location of structures during percutaneous umbilical blood sampling and amniocentesis, and volume of amniotic fluid.

Urine drug screening: Commonly available test in which the metabolic breakdown products of recently taken drugs can be identified in the urine.

US: *See* Ultrasonography.

Uterine atony: Failure of the uterine muscle (myometrium) to contract in the immediate postpartum period. A leading cause of postpartum hemorrhage.

Uterine dysfunction: Abnormal progress of labor due to uterine contractions that are inadequate in strength or occur in an uneven, uncoordinated pattern.

Uterine fibroids: Tumors of the uterus made up of fibrous connective tissue and smooth muscle. Also called *leiomyomas*. These myomas may become very large, occasionally interfering with implantation. Other risks, although uncommon, include placenta previa, obstructed labor, preterm labor, postpartum hemorrhage, and endometritis.

Uterine inertia: Inadequate labor caused by uterine contractions that are too short, too weak, and too infrequent to produce adequate progress.

Uteroplacental: Refers to the uterus and placenta together as a functioning unit.

Uteroplacental insufficiency: An inexact term suggesting a placenta that is functioning poorly, with inadequate transfer of nutrients and oxygen to the fetus, and used to explain some cases of in utero growth restriction or fetal distress during labor.

Uterus: A hollow, muscular organ in which the fetus develops, often called the *womb*.

Vacuum extractor (VE): An instrument used to assist delivery, in which a plastic cup is placed over the fetal occiput, suction is applied so the cup is sealed to the scalp, and then traction is applied to the cup. There are risks, benefits, and specific indications for use of vacuum extraction.

Vagus nerve: A major nerve with branches to the heart and gastrointestinal tract. Something that stimulates one branch of the vagus nerve may also affect another branch. *Example:* Suctioning deep in the back of a baby's throat directly stimulates part of the vagus nerve to the gastrointestinal tract and indirectly may affect the branch to the heart and cause bradycardia (termed *reflex bradycardia*).

Varicella-zoster virus: The virus that causes chickenpox in children. Adults who were not infected as children and, therefore, did not acquire immunity may also develop chickenpox, which, in adults, can cause life-threatening pneumonia. Infection in a pregnant woman early in pregnancy can cause severe fetal malformations and serious neonatal illness at term. *Note:* Reactivated infection in adults is herpes zoster. This occurs in a small percentage of individuals who had chickenpox as children and causes pain and the formation of vesicles along specific nerve tracks. These symptoms are known as *shingles*.

VariZIG: Varicella-zoster immune globulin. Specific antibodies to the varicella-zoster virus obtained from persons who have had the disease. Principally used to attenuate infection in the newborn of a mother who has the infection.

Vasa previa: An abnormality of placental development. Instead of joining together at a point over the placenta, the vessels that form the umbilical cord join some distance from the edge of the placenta. The vessels lie on the membranes and, if the vessels lie across the cervical os, are exposed when the cervix dilates. This is a dangerous situation because when the membranes rupture or are artificially ruptured, the vessels may tear open. The fetal hemorrhage that results is often fatal.

Vasoconstriction: Tightening of the blood vessels, allowing less blood flow through the vessels. *Example:* When a significant volume of blood is lost, the small blood vessels in the skin will constrict, thus allowing the remaining blood to be directed to the brain and other vital organs.

VBAC: Vaginal birth after cesarean.

VE: *See* Vacuum extractor.

Vein: Refers to blood vessels that return blood to the heart. In most veins, this blood is dark red because it has a low oxygen concentration because most of the oxygen from the arterial blood has been transferred to the body's cells for metabolism. The pulmonary veins, however, carry oxygenated blood as it flows from the lungs to the heart.

Vertex: Top of the head. A fetus in vertex presentation is headfirst in the maternal pelvis. This presentation is identified on vaginal examination by palpation of the posterior fontanel in the center of the birth canal.

Vital signs: Refers to the group of clinical measures that includes respiratory rate, heart rate, temperature, and blood pressure.

Vitamin E: A vitamin important for maintaining red blood cell stability. When a baby is deficient in vitamin E, the red blood cells may break down more rapidly than normal and the baby may become anemic.

Volume expander: Fluid used to replace blood volume, and thereby increase blood pressure, in cases of hypotension thought to be due to hypovolemia. Blood or physiologic (normal) saline solution are examples of volume expanders.

Woods maneuver: Maneuver for management of shoulder dystocia in which the fetus is rotated 180 degrees so the posterior shoulder becomes the anterior shoulder.

Zavanelli maneuver: Maneuver for management of shoulder dystocia in which the fetal head is replaced into the vagina and a cesarean delivery is done.

Index

Page numbers followed by *f* indicate a figure.
Page numbers followed by *t* indicate a table.
Page numbers followed by *b* indicate a box.